OTHER BOOKS BY THE AUTHOR

THE ARCHITECTURAL DOCTOR℠

Creating integrated solutions and systems for the fields of Architecture and Medicine to create healthy and healing places to live, work, and play. The Architectural Doctor – the liaison between Architecture and Medicine.

(Forthcoming)

INTEGRATIVE ARCHITECTURE

Integrating the processes between green, healthy, and sustainable Architecture methodologies for energy efficient, ecologically aware, and healthier built environments.

(Forthcoming)

SYMBIOSIS GLOBAL
NATURE IS THE MOST ADVANCED TECHNOLOGY
TECHNOLOGY & ECOLOGY : LIVING TOGETHER

How can we navigate the challenges of humanity while also striving for progress in the world of Technology? How can we create a future more aligned to the planet's Ecological systems?

Symbiosis Global outlines these topics with a focus on the premise "Nature is the Most Advanced Technology."

(Forthcoming)

ARCHITECTURAL MEDICINE^{SM}

BUILDING THE BRIDGE TO WELLNESS

CAN ARCHITECTURE BE HEALING?

TIMOTHY D. ROSSI

Copyright © 2020 by Timothy D. Rossi

All rights reserved.

No part of this publication may be reproduced, distributed, or transmitted in any form or by any means, electronic, mechanical, photocopying, recording, or otherwise, without express written permission of the author.

Architectural Medicine ᴿᴹ, Architectural Doctor ˢᴹ, and ARxMD ˢᴹ are all trademarks of
Timothy D. Rossi and
Architectural Medicine LLC.

Cover, book design, and graphics
by Timothy D. Rossi,
except where noted

FIRST EDITION

ISBN NUMBER:
978-0-692-99040-7

Library of Congress Control Number: 2020905146

This book is dedicated
to my Mother –

Francine E. Rossi

CONTENTS

Acknowledgements

Introduction

Part I

Chapter 1: What Is Architectural Medicine?

Chapter 2: Who Is This Book For?

Chapter 3: What Is Architecture?

Chapter 4: What Is Medicine?

Chapter 5: Architectural Medicine – Part 1

Part II

Chapter 6: Healthy, Green, and Sustainable Building

Chapter 7: Green Building Defined and Overview

Chapter 8: Sustainable Building Defined and Overview

CONTENTS

Chapter 9: Healthy Building Defined and Overview

Chapter 10: Introduction to Integrative Architecture

Chapter 11: How Do Buildings Affect Physical Wellness?

Chapter 12: How Do Buildings Affect Mental Wellness?

Chapter 13: How Do Buildings Affect Emotional Wellness?

Chapter 14: Architectural Medicine – Part 2

Part III

Chapter 15: The Architectural Doctor

Chapter 16: The Architectural Medicine System (AMS)

Chapter 17: The Healthy Building Inspector

Chapter 18: The Architectural Medicine Software Solution – ARxMD

CONTENTS

Chapter 19: The DNA of Cities & Parametric Architecture

Chapter 20: Wellness Centers

Chapter 21: Some Thoughts on the Future

Chapter 22: Follow up and Conclusion

About the Author

Notes

ACKNOWLEDGEMENTS

I first have to thank and give the highest praise to my mother, Francine Rossi. She was the biggest supporter of my life's path and believed in my ideas, concepts, and concerns — even when many others had doubts.

Without her support, I would never have been able to explore these varied concepts, fields, and ideas and have the courage to pursue these dreams.

This book is dedicated to her.

I'm also thankful to be able to draw on the lessons from my father, whose multi-faceted interests, from organic gardening and interests in the natural world to music and sports, gave me a wide range of topics to learn and develop in my early years into adulthood. I can also be thankful for his discipline; without which I am not sure I could have navigated rough seas when they've occurred in my life.

Through the years, some friends and family have encouraged me, have been supportive, and have shown interest in my ideas that have given me the courage – especially at times when needed the most – to keep going. Thank you all.

Special thanks to my Aunt Valerie and Uncle John, who planted many important and helpful seeds in my childhood in which, I think, has brought thriving blossoms forth. Also, special thanks to Bernadette Soon, whose support during challenging times in my life gave me tremendous support.

I would like to thank a small group of people whose inspiration, dedication, and support on my path have been extremely important. Their knowledge and wisdom in which I have learned over the years, set a path for me to explore in an inspiring and hopeful way. This includes Bosco Büeler, Cedar Rose Guelberth, Christi Graham, Mary Cordaro, Richard Scarborough, Helmet Ziehe at the International Building Biology Institute, James Hubble, Professor Robert Blank, Nancy Sheinbein, and the Yestermorrow Design/Build School in Vermont.

I would also like to thank those who I have never met who have been incredibly important to me in my life. This includes the lyrics and master teachings of the late Neil Peart of Rush – on the drums as well as in the wisdom of words. Even while I never met him, his mentorship provided many vital topics to ponder for a lifetime.

The courage and pervasiveness of Buckminster Fuller, and the inspiring designs of Frank Lloyd Wright, as well as the pioneering perseverance of Rachel Carson and Florence Nightingale have been motivating factors in my life. I will also include in this list the inspiring messages and life of Henry David Thoreau.

A thank you to the Pixar animation company and the life and visions of Apple icon Steve Jobs. There have also been the spiritual quests of Gandhi, Krishnamurti, and Alan Watts, which have been of great value. I'm also grateful for the inspiration of Martin Luther King Jr. and the life and lessons of lacrosse legend Oren Lyons of the Iroquois nation.

And finally, I'd like to show my thanks for the inspiring designs and developments of Zaha Hadid, Santiago Calatrava, Sim Van der Ryn, James Hubble, Frei Otto, Eugene Tsui, as well as the pioneering work of Janine Benyus and Neri Oxman.

INTRODUCTION

I first began writing this book in my mind soon after I came up with the concept of Architectural Medicine. In all honesty, while I had not arrived at the name Architectural Medicine until around 2011, the road to this project started many decades ago. I have spent a lifetime seeking the end goal of what a healthy built environment might be defined as, and this process has brought me on quite a journey.

I state this because the process was not exactly clear when I first began. Yet, for me, the ideas of architecture as a structure that is enjoyable to live within and architecture that is energy efficient, ecologically aware, and properly supporting health seemed to be a no brainer to me. Yet as I began my adventure into the field of Architecture, I quickly realized that, especially when I started on this path in the 1980s, this was not the case.

Therefore, this interest in achieving these goals has led me on a path of reverse-engineering the goals and converting this into a structural system. In this way, I've worked to provide a pathway leading towards these goals. There is still much work to be done, and as such, it is a work in progress.

Growing up in the 1970s in the USA, where topics such as the energy crisis and environmental degradation issues were regularly in the news, was a powerful education to begin life. And, of course, the warnings of health in buildings related to lead paint, asbestos, and other building concerns was a strange juxtaposition to the construction world that I would eventually work in.

I did have some idea and ideal as to what kind of world of architecture that I thought I'd like to live in and how this world might be built. Yet while many of these ideals were influenced by my upbringing, the challenge in this process was that it didn't begin to come into some form of clear vision until I was in college in the late '80s.

I had many questions and concerns about architecture and the built environment, and this questioning process has brought me on this long journey.

Standing on the Shoulders of Giants

Let me be very clear with this statement; this book would not have been possible without the ability to "stand on the shoulders of giants."

While some of these people who I have mentioned in the acknowledgments have been my personal teachers in terms of working with them or learning from them, in other cases, I have learned from them via books or from afar. Either way, they have all been great and tremendous teachers. They deserve a tremendous amount of credit.

A part of this book will give credit where it's due by discussing the history of those whose work over the past decades has enabled those such as myself to gain from their knowledge and wisdom through their trials and tribulations.

A hope of this book is to pass on this information and knowledge, as they have passed on their knowledge and wisdom to me.

It is challenging to summarize all they have done, but I will do my best to highlight their work. I highly encourage you to explore their work and what they have learned and to utilize their wisdom as we all move forward as a global humanity and civilization.

While humanity has always been global, it has never been in a way in which recorded history has been known in today's day and age. We have never had the capability or capacity to have such a significant impact on this planet's environment. And we have never had the means to make massive changes to our environment and the biological world – either positively or negatively – as we have at this time in history.

It is with great hope that we can navigate these challenges and opportunities with wisdom, compassion, and intelligence.

How This Book Came to Be

This book came to be over many decades of research and questioning, and at times, not knowing I was on this specific path to writing this book. The term "Architectural Medicine" itself came to be after several decades of striving for a process to define a better built environment.

The term "better" can be defined in this manner as healthy, green, and sustainable – while also being described as places and spaces that I wanted to live and work within.

This includes the scientific understanding of topics such as the toxicology of materials and other material information related to data and informatics.

Yet, it also includes the less formulaic and more "felt" topics of how spaces feel and how people respond to places emotionally and psychologically.

Both Architecture and Medicine have aspects of their field defined by both the "arts" and the "sciences" of their professions, which means that data alone may not be enough to determine best practices.

An excellent example of this topic of the arts and sciences being integrated is discussed in Chapter 12: How Do Buildings Affect Mental Wellness? As the emerging field of Neuroscience of Architecture can view the brain and body responses to visual examples, this can show the impact this has on our bodies' various systems. This includes, for example, the impact that a visual image or design has on the brain center and whether or not the image is seen as a threat to the body – or a nurturing, safe design element.

This new capability to "see" how the body responds to designs in a physiological format through neuroscience is helping to merge the sciences with the arts in the human experience.

In having this form of understanding, future architecture and designs can better understand the pleasing sensory aesthetics of places and spaces. They can also have more insight into the body-mind physiology and how humans respond to these built environments.

In utilizing this type of information and learning, both the design and the health fields can add this to their toolkit to apply to future designs that support better overall health – from rural areas to highly populated cities.

In places and topics that include data, I will add relevant information, and in other areas where the senses and art are part of the process, this will be highlighted.

After years of questioning and analysis, I finally realized that at the core of these developments of health in the built environment are these two central concepts and fields – Architecture and Medicine.

Time and again, when I began to unfold the many layers of these topics, inquiring as to the centroid for hopeful solutions, I ended up at the core foundation of both Architecture and Medicine.

Since 2011, when I first came up with the term "Architectural Medicine," I've continued to build upon this concept. And each time I've built and updated these ideas, the core has remained steady. Architectural Medicine has remained a core as both a foundation and an umbrella term that seems to cover the many, multi-faceted aspects of the healthy, green, and sustainable built environment for a future that I dream of.

Credentials

You might be wondering what my background is to write such a book, and that's a fair question. To be clear, I'm neither an Architect nor a Doctor, yet as I set out in my early career to work towards many of the goals that I've outlined in this book, my research, study, and work in the fields led me to a hands-on education. It also showed me the many gaps that exist, and since none of these systems existed in the past, my path has been to create and define them as I thought they might benefit these developments.

Essentially, I've spent most of my professional life working towards achieving these goals or working in many different fields to gather the knowledge to develop the Architectural Medicine System (AMS) and the ARxMD software and processes. All of these topics will be discussed later in this book.

While much of my research and development has provided me with this integrated solution called Architectural Medicine and the Architectural Doctor, I've had many decades of learning from some great pioneers in these fields. It has helped me provide an overview of these many facets and given insights into the gaps. I've also been involved in co-forming companies in my career, striving to provide professional solutions for these fields, which has also provided a greater understanding of best practices working with those across different professions.

A Bit of My History – How I Got Here

One of the first green, eco-building events I attended was in 1993 at the Eco-Design, Environmental Building event in New York City with William McDonough, James Wines, Paul Bierman-Little, Mary Cordaro, and Katherine Metz.

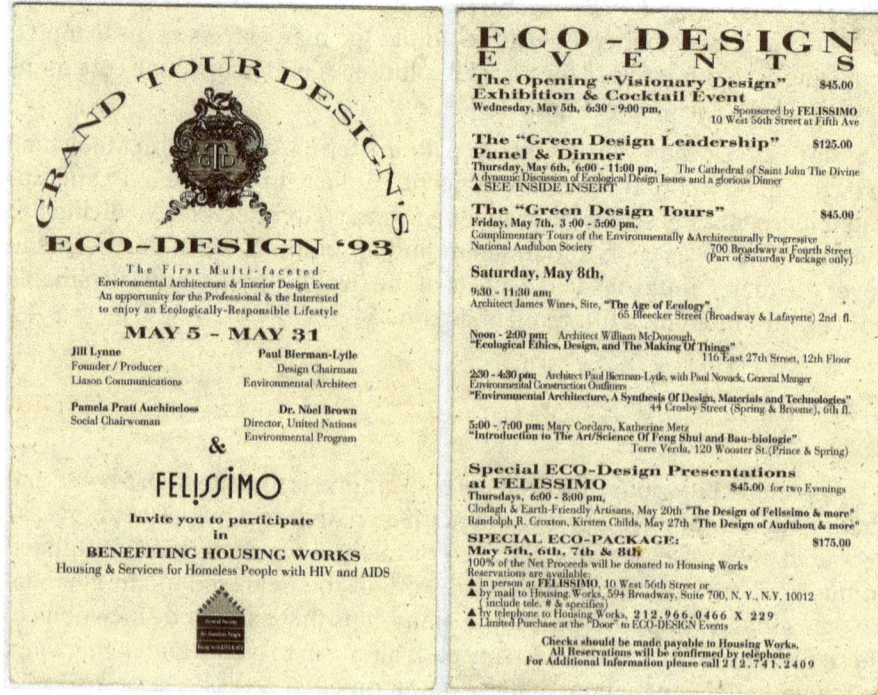

Introduction

All pioneers in the green, sustainable, and healthy building movements. This is where I first met healthy building consultant Mary Cordaro, with whom I spent many years discussing and working to create solutions to these issues in the built environment.

I first attended an organized event on Healthy Building in 1996 titled "Building For Health," with teachers who have also been pioneers in the field. This includes Cedar Rose Guelberth and Carol Venolia, as well as Paula Baker-Laporte, who told me years later that this was her first event in which she presented. Her book *Prescriptions for Healthy Building* has been a guiding source for many in the building professions, along with the general public, in striving to create healthier buildings.

While the topic of healthy building is new to most, there have been many people and groups working to create healthier built environments for many decades.

It's also a huge topic for many to grasp as they are often introduced to the concept of healthy building, along with green building and sustainable building, all at the same time.

Often, the average person's introduction is either buying, building, or renovating their first home. Much too often, they are brand new to building topics in how structures function, and the many details of what they need to know to make decisions are often overwhelming.

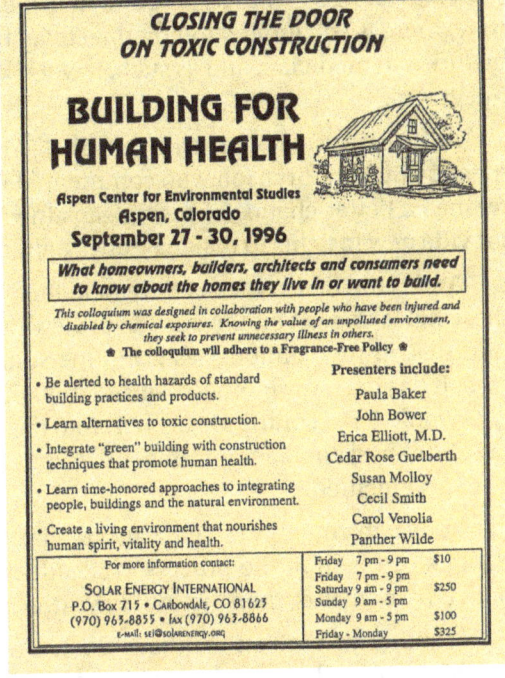

In many ways, this is tremendously unfair for the average homeowner, as it often takes a lifetime for the professionals in the building fields to understand these topics. It is often the case that even these building professionals are not fully aware or comfortable making decisions to create healthy, green, and sustainable built environments.

This, in part, is why this book is being written with all three main groups included, which are the General Public, the Architecture fields, and the Medical fields. Without an integrative understanding of these topics and an interconnected process, these solutions are tremendously challenging to achieve.

Perhaps, this is a big reason why the field of healthy building has been slow in progress and less understood. Even Green Building, which has gained popularity as a public term in the past two decades, is mired in confusion about the definition.

What You Should Know

This book is a work in progress in these emerging developments. At this time, there is still limited interconnectivity between the professions of architecture and medicine, and as such, it will take time for these to become more integrated.

At first, I hesitated to write this book. Yet, one day I was reading a comment by Richard Branson who commented that a person on the "outside" often has a better chance of seeing gaps in various fields and can sometimes provide new insights to making things better.

And through the years, I have benefited from being on both the inside of these fields and yet on the outside to view them from both close-up and afar. And this, in my opinion, has given me some insights that are uniquely my own. It has been my intention since I thought about writing this book that my goal would be to contribute my part into the cohesive whole of what seems to me either broken fragments or new systems that haven't yet been considered nor implemented.

In recognizing this reality, I also realize that I can't do it all. If my contributions can help in the process of healthier, greener, and more sustainable built environments, then I know I have done my part.

Whether you are an architect, doctor, or a member of the general public, this book will provide an outline of the many topics involved, as well as information as to how these fields can become more connected. It will take a multi-disciplinary effort to supply these solutions and the general public's demands to achieve these goals.

Why Have Interest in This Book?

If you are wondering why you should read this book, I will offer this as a reason in the question format:

"Are you wanting a better world in which to live, work, and play for both yourself and future generations? Are you concerned about the future of your health and the health of your children, grandchildren, and the many other creatures and animals that live on this planet?"

While I can't promise I know all of these answers, I am certainly asking these questions with great concern, and this book came to be after my many years of seeking these solutions. It has come to be after years of learning and years of being involved hands-on with these developments. My direct experience was either for work or merely exploring this on my personal time as a pathway towards knowledge.

This book will provide a framework for the many topics related to health in the built environment and the trajectory of solutions from where it has been to where it may likely be going.

A Systems Approach

A key facet of this book is that, while there have been great strides in the emerging fields of health in the built environment, a big part of what makes this book a bit different is the focus on systems.

As will be outlined in this book, a cohesive systems approach in a multi-disciplinary format is, in my opinion, a key to providing healthier built environments for current and future architecture.

And by systems, I am specifically talking about the fact that in most of the world, in today's modernity in the worlds of medicine and building, there is very little integration between the medical and architecture fields.

The fact that most people are spending from 60 to 90 percent of their lives inside of architecture, and we as a society are rarely factoring in building health into the equation of wellness and well being in life, is to me strange.

The fact that so much time is spent indoors with so many potential pollutants and impacts that buildings can have on health is often a perplexing scenario for me to understand. The fact that there are no standard processes that consider the built environment in evaluating health to help with diagnosing ailments seems odd.

In chapters 14 and 16, we delve into these system approaches and solutions.

When you begin to think about all of the steps and procedures required for this process to happen as outlined in this book, you will soon find many processes that do not currently exist, along with integrations needed between professions that also do not exist.

This process also requires at least two new professionals – the Architectural Doctor and the Healthy Building Inspector. The Architectural Doctor, which in many ways can help to build these bridges between professions to support the multi-disciplinary process required, is a central focus and an essential part of Architectural Medicine.

As we discuss in this book, a part of this process will be to create integrated solutions to achieve these goals.

Right now, as I am finalizing the writing and editing of this book, it is the year 2020, and the world has come to a standstill with the novel coronavirus pandemic. The stay at home initiatives have become common, as COVID-19 has added to this building health complexity.

However, what we can see in this pandemic is that the health of our built environments has a huge impact on our health – both on the micro-level as individuals and separate households, to the larger macro-level of worldwide health.

This is a perfect time to begin these processes and to put into place many of these systems to help with better health in the built environment — physically, mentally, and emotionally.

Florence Nightingale-200th birthday (1820-2020)

As mentioned in the previous paragraph, this book is being edited and revised in 2020, and as I write this, today is Florence Nightingale's 200th birthday. She was a pioneer in nursing, but also in the development of health in the built environment at large.

She was a nurse who cared for people and their health, and she is an icon today of someone who cared about people and utilized the benefits of science. This embracing of both science and human empathy is also a mantra for the current-day scenario where work on this subject still needs to be done.

As this book is based on health in the built environment, it is essential to recognize those who have strived to create better health for the public, and she deserves to be given high accolades and credit as a pioneer for doing so.

And with her work and the many decades since her time of bringing to light the importance of health relative to the built environment, this segues nicely into the first chapter...

> "The connection between the health and the dwellings of the population is one of the most important that exists."
>
> – Florence Nightingale

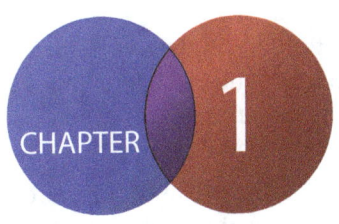

WHAT IS ARCHITECTURAL MEDICINE?
AN OVERVIEW OF THIS EMERGING DEVELOPMENT

Perhaps the words "Architecture" and "Medicine" next to each other is a new idea, yet a goal of this book is to discuss this potential for overlap with the result of a better built environment for health and wellness.

The fields of Architecture and Medicine have changed quite a bit in the past fifty to one hundred years, and while there have been many beneficial developments in each of these very large fields, there are still gaps relative to health in the built environment that can benefit humanity at large.

This also includes the increasingly important issues of building energy use, and the impacts buildings have on the ecology, focusing on a more sustainable future. As climate change is on many people's minds, the issue that buildings consume and utilize a substantial percentage of energy and have a large impact on the environment is becoming more of a focal point. A question then becomes, "what can be done about it?"

"Building" the Bridge to Wellness

While there are great developments occurring in each of these professions, from evidence-based design, green building, environmental psychology, and building science in Architecture to integrative medicine and environmental health in Medicine, these fields continue to be increasingly complex with many facets within each field.

The intent of Architectural Medicine is to help integrate these various fields for the improvement of health and wellness in the built environment.

A key to Architectural Medicine, as opposed to other fields such as Healthy Building, is that it considers all facets of human health – physically, mentally, and emotionally.

This focus is inclusive for the entire General Public and the overall fields of Architecture and Medicine. A main goal is to help define these integrations between these various fields and create bridges between these fields in how they might all work together. This is discussed in more detail in later chapters.

In this way, the average person as the General Public can feel empowered to make best decisions in their built environments for the health of themselves, their families, and their futures.

Yet, it's also important to recognize that the professionals in these fields also deserve to have an integrated approach properly defined for them to address client and patient issues and utilize best practices towards health, healing, and wellness.

Can Architecture Be Healing?

The impact that the built environment has on human health and well-being is becoming a topic of increasing study, interest, and recognition. Both the Medical fields and the many fields connected to Architecture are learning of this influence on human health, particularly with recent research in the past twenty years.

As the integration between Architecture and Medicine continues to develop, there becomes an increasing need for these often independent fields to connect the "dots" of their research to the bigger picture. The collaboration of this research can benefit both the professions involved in the built environment and health and the general public who are influenced and affected by the built environment.

Architectural Medicine works to connect these dots to provide updates on the latest information related to these fields and help build bridges for a healthier, greener, and sustainable built environment.

I've chosen to discuss this topic with the simple question:
"Can Architecture Be Healing?"

This book is based on both Architecture and Medicine as a foundation of what's required to achieve a healthy built environment and how these two fields can work together to accomplish this goal.

This is no small task, yet at the same time, many facets can be connected to help support this development, which eventually can create built environments that are healthier places to live in.

Architectural Medicine can be both a foundation on which to build upon and an umbrella term to include the many different fields and sub-fields of both professions. There are a considerable number of fields that are involved, and these will be referenced to show the potential for an interconnectedness in achieving a "whole" picture viewpoint.

Architectural Medicine Defined

The term Architectural Medicine came to be after many decades of my pondering, evaluating, and processing the large amounts of information that each of these professions addresses on a very wide scale. As I considered all of these many facets, I began to see a pattern that emerged, showing a core essence that related to health in the built environment. This research resulted in the idea that at the core and at its heart were these two topics of "architecture" and "medicine."

When we view these worlds of architecture and medicine, there are two core principles that this focus is based upon. And these core principles are that the world of architecture and the built environment can be seen as the "external world," and the world of medicine and health is based on the human "internal world."

When pondering these two concepts, while they may at first seem very simple, they can lead to extremely complex topics. You can easily get existential about these topics, and while that has its place, a key part of this book is to discuss the practical facets of these fields having more overlap and integration. The health impact of buildings on the general public has an often unknown yet large effect on people.

If you take time to ponder this idea of Architecture as the exterior world and Medicine as the interior world, you might find something interesting in terms of the questions of where one begins and the other ends.

After all, if you take the example of sight, you will quickly notice that what you "see" in the world outside of you is technically "seen" inside of your brain. When the light of the exterior world enters your eyes, it is to say that you see this exterior world inside of your mind. And when you take it a step further, you can recognize that this light enters your eyes, is transferred into digital signals, and then becomes an electric signal that enters your brain and is processed and experienced internally. So technically speaking, you "see" and experience the exterior world internally.

In addition to sight, sound has a similar process. The sound waves from the exterior world come into contact with your eardrum and inner ear, which in turn converts this analog wavelength into a digital signal that again goes to your brain and is "heard" by you internally. Again, the sound in the external world is experienced inside of your brain and body.

Your sense of smell, taste, and even touch is also processed in the same manner, and so it can be said that the exterior world that you see, hear, smell, taste, and touch is actually experienced internally – inside of your body.

So what does this have to do with architecture, and what's more, what does that have to do with health?

We dive into these questions throughout the book as we discuss the many facets of these wide ranging topics. We'll discuss how the built environment can impact health and wellness and address solutions to help evaluate buildings for health. And we'll review the potential for new systems that connect the fields of architecture and medicine.

A Quote From Vitruvius and Commentary on Architecture and Health

For many people, the concept of the buildings they live and work within might be so familiar that they don't often consider how these spaces are impacting their health. And not just physical health, but also their emotional and mental wellness.

Unless you are a designer or architect or in some fashion connected to architecture, the spaces and places you live and work in might be off the radar in terms of how these places are impacting one's life.

This is understandable, as the topic of a building's impact on one's life is not common and certainly isn't a popular topic in general society. Yet over the past few decades, with larger populations moving to cities and spending more of their lives inside and around buildings, these topics have gathered more interest.

With the focus of Architectural Medicine on health and wellness in the built environment, there is a viewpoint in the built environment that might begin the thought process of how architecture can impact health.

The concept of medicine being involved with architecture is not exactly new. As the architect Vitruvian stated over two millenniums ago:

"The architect should also have a knowledge of the study of medicine on account of the questions of climates, air, the healthiness and unhealthiness of sites…without these considerations, the healthiness of a dwelling cannot be assured." [1]

Below is a concept that can be applied to this thought process. Viewing the topic of health as internal medicine, and architecture as impacting health as external medicine, this might provide initial insights into these concepts:

Internal Medicine (Medicine) – External Medicine (Architecture)

External spaces (Architecture) – Internal space (Health/Medicine)

As you view the concept of architecture as external medicine, this might be curious and surprising. How can the exterior world impact your health and be considered as external medicine? What does that mean?

In the next few chapters, we'll discuss this as we outline both architecture and medicine definitions and dive into these details with more specifics. In fact, in the next section, I'll provide an overview of what to expect in this book.

What to Expect in This Book

In this book, I will review how the shapes and forms that we see and experience in architecture, the external world of our lives, can significantly impact our internal world and how this impacts our health. The built world that we experience — that which we hear, smell, taste, and touch all significantly impact our everyday health, which we are often not aware of.

We will discuss how these shapes and forms, as well as the materials and the components of buildings, can impact human health.

In chapter 5 we'll review the many facets of the built environment for context. In chapters 6 through 9, we'll discuss the topics of green, sustainable, and healthy building and how they relate to health. Chapter 10 will discuss the new concept of Integrative Architecture and how it relates to green, sustainable, and healthy building. Chapters 11 through 13 discuss how the built environment affects physical, emotional, and mental or psychological wellness.

The first few chapters begin with the topics of healthy building, green building and sustainable building, how they are both similar and dissimilar, and why I'm adding another term of Integrative Architecture to this development of Architectural Medicine.

In chapter 14, I put all of these topics together to discuss the big picture overview and how they interconnect with the fields of both architecture and medicine. We'll discuss how these three main topics of healthy building, green building, and sustainable building, can combine with the topics of physical, mental, and emotional wellness in the built environment.

These are critical topics to discuss when viewing the big picture of health in the built environment because without considering these different facets, there can be missing pieces in this big jigsaw puzzle.

It also provides a foundation to discuss the topics relative to later chapters discussing the Architectural Doctor and the importance of systems involved in achieving the goals of Architectural Medicine.

Without a foundation of these topics and an understanding of the many systems involved, the result of healthier built environments will be difficult to achieve.

And I state the above as part of my own personal experience. My experience over the past 30 years has led to this development of Architectural Medicine. When I first came up with the idea of striving to integrate architects and doctors in 1999, it was based on my frustration in architecture trying to create and support healthier built environments – for myself and others.

And as a result of striving to achieve these goals, Architectural Medicine's seeds began, leading to this very book.

But before we get into those details, let's start with a few basics first.

What Is Architectural Medicine Striving to Achieve?

When thinking about the origins of Architectural Medicine, I can say that this formation developed from the goal of striving to achieve healthier built environments. And this included the concept of what the path would be to get "there" and how this would look.

This path of "there" discusses the "here" as places and spaces that you live, work, and reside within. And the goal of this path is to re-search the many parts required to fit together in striving to arrive at these goals for better health and wellness.

Many years ago, as I began my venture into the world of architecture, I began to question specific processes. Honestly, I did not understand how certain processes were acceptable, which others just ignored.

For me, these processes included a focus on health, green building, and energy efficiency. It also consists of the considerations of the impacts that our buildings have on the environment. While I delve into each of these in the next few chapters, the key for me in this writing is focusing on the big picture. How the many facets of this big picture as smaller segments create the whole is critical to comprehend.

In particular, I've had questions about how buildings are not studied and evaluated on a greater level focused on occupant health and societal health.

For years I read about the importance of health and taking care of your body, eating healthy foods, and in the past twenty to thirty years have heard over and over the importance of mental and emotional health. These topics include eating healthy and exercise such as yoga and meditation, to name just a few of these emerging focal points for overall health and wellness.

Yet, for me, I have been confused as to how the built environment is almost totally excluded from these conversations. Until about a decade ago, I rarely, if ever, heard or read about a doctor discussing their patient's built environment. And even less so about any processes to include the built environment in their patient's evaluations.

In the past decade, the topic of social determinants of health have become more common, and we'll discuss this topic relative to Architectural Medicine in later chapters.

Yet with people spending from 60 to 90 percent of their lives inside buildings, and with this number is increasing, I still cannot fathom how the medical professions are not including the built environment in their patient's health.

However, it's also important to state I likely wouldn't understand these comments myself if I hadn't been involved in the fields of architecture and construction with a focus on inspecting structures relative to health and wellness.

I began to see how complicated this process is firsthand. Over the past twenty years, I have also learned more about the complexities of the medical fields and functions.

This, of course, also includes the very complex profession of architecture. The Architecture, Engineering, and Construction (AEC) fields have similar complexities to the medical fields, and each has a tremendous amount of education required for their professions.

There is also one other important lesson that I've learned over the past few decades, and that is this – if these complex fields do not have systems in place to support processes, procedures, and integrations, it will likely not work for each professional. Adding other processes into their workflow without training or systems will create too many variables and challenges for any fluent methods to function.

And this is very important to address as, in my opinion, the addition of information for these professions is only a piece of the complex puzzle. What is also required is for this information to be made into an actionable process. And to achieve this integration, there is a need for systems to be in place to ensure these goals can be manifested.

A big part of this book is discussing the various systems that need to be put into place to support the process to be applied for real-world solutions for health and wellness.

In terms of the book's subtitle, "Building the Bridge to Wellness," what exactly is being bridged?

Yes, this is a play on words in terms of the Building and Construction fields. What is being bridged are the professions of Architecture and Medicine, with the goal for each professional to have systems in place to work together to support the best health of the occupants in buildings.

Basically, it is to create and support new systems that allow the built environment to be included in the patient's health evaluations and provide the necessary processes to achieve these health and wellness goals.

This includes the development of two new fields or the support of two professionals – the Architectural Doctor and the Healthy Building Inspector.

I say new as a term loosely because there have been people who have been doing a type of this work along these lines. This includes those such as the environmental inspector and consultant. Yet to the extent that this includes systems that are agreed upon or having common standards, procedures, and protocols between professions has been missing.

And this missing part of the puzzle is, in my opinion, a key to why these processes do not exist for the Doctors and Architects in their professions.

And so, these missing pieces and the filling of these gaps are that which are being built to bridge these pieces to provide better and more complete solutions for health and wellness.

Tuning in to the Needs of Children and the Elderly

When evaluating the built environment and its impact on health, children and the elderly are particularly vulnerable to adverse health environments. Children, as an example, are not smaller versions of adults. Their systems are more sensitive, and I'm not just talking about their emotional states of being. They have more sensitive nervous systems, more sensitive endocrine systems, and their overall sensitivity in their growing process is more affected by toxins, pollutants, and their environments overall.

Similarly, older generations are also more sensitive, and in many ways, more highly influenced and impacted by their built environments. Their bodies may not regenerate as easily, and often their healing is not as rapid in responding to disease. Therefore, they are more sensitive to their built environments as well as any toxins or toxic built environments they reside within.

Often, issues in the built environment do not impact those who are young adults and healthy, as much as they can negatively impact children, elders, and those with compromised immune systems at any age. And unfortunately, these issues in the built environment are not as easily recognized by those who are healthier.

Those who are healthy young adults, typically in my experience adults in their 20's to 40's, may accuse or infer that those who are not as healthy should learn to ignore possible health issues and get over the fact that nothing in life is perfect.

That is true. Nothing is perfect — yet can't we do better?

What happened to striving in life for the better? And shouldn't better built environments for optimal health and wellness be a goal?

A Changing of the Guards in Buildings

What is also of interest in the context of the built environment is somewhat of a changing of the guards from previous centuries. In the distant past, the women of the hunter-gatherer communities seemed to be most involved with building and creating the home.

This would make sense as the process for mothers would be to nurture and take care of the children, as the men went out to hunt. At that time, the women were known to be the gatherers as well as the caretakers. They created places as homes as nurturing spaces that were likely more similar to the womb – in that they were designed to create comfort and embrace the needs of the children and the family.

This is not at all to state that women should have this role as builders, nor should it state that men cannot attend to emotional, nurturing needs. Yet, in my opinion, there is a need for more nurturing environments to be created that are attentive to the needs of the whole person, including one's emotional wellbeing.

The process of creating, building, and updating the home should include taking care of the children and elders with a goal of wellness and well-being. Structures should be made as shelters for the world's dangers, yet also nurturing for a healthy life.

However, in today's modern-day and age, some of the structures as homes and places of work are creating dangerous environments in which to live and work.

After working for a decade-plus in the construction field, I can tell you that I rarely, if ever, heard a conversation about how the workers must respect the spaces being built for the optimum health of their families and the planet. And I never heard a conversation that these structures must be built like a nest or womb to help shelter and protect the children and elders in all facets of their lives – mentally, physically, and emotionally.

It's a badge of courage for many men to push through the emotions and senses and overcome these so-called weaknesses. Although they are typical of construction job sites in my experiences over the years, these are not my words alone.

However, this is not to say that everything has to be emotionally based. It doesn't mean that this masculinity has to be removed. Still, as more and more of the built environments affect the daily lives of hundreds, thousands, millions, and even billions of people, there must be a little more attention placed on the nurturing aspects of human beings.

This is particularly important as the number of people getting older is increasing, and the time that the average person spends inside of buildings is increasing. The current trend of populations moving to urban environments means that the average time spent inside will likely increase. If anything, this will require more nurturing environments to be developed into the future if health and wellness are going to be important moving forward.

In my experience, many tough construction workers would scoff at comments made on the job site, which mentioned that buildings need to be more nurturing.

However, few would say that their children and their elders should not be protected and cared for with more respect, sensitivity, and nurturing in terms of their shelter and home.

It may be funny to discuss for those who are healthy and able to push through these more toxic environments. Still, when it comes to babies, small children, elders, and those who are negatively impacted by their built environments, it is not very funny.

Seeing someone we love and care about being negatively affected in their health is terrible to see and is not very funny.

Knowing that we can do better by paying more attention to the senses and the many facets of a healthy human life by recognizing how the built environment affects us – mentally, physically, and emotionally – is not a joking matter, at least not to me.

What's strange to me is that while many of these tough people work hard jobs and long hours to protect their families, they might be creating toxic buildings and contributing to construction that can create and perpetuate unhealthy environments. And this is doing the opposite of their goals of protecting their families and those they care about.

While I don't think that they are intentionally doing this, the irony is that they are strong and stoic to be protective for their children, partner, and elders, yet in this process of being stoic, they are detuning their senses from these types of construction dangers. And this could be detrimental to the health of those whom they are striving to protect by ignoring the senses that could be the canary in the coal mine recognizing such issues in these built environments.

This kind of backward thinking, or lack of critical thinking on these topics, has been something I have navigated and viewed my entire life. Over the years, I have gained a better grasp of the psychological understanding of why some may do this, which I've found is often to focus on making a living to provide the monetary needs for their families. However, even having some understanding of this does not make it easier to digest in terms of the potential negative health issues that can result. What it should note for us as a society is that we can do better in terms of solutions for the workers as well as the inhabitants of these buildings.

However, if we are to combine this masculinity and femininity in the process of building structurally sound and nurturing, healthy environments, then the result is a win-win.

Growing up Sensitive

As a child growing up, I was always very sensitive to the surroundings I was in, from the objects around me and the clothes that I wore to the spaces and places that I lived and spent time within.

While being sensitive is not atypical, I later learned that a heightened sensitivity to my exterior environments as spaces and places was not common, especially for those involved in the construction fields.

This sensitivity was often a result of reactions to the colors, sounds, textures, shapes, lighting, smells, and the many other features of the natural and built environments. It led me to explore these topics in more depth and inquire about how these built environments impact human health at large.

While this sensitivity as a child was both perplexing to me and those around me, it became a part of the reason that Architectural Medicine exists today. Due to my sensitivity, I became a bit of a canary in the coalmine in my life. And while I could tell when I was in a toxic or stressful built environment, I learned as I got older that this was not typical for others to recognize.

This writing about being sensitive may sound like a specific personal experience in the built environment, yet I write this for two reasons.

One is to discuss topics related to my built environment experiences and how this led to the development of Architectural Medicine. The second is to provide context to the next segment...

The Importance of Emotionally Intelligent Architects and Doctors

And while these comments in the previous paragraphs are focused on the emotionally desensitized construction workers, the world of architecture requires architects who are more in tune with the emotional intelligence of their designs. In my experience, some architects are either happy to focus on the intellectualism of architectural design or are those who are logically and rationally driven with little focus on emotional intelligence.

What is Architectural Medicine?

In too many experiences in my life around the field of architecture and construction, the senses are either something to overcome or often the case has been that workers are desensitized to the emotional realms. I experienced this firsthand in both my studies and in the world of construction.

To be clear, this is not to state that logic should be ignored and that emotions should lead to all decision making. Obviously, the structural integrity and intelligence of the design process is an essential component of architecture and medicine.

Instead, it is to state that these fields are more than just a group of logical analysis and processes.

Buildings can be simple shelters to support life in the physical realm and can also transcend the basic building into architecture. And it can do so by supporting the emotional and psychological experience of the occupants of these built environments.

Otherwise, buildings are just storage containers for humans to survive or exist within. And architecture should be more than just shelter. It should support thriving in life and lift one's spirits.

As well, as anyone who has been rushed to the hospital or has been sick or injured can tell you, being supported by a doctor whose intellectual capacity and understanding or how to evaluate and analyze your illness is not only critical, it is literally lifesaving.

And when you find a doctor and health practitioner who are emotionally intelligent, they can recognize that you are probably scared and feeling extremely vulnerable. Providing better emotional support can be the difference between absolute panic and the comfort of facing the scenario, knowing that those helping you have empathy and compassion during the crisis.

Being that this is a critically important reality, many people working with their doctor may wish for better emotional and empathic support in times when they are most often helpless. This is not to discredit the doctor and not appreciating their incredible abilities on an intellectual, rational, and logical level. It is instead a call to request that this empathy be added to medical professionals' intellectual capabilities, as patients are fragile during times of their health conditions.

I am stating that because many people go to the doctor under very vulnerable circumstances, feeling emotionally supported in this very weakened state can make the circumstances more comfortable for patients to navigate. And this mental, psychological, and emotional support can do wonders during times of angst and high stress.

With this viewpoint, I would state that an architect and doctor's emotional factor and emotional intelligence is critical.

In situations that I've experienced or witnessed in my life, a doctor who was emotionally supportive was a special type of person that provided the rational, cognitive capabilities along with the emotional support to help through very stressful events.

For me, it made all the difference in my suffering, and to have such reliable emotional support allowed me to relax in a way that provided the state of mind to trust and let the healing process to begin.

And the locations in which this care is being provided, which includes the design elements of the rooms, the medical devices, and the overall hospital or health care environment design, can also make a significant difference in how the patient experiences their health issues.

While many view a doctor or the medical professional's support as direct formats of acute or emergency care, there are also long term scenarios that the built environment has on human health. The architecture of where you live and work, over time, can impact your health significantly.

And to not have the medical professionals include the built environment in both analysis of conditions, and as a potential cause of these conditions, in my opinion, is a gap in analysis for their patient's health.

There will always be varying degrees of emotional intelligence, and this is a human reality. However, for those practicing architecture and medicine, the ability to have this emotional intelligence added to their intellectual logic and reasoning is critical for the current and future health of human and planetary wellness.

The mindset of paying more attention to these emotional intelligence topics would require a need to balance the logical and the rational mind with the world of the senses and emotions.

We don't have to throw away our logic. This is not about removing the facet of life that requires humans to be strong. It's about adding the more nurturing aspects of life to ensure that our strength is not ignoring critical human characteristics that equally protect humanity.

Many have seen the emotional life as something to overcome, but this is something that can be *utilized* in order to survive. Once this survival has been achieved, then you can spend time thriving, and this requires that we pay attention to the whole person.

If we are focused on overcoming the emotional world, then what happens when we have worked to be at a place where we are thriving and can now enjoy life? Enjoyment is connected to the senses, and this means that we have to sense and to emote to then allow this "joy" in "enjoy" to be experienced.

Without the senses, joy cannot be experienced, so if we destroy the emotions to overcome them with logic and reason as a goal, then there can be no joy when logic and reason overcomes the process. What's left is a robotic machination of life that cannot then experience this joy and appreciation.

Doing so also is extremely dangerous, as removing emotional connections can sever ourselves from human experience and suffering. And when this is "overcome" or ignored, then we become machines of life, having no empathy or compassion for others, including young children and the older generations who are more susceptible to being negatively affected by their environments.

These groups are more susceptible to being "less at ease" and can be more "dis-eased" by these factors of life. To overlook this and ask them to ignore or push through these states of being is not only cold and cruel, but it is also inhumane.

While there are many times that the logical, rational minds of architects and doctors are not only desired but required, there is also a critically important component of the human experience to have their patient's emotional wellbeing recognized and supported in the human experience.

To lack compassion and empathy as an architect and doctor, especially during times of sickness when people are often most vulnerable, is to add insult to this very injury.

The everyday built environment of home and work needs to nurture and support well-being, which requires a recognition of how the built space is impacting human health.

Again this does not mean that we need to be less logical, but instead to add the senses, emotional intelligence, and the emotional life of being human in recognizing our humanity, and in essence, becoming more humane.

We need to spend as much time on the creation of the healthy built environment as we do the structural engineering of the built environment. By doing so, we are integrating the many facets of life for a whole solution.

The Significance of a Multi-Disciplinary Approach Between Architecture and Medicine

An essential part of my young adult life was learning a key process of learning itself. While both of my parents were teachers, an essential connection to learning occurred during a semester of college where several of my courses on different subjects – calculus and physics – came together into realization during my design and engineering classes.

The light bulb went on when I had a calculus class in the morning, a physics class at noon, and a structural engineering class in the afternoon. What I learned in calculus was applied in physics, and together were applied in my architecture and engineering courses.

I first began to see how important it was to have this integration between subjects and recognized the synergy of these different topics to eventually supporting the cohesive whole.

With my interest in architecture and my desire to learn, I was able to see how the math and science courses fit together to achieve these goals. And through this process, I became aware of the "why" of how these courses are interconnected.

Thus began my lifelong process of multi-disciplinary learning, which I knew was critical to my lifelong education. While many benefit from diving deep into one subject, focusing on one subject and one topic can sometimes limit progress in life.

While my experience 30 years ago was to focus on multiple subjects, today I'm happy to see changes for the younger generations, focusing on multi-disciplinary learning and STEM courses for all students. This, along with the STEAM approach adding the Arts to this integrative learning, can benefit society as a whole.

The process of writing this book and working to support these initiatives has helped me to have a feeling that I can contribute to these healthier building developments. And in this way, it has provided benefits to my own professional and personal development.

So for me, it's been a win-win that took several decades to truly live with and accept as a part of my journey. There have been many challenges and bumps along the way taking this multi-disciplinary path, yet Architectural Medicine would not have come into existence without this approach.

"Without health there can be no happiness."

– Thomas Jefferson

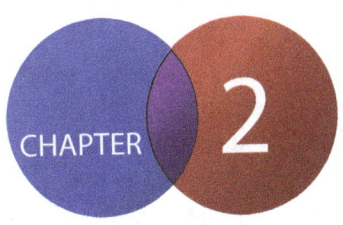

WHO IS THIS BOOK FOR?

A FOCUS ON THREE MAIN GROUPS

This book is written in three main parts. The first is focused on an overview of the many topics discussed in the book. The second part is geared towards the integrations between these fields. And the third part is focused on the details of achieving these integrations.

I've written this book in both the macro for the big picture, as well as the micro aspects of achieving the steps to these goals. Typically, books of this nature either address the general public in large picture formats or focus on one specific profession with a micro-focus on the small details.

However, I've chosen to write about these topics for both the general public on the macro level, and the professionals in the architecture and medical fields on a more micro level.

Why have I done this?

I'm writing this book for all three groups because the solutions to providing better health and wellness in the built environment will require an integrative approach.

This means that medical professionals will need to have an awareness of the health implications that the built environment has on their patients.

It also means that the architecture professionals will also need to have an understanding of health in buildings.

And last, yet definitely not least, is that the general public will need to understand how their built environments are impacting their health.

When all three groups have a baseline of understanding, then forward movement can proceed. All of these groups are involved in evaluating, analyzing, understanding, and providing solutions to creating healthier built environments.

By viewing these connections between the macro and the micro-details of both professions, the gaps that are currently preventing better solutions become evident. This approach has provided insights that have led to the development of Architectural Medicine.

I had chosen this path of integrating these multi-disciplinary topics many years ago and have never looked back. Although, in truth, I had to look back to understand and reflect on my path's trajectory, which has led to this concept of Architectural Medicine.

The path has been long and challenging, but I felt it necessary to stay on this path to gain insights into the many different health and wellness topics in the built environment.

I did this by seeing a lack of integration between these fields and the gaps between them. This resulted in a better understanding of why architecture and medical fields were not working together in a more cohesive format to achieve better health and wellness.

For me, the end goal became clear, yet I needed to reverse engineer this goal to provide steps to achieve these results. While this journey has often been very challenging beginning in the late 1980s as an architecture student, I've seen more discussions on these topics in the past several years. The momentum of this movement has become more common, and better solutions are beginning to appear.

As someone who has felt the impact of spaces and has been impacted by buildings in ways that often seemed different from other's experiences, the process of defining and discussing what I was experiencing was a challenge.

Eventually, particularly in the late 1990s, when the internet allowed these topics to become easier to discuss with other like-minded people, the process became easier to navigate and share these concerns with others.

However, a key to the process of solutions, which is still disconnected today and could genuinely support better health in the built environment, is, in my opinion, based on systems.

And in this book, this topic of systems will be an essential issue discussed and evaluated.

Three Reasons for This Book and Main Goals

The actual building of a house can take a long time when you slowly, over the years, pick up pieces needed to create a structure and then slowly sort these pieces to build a home.

In today's modern world, when you build a house or structure, you design the structure, itemize a building list of materials, and then go out and buy these materials and begin building.

Often you are hiring someone to do this work, but essentially these are the typical steps taken. There is also a timeline that you will follow. And most of the time, when building in this process, you buy what you already know you need for building the home and then complete these tasks.

I state this because when you are building a structure, whether an actual building or a system of some sort and don't know exactly what the final design will look like, you don't have a clear set of blueprints and materials to build this system. And for me, this has been the process of building Architectural Medicine.

In this process and journey that I have been on for most of my adult life, I have been slowly picking up pieces for a structure that I have been building, yet I have not always known what the finished product would be.

Therefore, through the years, my process has been to pick up pieces of knowledge in different places and then put these topics together to form a blueprint for a new system.

This process has led to the eventual creation of this project called Architectural Medicine and this book's writing.

When I first began on this journey several decades ago, I knew I wanted to be involved in architecture. Yet, I was unsatisfied with how typical architecture was structured and chose to take a path of exploration to find what I was looking and searching for.

The process of this book has come to be based on this journey, and I write this book for three main reasons:

1. **Context is critical for the future of Architecture:**

I grew up in the '70s and '80s, where there was no internet, and the local library and the people you knew were the extents of what you typically knew in life. When I was going to school for architectural engineering, I had limited knowledge about current developments in healthy, green, and sustainable building. It was not in the libraries, nor was it known by my professors. This writing for me is to share what I have learned and possibly provide the knowledge I wish I had as a student.

2. **The process of writing this book is an exploration:**

It is my hope that more people will become aware of built environment topics and focus on building solutions for better health and wellness. It is a topic that I continue to develop and strive to learn more about. As it is in its infancy and just developing, I continue to learn as I write this. Contributing to the development of this field that I believe in and want to participate in to create beautiful, healthy, green, and sustainable architecture is a main goal.

3. **The third reason is to support an integrated systems architecture for healthier built environments:**

In my opinion, these different fields and professionals will need to work together to weave together the many facets required to make this happen. It will require both the general public's demand and the many professionals' support and supply to help this integrative process to function. These integrations can create beautiful, inspiring, and supportive built environments that are also healthy, green, and sustainable.

That is the goal of this book. It is about exploring this process, researching the many facets involved, and contributing my part with new systems.

This includes the Architectural Medicine System (AMS), new procedures and software such as ARxMD, and new professionals such as the Architectural

Doctor and the Healthy Building Inspector. By establishing these pieces of the puzzle, a path can be provided to achieve these goals.

In order to achieve these goals, it requires that many different professionals from the architecture and medical fields work together for the benefit of the general public.

And so this brings the focus on these three main groups:

- The General Public
- The Architecture, Engineering, and Building/Construction Fields (AEC), and
- The Medical and Health Fields

While this may seem to be an extensive range to discuss for one book, it's pivotal that all three are included to address the interconnected and interdependent processes involved for whole systems solutions.

What Is the Purpose of This Book?

While the book is ideally written for these three groups – the General Public, Architects, and Doctors – in reality, the latter two are obviously included as the general public.

As stated earlier, it may sound like too broad of scope or range to have any consensus and clarity on these topics. When you view the steps and requirements for solutions, you will see how important that all three groups are involved.

You will soon see in future chapters that these are merely the big three groups involved. To achieve the goals of health in the built environment, many different groups will overlap. In the future, there will likely be many groups and professions that will be more directly involved than there are today.

And if these many groups are not currently involved, they will need to be engaged if cohesive, whole system solutions are to be achieved.

It will require a multi-disciplinary integration process for the goals of health and wellness in the built environment to be reached.

And this is not just the topic of healthy building. In defining the process for healthy building, the topics of green building and sustainable building will also need to be included. It is my opinion that all three are required to be considered a complete equation.

Why Have Interest in the Topics of This Book?

If you are wondering why you should read this book, I will offer this as a reason in the question format:

"Are you wanting a better world in which to live, work, and play for both yourself and future generations? Are you concerned about the future of your health and the health of your children, grandchildren, and the many other creatures and animals that live on this planet?"

While I can't promise I know all of these solutions, I am certainly asking these questions with great concern. And this book came to be after many years of seeking, reading, and learning about these topics along with hands-on involvement. My direct experience was either for work or merely exploring this on my personal time as a pathway towards knowledge.

My viewpoint and intentions are that this book will strive to define a history of these developments and potential integrations, and in turn, it may help clarify the why's of this work. Perhaps this may inspire others to seek these solutions and co-create them.

Yet without context and an understanding of the history of these developments, it may leave significant gaps in understanding. However, if there is more context and clarity about this trajectory, it can help clarify the next steps and pathways toward these goals.

As I wrote above, the intention of this book is a lifelong process to seek a better world in which to live, work, and play – literally. How can the built environment support a better world and a better life? How can we, as a society, both locally and globally, find healing where this is needed?

I've often found the definition and etymology of the word "healing" very interesting:

healing (n.)

"restoration to health," Old English hæling, verbal noun from heal (v.). Figurative sense of "restoration of wholeness" is from early 13c.[2]

heal (v.)

Old English hælan "cure; save; make whole, sound and well," from Proto-Germanic *hailjan (source also of Old Saxon helian, Old Norse heila, Old Frisian hela, Dutch helen, German heilen, Gothic ga-hailjan "to heal, cure"), literally "to make whole" (from PIE *kailo- "whole;" see health).[3]

If healing is "putting together the pieces of oneself to become healed, or whole," then to become whole individually and as a global community, we will need to have some paths to this healing and the support necessary to achieve this. The built environment has a considerable impact and influence in this healing, yet few are even aware of this influence or healing potential.

And if there is to be a "restoration of wholeness," then this wholeness must first be recognized in all of its facets. There must be some awareness where this wholeness is lacking or where wholeness is broken. With this awareness, the broken pieces can be placed back together, and it is this wholeness that can then bring healing.

The built environment, and in particular, our homes, are a key ingredient to this healing process. With up to 90 percent of our time spent inside in the modern-day world, it becomes critical that these interior environments are healthy and support our health and healing.

Why Is This Book Important Now?

As the world becomes more multi-faceted and seemingly broken or troubled, it becomes more evident that healing and health become a path that more people are seeking. While a specified solution may not be formulaic, my hope and intention is to provide frameworks that may support this healing and contribute to this process.

This information has been a big part of my life's work and has taken a lifetime to put together.

While it's becoming easier to find the information, where in the past, the challenge was to find the content, the challenge in today's day and age is "context."

While it used to be that information was King, in essence, the truth of the matter now is that *context* is King. Without this reference to the whole, the information is merely data without deeper meaning.

Context is key, and in this age of information, without context and knowing the interconnections of how topics fit together, there is a chance for large holes of knowledge to prevent wholeness.

This can often create more problems as one facet of these problems may be solved, yet many others are made.

Chapter 5 will discuss more details about this context being key, yet a simple version can be provided for now. With the plethora of information being available in today's 21st century, the key to information as knowledge is to have context. This means that information relative to other information can provide meaning and can be recognized as integrative sourcing. This contextual content can weave together many different topics, along with how they are interconnected.

In the past, hierarchal information would define solutions without a shared process. And now and into the future, a more nodal or multi-disciplinary approach will be required.

An essential purpose of discussing context is that larger problems can be created when the many variables involved are not factored into the entire equation.

This is a critical concept to keep in mind when navigating the content throughout this book and Architectural Medicine as a whole.

While there are many other books written about the healthy, green, and sustainable built environment, this book strives to provide a framework for these many fields. This can provide insights into what the future may hold in creating these healthy, green, and sustainable built environments.

It is also intended, as I've mentioned earlier, to give credit where it's due and to provide links to more details should the reader have an interest.

This process is intended to create context to the various, and now numerous information sources that exist. This information's complexity can often overwhelm and leave people without direction or a positive, hopeful feeling.

Empowerment of information that is contextual can then lead people to have more confidence and more hopefulness in the solution process.

And while all of these reasons are great, in my opinion, all of these reasons are secondary to the real reason why I'm writing this book.

And the real reason is to support and contribute to creating built environments and architecture that supports physical health beyond surviving and survival. It is to support architecture that can support thriving for human beings in health and wellness – mentally, physically, and emotionally – and, dare I say, spiritually.

To achieve these goals, there has to be a focus on three main topics in architecture, which are becoming topics more recognized and seen as more critical each year.

These are the three topics of *healthy building, green building,* and *sustainable building.*

And this, along with the three topics of *physical, emotional,* and *mental or psychological wellness* in the built environment, can combine to form a foundation of architecture to support human thriving in the current day into the future.

These six topics are very important threads in creating the healthy built environment, which have had an interesting path over the past 30 to 50 years. And when placed together, it has the potential for an even more interesting trajectory in viewing this past relative to the future.

It is my thought that these threads in the building and health worlds are going to merge with a significant result. And while they are currently merging in some ways, their ability to connect with an integrated format with ease, or lack of integration and dis-ease, may determine the whole of life on planet earth as we know it to be.

It is my thought and concern that if we don't find a way to attend to all of these topics in an integrated and mutually beneficial format, our built environments and human developments will become the downfall of humanity and the sentient world as we know it.

This is not a light topic, nor a subject that can be discussed over light conversation. Yet, if we do not begin talking about this and creating a demand for solutions with sufficient supply, we will not make it easy for life on planet earth for ourselves and for future generations.

And I personally don't think this is fair to create such problems for later generations and even for the current generations that live on earth right now. It's also highly illogical and unreasonable as civilized beings to live life in this form of uncivilized mannerisms and actions.

Our current or at least our "up until recently" mindset about the built environment has been very concrete and unmoving, which ironically has been the purpose of these endeavors. Yet in the process has also created these concrete problems that we now encounter.

Many groups will need to be involved based on the complexity of achieving the healthy, green, and sustainable built environment. At this time in history, it is going to be a requirement that we work together as a collective humanity to accomplish this.

This demand for building these updated forms of healthier architecture will require the supply of the needed tools, materials, techniques, and solutions to fill these demands.

You cannot have one without the other in terms of a whole or holistic approach to the process. This approach will be a requirement as a collaborative process to accomplish the many steps involved.

An important key to these steps is that they cannot be merely linear steps with a start and end, and will have to be cyclical and iterative. This means the process will require a process from start to finish and then a return to the beginning to implement updates with new enhancements.

This cyclical process allows proper evaluation of the processes outlined in this book focused on health and wellness. And an ideal method of achieving these goals will include the professionals involved and the public at large. When the public has information to empower themselves to learn about their surroundings and buildings they live and work within, they can make educated and informed decisions for their own best health.

To return to the initial question of who this book is for, the answer is that it's for the general public seeking a healthier life and those directly involved in the architecture and medical fields.

What Is a Spiracycle?

As mentioned in the previous paragraphs, when the building process is improved upon for health, lessons can be learned to provide adjustments as an iterative process with updated content.

This can be continually updated for forward progress for better solutions. When this cyclical process is implemented, it can allow for iteration that is synergistic between all of the many professionals involved for the best solutions.

The term Spiracycle is a word that I use to describe this cyclical iteration – the process either spirals upwards in a positive cycle or downwards in a negative cycle.

The point is not to always expect there to be a positive upward direction, as the attempts to make it better will yield some negative or failed results. With the overall focus on progress, failures can be learned from to iterate towards a hopeful, positive direction with eventual success as a key goal.

Some may say this meliorism viewpoint, somewhere between pessimism and optimism, is also considered idealistic, yet it seems more practical to me than anything. If we are not focused on striving to make things better, we've quit striving to make things good.

This concept of a cyclical process with the terms cyclical economy and circular economy have become more common topics in the past few decades. By evaluating nature's cycles, which are often seen as forming in circles, the added process of time can add another dimension to this two-dimensional concept. The result is a third dimension as a spiral.

And this spiracycle process of iteration supports a positive movement forward, where many topics can form better solutions for health and wellness in the built environment.

How Is Medicine Connected to Architecture?

Up until now, this writing has been discussing healthy building and green and sustainable building, yet there haven't been any specific definitions of what all of this really is.

In the next section, we'll get to a few reasons why these topics can be viewed as valuable, and then in future chapters, we'll dive into more details on each of these topics.

If you wonder how and why medicine and the medical fields are involved in this process of healthier built environments, this may be a new facet for many in connecting health to the built environment.

I would also be wondering why and how medicine and the medical fields are involved in architecture if I were reading this book, had I not been involved as I have in the trajectory of this field over the past twenty-five years.

While I go into details in the chapter "healthy building", I can comment that this might be surprising to many because it has often been the most overlooked or underseen if that definition works better.

I can comment that this might be surprising to many because we are often not aware of how the exterior environments, as built environments, impact and influence our health daily.

Most people do not connect their health relative to the public spaces and architecture as the built environment. Still, the reality is that there are many layers to how the built environment affects human health – and not just physical health.

With many people spending up to 90 percent of their lives inside, the built environment is having an increasingly large impact on human health. This includes an impact on physical, emotional, and mental or psychological health and wellness in ways that many do not consider.

Most people have become accustomed to buildings as familiar places they spend all of their time within, yet do not spend much time contemplating these impacts.

The built environment has, for many, become a natural part of their lives that they don't even question. And perhaps it is not essential to spend too much time analyzing as a huge part of one's life that people ignore in many ways, it might be a good idea to contemplate this on at least some levels as an occupant.

When you begin to evaluate the built environment, there can be many facets of knowledge attained or adjustments made to benefit wellness and achieve a better quality of life.

Architectural Medicine – Building the Bridge to Wellness

These evaluations and research of the built environment on health is also an interesting dynamic to follow. This is because many of the issues related to the unhealthy built environment, which historically have been brought up by environmental and ecological groups, have more recently become issues raised by public health, epidemiology, and toxicology fields.

Environmental groups have flagged such health issues in the past, yet these groups are often seen on the extremes, and all too often, they go unnoticed or are not taken seriously.

While the voice of the environmentalists has often been loud in signaling concerns, in the past decade, many of these similar concerns of health in the built environment have been coming from those in public health.

These professionals have been studying the negative toxicological impacts on human, biological, and ecological health and recognizing the detriments of such materials. They are now making more waves and bringing awareness to the general public about topics related to health and the built world in which we live.

When reading about these toxicology issues from the top science fields, it can often be a surprise that these negative issues can be true. The impact of BPA and phthalates on allergies, asthma, and immune function[4], for instance, can be materials found in common building materials in modern structures.

And perhaps this should provide more information for the general public to not only be aware of, yet demand that better solutions are created for their homes and workplaces.

If you read *Silent Spring* you may have noticed that Rachel Carson was herself a top scientist at the time of her research on the topics of the day, and that was 50 years ago. She was a voice of reason that was chastised and criticized at that time, yet her research was focused on human concerns and the health and well-being of biological life.

Only in today's day and age, this voice of one person from the past, and specifically a female voice, has been combined with many more voices of the current day with an increasing amount of data to back up these metrics as knowledge and facts. Today's voices include a wide range of backgrounds and professionals, which is much harder to ignore than one female voice half a century ago.

And this focus on science and data defined as Evidence-Based Design and will be discussed in other chapters in this book.

Yet being that this book is titled Architectural Medicine, there is also an emphasis on the medical fields. In many ways, it is as important as the field of architecture – if the topic is health in the built environment.

The truth is that both fields of architecture and medicine require a mutual interconnection and interdependency to make the whole jigsaw puzzle fit together.

And that is precisely why the medical fields are being discussed because the built environment that we currently live within has become more of a puzzle of unknowns than any other time in recorded history.

In the past 50 years, we have created more new products, mostly synthetic, where there is little information about how all of these various materials combine in the real world and impact health. How these combinations impact human, biological, and ecological health and well-being in many ways is still unknown.

And as I'm finishing the writing of this book in 2020, the pandemic of the novel coronavirus is affecting the entire world's health. And the focus of health in the built environment has, perhaps, never been as focused on this topic, particularly the attention from the masses.

The House Doctor of the Past and Future

It is also interesting to recognize that, in the past, the traditional process of the "house doctor" or the doctor visiting the patient's residence in the past was not uncommon. The idea that a doctor would travel to the patient's house when they were sick has become a forgotten notion.

And perhaps it is a misunderstood factor of importance in previous evaluation processes in the doctor's medical evaluations at that time. Viewing the patient's built environment may have provided insights into potential health issues and solutions.

In the manner that Florence Nightingale provided insights into natural lighting and fresh air for patient's healing processes, perhaps it was more common for the house doctor in the past to utilize this knowledge to help in their patient's healing.

Few if any doctors of today factor in the built environment in evaluating their patient's health, even though most people are spending more of their time inside the built environment, both at their homes and at work.

And in this manner, the future doctor may return to the concept of a house call to evaluate their patient's health, although this process may be a bit different from the past, as is discussed in later chapters. These future house calls may include the concept of an Architectural Doctor and a Healthy Building Inspector.

This is described in more detail in later chapters and will inevitably or potentially include the facet of telemedicine as it is becoming increasingly popular in today's modern medical development.

Up until this point, there are topics that have been discussed that right now are a bit vague, yet we will get into these specifics in later chapters.

What's critical at this time is to discuss the topic of context because much of these topics are relative to the interconnections between these subjects. And context is crucial to gaining insights into how these are all connected. Without this contextual understanding, the essential systems for solutions cannot be appropriately architected.

This brings us back again to the three main topics of Healthy, Green, and Sustainable Building. What do these mean, and why are these three so important in the built environment's future?

Before we discuss the details of these topics, I think an essential factor in grasping the many topics related to Architectural Medicine is to talk about these two words themselves – Architecture and Medicine.

These big topics and fields will be discussed in the next two chapters, ensuring a baseline of understanding. This way, there can be clarification on these terms in how they relate to this book and, eventually, to the concept of Architectural Medicine and health in the built environment...

"We are called to be architects of the future, not its victims."

– R. Buckminster Fuller

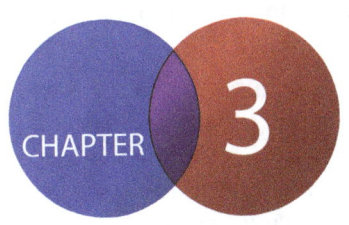

WHAT IS ARCHITECTURE?
THE EXTERIOR WORLD – THE BUILT ENVIRONMENT

The topic of architecture is sometimes very matter of fact, and other times can be very abstract. Some may define architecture as the same as that of any building, and others may see architecture as much more — differentiating itself from the simple shed in a backyard to that of the great ancient pyramids or modern-day skyscrapers.

Before we go into more details about Architectural Medicine, there needs to be a foundation to build upon in defining this word architecture.

So, what exactly is Architecture?

The Oxford English Dictionary (OED) defines Architecture as:

"The art or science of building or constructing edifices of any kind for human use."[5]

And the OED defines edifice as, "a building, usually a large and stately building, as a church, palace, temple, or fortress; a fabric, structure."[6]

While this certainly describes the basics of Architecture, a bigger scope expands on this definition from the simple building into architecture. While there are many different definitions of architecture, at the core of this topic is shelter, combined with creating a safe and enjoyable space and place to live and work.

For centuries, architecture served as basic structures for homes that shielded humans from the elements, whether hot, cold, wet, or dry environmental conditions. In today's modern world of the 21st century, it can be easy to forget that it's only been the past century that humans have become adept at building and sheltering in the way we can today.

The modern type of building has the capability to shelter us from the natural elements. It can also provide temperature control and electricity and plumbing resources that allow for the comfort and tempered indoor environments that many come to expect of the built environment.

Before the mid-20th century, this was still uncommon in many developed areas of the world, and the battle against nature's elements was still a challenging feat for even the best architects. In many parts of the world, we may find it commonplace in buildings that these amenities are a given in the modern world, while other parts of the world still do not have these modern services.

The etymology of the words "Architecture" and "Architect" can give some insights into what exactly the profession is along with its purpose:

architecture (n.)

1560s, "the art of building, tasteful application of scientific and traditional rules of good construction to the materials at hand," from Middle French architecture, from Latin architectura, from architectus "master builder, chief workman" (see architect). Meaning "buildings constructed architecturally" is from 1610s.[7]

architect (n.)

"person skilled in the art of building, one who plans and designs buildings and supervises their construction," 1560s, from Middle French architecte, from Latin architectus, from Greek arkhitekton "master builder, director of works," from arkhi- "chief" (see archon) + tekton "builder, carpenter," from PIE root *teks- "to weave," also "to fabricate."[8]

The definition of architecture can be defined as, "structures that are technically and artfully created to support human life and to provide shelter." However, architecture is not just for surviving. At the highest level, its purpose can be focused on human thriving.

It can strive to support health and wellness in an optimal format. Not just for physical comfort but also for emotional and mental or psychological wellness.

Buildings may exist for basic shelter, yet architecture can support human thriving.

What's important to outline, relative to the topics of Architectural Medicine, is to recognize that Architecture is the external world in which we live, work, and spend much of our time within –particularly in the suburban and urban environments. It may sound basic to state this, but as we delve into the definitions of Medicine in the next chapter focusing on our internal world, it becomes relevant to keep this in mind.

Modernism and the International Style

Creating shelter that goes beyond the basic protection from the elements, which can avail the ability to control the temperature and humidity, and provide indoor plumbing is actually a relatively new capability. And more recently, in the late 19th to early 20th century, has been the addition of electricity to modern structures.

I state that this has occurred *recently* on purpose – because architecture has been around since the origins of humans and the timeline of architecture of the past one hundred years is not very old. To be more exact, architecture has been around since the origins of biological creatures, as humans are not the only beings on this planet that build. Let us not forget that the architecture of animals, insects, birds, and many other living beings on this planet have been creating architecture much longer than humans.

You can view these designs and building processes, such as a bird nest and a beaver dam, as well as the nautilus shells and the termite skyscrapers. As the field of Biomimicry is showing, much of human inspiration in architecture can stem from our fellow living creatures on this planet. These designs can continue to inspire with the wisdom of biological approaches to building solutions.

And getting back to the topic, a goal of human architecture has been to live beyond the negative impacts of the natural elements and to be able to overcome the potentially harmful impacts of the natural world.

In fact, this architectural process can be seen in the International Design style movement, which worked to create shelter that could protect humans from the elements. The method of creating a building that could exist in any place in the world, from the polar cold and the hot deserts to the wet rain forests and the open plains, would be a solution to a human issue since the beginning of time.

And that issue was to overcome the harsh impacts of the natural elements.

In the mid 20th century, architecture was able to overcome many of these challenges, and building in remote locales became a reality. No matter what the natural environment is, the design of modern architecture can supply a controlled environment, with electricity, plumbing, and all of the essentials for shelter and safety in almost any environment.

In many ways, this process has also disconnected us from nature and the natural environment. It is understandable that over the centuries, the goal has been to remove humans from challenging natural conditions and not be at the mercy of these harsh environments.

Yet as we are now discovering, you cannot separate yourself from nature, as humans not only exist in the natural world – we are a part of the natural world. We depend on the natural world in an interconnected and interdependent way. And this is a big part of human health and wellness that we will discuss in subsequent chapters.

There is a tradeoff that we are now beginning to seriously recognize, which is to see that there is a cost to this style of architecture that removes us from the natural world, and eventually, there is a price to pay. This cost is often challenging to determine, as it means an evaluation of costs in energy use and the long term costs of the production of these building materials and their use in creating the modern built environment. And it also has a cost to human health, wellness, and quality of life.

A challenge is that this cost is something that happens over time. The impact this has on the ecological and biological world can often take decades or longer before the results become evident. And in today's fast moving world, for societies that are only looking at the short term processes and impact, there is becoming a massive wake up call to this impact that has now been ongoing for over half a century.

Much of the ecological impacts and energy awareness topics in the architectural world did not become common, at least in the US, until the energy crisis of the 1970s. This awareness resulted in alternative building developments to find solutions, which has created a strong foundation on which the past several decades have built upon.

Modern architecture can be seen as a positive on many levels and a negative on other levels. And if we can work towards more balance and harmony in achieving both the modern-day comforts with the capability to maintain the fragile balance of the planet, there is hope for a better future.

Much of these newer viewpoints towards these solutions have been an unfolding process of learning over the past few decades. While some of these efforts have been to reduce energy costs and reduce ecological impact, there has been another issue that has arisen from these newer, modern styles of building. The goal of controlling the interior environments from the harsh natural world has caused new problems – and this has been a negative impact on human health.

We will discuss this in more detail in the next few chapters, yet for now, this is a good segue into the next topic…

> "Wherever the art of medicine is loved,
> there is also a love of humanity."
>
> – Hippocrates

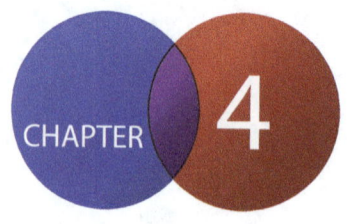

WHAT IS MEDICINE?

THE INTERIOR WORLD OF OUR LIVES

What exactly is Medicine? The Oxford English Dictionary (OED) defines Medicine as, "The science or practice of the diagnosis, treatment, and prevention of disease."[9]

"A substance or preparation used in the treatment of illness; a drug; esp. one taken by mouth. Also: such substances generally. To treat or cure (a person, condition, etc.) by means of medicine; to give medicine to."[10]

As the definition of architecture has a varying level of definitions, the term Medicine also has varying definitions and meanings.

If we look into the etymology of the word Medicine, there are a few key features that define the term that is relevant to how the word is used in this book:

medicine (n.)

c. 1200, "medical treatment, cure, remedy," also used figuratively, of spiritual remedies, from Old French medecine (Modern French médicine) "medicine, art of healing, cure, treatment, potion," from Latin medicina "the healing art, medicine; a remedy," also used figuratively, perhaps originally ars medicina "the medical art," from fem. of medicinus (adj.) "of a doctor," from medicus "a physician" (from PIE root *med- "take appropriate measures"); though OED finds evidence for this is wanting. Meaning "a medicinal potion or plaster" in English is mid-14c.[11]

healing (n.)

"restoration to health," Old English hæling, verbal noun from heal (v.). Figurative sense of "restoration of wholeness" is from early 13c.; meaning "touch that cures" is from 1670s.[12]

heal (v.)

Old English hælan "cure; save; make whole, sound and well," from Proto-Germanic *hailjan (source also of Old Saxon helian, Old Norse heila, Old Frisian hela, Dutch helen, German heilen, Gothic ga-hailjan "to heal, cure"), literally "to make whole," from PIE *kailo- "whole" (see health). Intransitive sense from late 14c. Related: Healed; healing.[13]

health (n.)

Old English hælþ "wholeness, a being whole, sound or well," from Proto-Germanic *hailitho, from PIE *kailo- "whole, uninjured, of good omen" (source also of Old English hal "hale, whole;" Old Norse heill "healthy;" Old English halig, Old Norse helge "holy, sacred;" Old English hælan "to heal"). With Proto-Germanic abstract noun suffix *-itho (see -th (2)). Of physical health in Middle English, but also "prosperity, happiness, welfare; preservation, safety.[14]

Medicine and Healing

As the above word origins show, the concept and essence of medicine has been based on "medical treatment, cure, remedy - medicine, art of healing, cure, treatment, potion," and "the healing art, medicine; a remedy."[15]

The term medicine references "a remedy" and a "treatment, potion" and an "art of healing". And from this we see that the origins of healing and health are based upon:

healing (n.)
"restoration to health," Old English hæling, verbal noun from heal (v.). Figurative sense of "restoration of wholeness" - heal (v.) Old English hælan "cure; save; make whole, sound and well," health (n.) Old English hælþ "wholeness, a being whole, sound or well."[16]

So if you put the two terms of medicine and healing together, you will find that medicine is the process, treatment, and remedy to a "restoration to health," and a "restoration of wholeness, a being whole, sound or well".

If medicine is seen as your internal world, that which is based on "Health," which is focused on a "restoration to health, restoration of wholeness", then the concept of "being whole, sound or well" can relate to the concept of wellness and well-being.

In later chapters, we get into how this relates to the world of architecture, yet as mentioned above, if good health is based on wholeness and being well, then there is another facet of this equation that should be included.

And that is the concept that you experience the exterior world internally. Therefore, the environment that is outside of you, including the built environment, is mostly experienced internally.

And if your exposure to the world is actually experienced internally, such as your vision, hearing, taste, smell, and touch, perhaps it is not as far-fetched to think that the exterior world has an impact and influence on your overall internal well being.

And the word "Medicine" is defined as the interior world relative to a "restoration to health, restoration of wholeness, and of being whole, sound or well". Referring to the two terms of medicine and healing together, the term "Medicine" in "Architectural Medicine" is focused on the process, treatment, and remedy to a "restoration to health, restoration of wholeness, a being whole, sound or well."

Chapter: 4 — What Is Medicine?

Medicine's true focus is to help the patient to achieve this "wellness" and "well being."

In this book and the work of Architectural Medicine, the term "Architecture" is defined as the exterior built world. It includes "the art of building" and the "tasteful application of scientific and traditional rules of good construction" as a definition.

The Latin architectura, from architectus as "master builder, chief workman," is also a key to the concept of what a master builder is responsible for and how this definition has evolved over time into the modern-day world of materials and methods. We dive into those concepts on a deeper level and explore what the current and future architect will navigate in a future chapter. That said, the future of architecture will have to include modern-day concerns of health in this ever-changing profession.

What these word origins also describe is a "return to wholeness", and so the next question may be, how are we as humans disconnected? If being ill is a lack of being whole and requires a restoration of wholeness, then the question might be, how are we disconnected or separated?

And how can we put these pieces back together to achieve wholeness?

The discussion of wholeness and how the modern-day world has disconnected us from wholeness, is again part of the discussions throughout this book.

This leads us into the next chapter, Architectural Medicine -Part 1: Reviewing the Many Pieces of the Puzzle...

"The architect should also have a knowledge of the study of medicine on account of the questions of climates, air, the healthiness and unhealthiness of sites...

for without these considerations the healthiness of a dwelling cannot be assured."

– Vitruvius

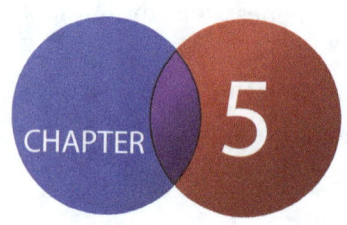

ARCHITECTURAL MEDICINE - PART 1
REVIEWING THE MANY PIECES OF THE PUZZLE

An essential component of Architectural Medicine is the integration of many facets of both architecture and medicine. When referring to the chapter subtitle of a "review of the many pieces of the puzzle," what puzzle pieces are being referenced exactly?

The fields of architecture and medicine are wide-ranging, so the facets discussed in this book are a start yet do not include every facet. That said, with a focus on health in the built environment, Architectural Medicine includes the fields of green building and sustainable building, as well as healthy building as "pieces" of the puzzle to fit together.

The reason why these other fields are included is based on biological health.

Human beings require clean water, clean air, and clean soil for food to support good health. Sometimes people forget that you are not only living in the natural world; you are a part of the natural world.

Your body consists of around 70 percent of water and is composed of many other natural elements. The calcium of your bones, the silicon of your skin, hair, and nails, and your organs and cells are composed of many various minerals and natural substances.

The architecture of your body is composed of natural elements, and if we pollute the natural environment, eventually, our bodies are then polluted.

And when your body is polluted, this causes dis-ease, just as polluting the environment will cause disease for other biological beings that we share this planet with.

Therefore, if we are to focus on human health, there needs to be a focus on biological and environmental health as well. You cannot separate the fact that we are a part of nature. So if we ensure that we do not pollute our natural world, it can help ensure that our bodies are not polluted.

This can be a tremendous support for promoting good health and wellness and cannot be overlooked.

Why Are the Three Topics of Healthy, Green, and Sustainable Building So Important to Include Together?

As written in the previous chapters defining architecture and medicine, the next step and question might be to ask, "how does the built environment impact human health and wellness?"

And that's a perfect segue into this chapter to discuss the integration of these three fields to help put the many pieces of the jigsaw puzzle together. In this approach, evaluating "how" the built environment impacts health can lead to "what" can be done about it for better health.

And this process requires a lot of topics to be evaluated either at the same time or in similar time frames to see the whole picture of a patient's health. In this manner, there will be new processes and systems that are required to achieve these goals, as well as education and information for each professional involved.

As we venture into the details of this book, there are graphics that will be used to define these discussions. These images can provide road maps as to where these discussions will lead. And to start this description of the many pieces involved below is a graphic of the final result:

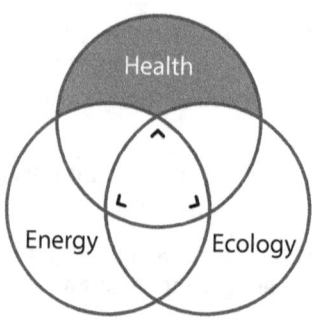

Health/
Healthy Building

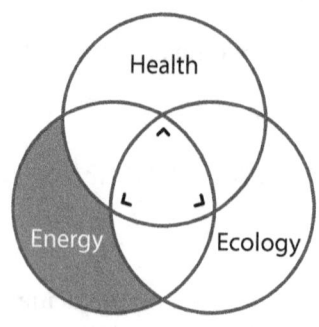

Energy (Efficiency)/
Green Building

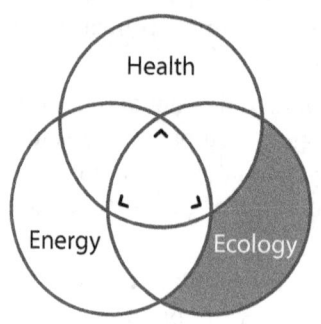

Ecology/**Sustainable Architecture-Building**

The Intersection of Energy, Ecology, and Health in the Built Environment

Health

Issues related to physical health, removing toxic materials and improving occupant health. Groups and organizations with a Health focus in the built environment include: Healthy Building Network, Bau Biologie and Biophilia

Energy

Issues related to optimizing Energy use, sourcing more sustainable energy options, striving to reduce pollution, and working to reduce carbon footprint. Groups and organizations related to this Energy focus include: Architecture 2030 and the US Green Building Council (USGBC)

Ecology

Recognizing and designing for the Ecology, creating more sustainable solutions with materials and methods. Considering Life Cycle Assessment (LCA) in all designs. Groups and organizations with an Ecological focus in the built environment include: Biophilic Design and the Permaculture Institute

This graphic includes the segments as an integrated whole, along with separate components with more details on each topic.

In chapter 14, we put all of these facets together with the professions of architecture and medicine in an interconnected format, including the general public as the building occupants. We'll discuss these integration details in later chapters, and for now, we'll focus on the three facets of healthy building, green building, and sustainable building as the first triad of topics.

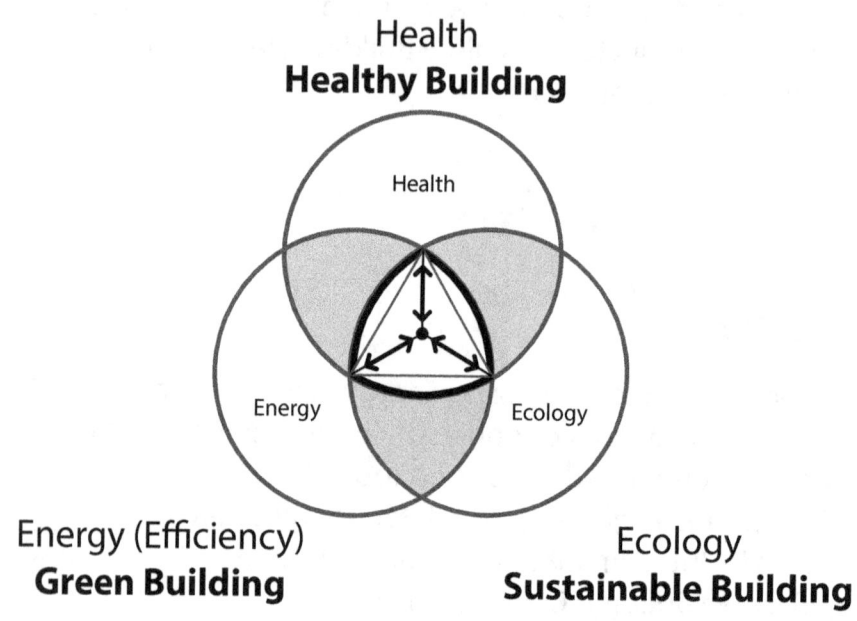

Whether you are new to these topics in the built environment or have spent decades involved in these fields, an essential part of the topics of Architectural Medicine is *integration*.

Now, this word integration is being used quite a lot in the past few decades, so I'd rather this not be as much a buzzword and have it more focused on its base definition:

integration (n.)

1610s, "act of bringing together the parts of a whole," from French intégration and directly from Late Latin integrationem (nominative integratio) "renewal, restoration," noun of action from past participle stem of Latin integrare "make whole," also "renew, begin again" (see integrate).[17]

Yet as this definition defines "bringing together parts of the whole," the question is, what parts are being integrated?

And this is where the concept of *Integrative Architecture* enters into the lexicon of this book.

A Brief Introduction to Integrative Architecture

In the past century, medicine has seen significant changes. In the world of modern medicine, these changes have included the technologies of X-rays, MRIs, and the many testing capabilities, including insights that can be gleaned with blood tests. These technologies include the pharmacological developments of prescriptions, yielding powerful medicine for better health.

Over the past several decades, these technological developments have been merging with what's known as traditional therapies to form *Integrative Medicine*. And this has often been differentiated from the growing developments of Complementary Medicine (CM) – also known as modern medicine.

Even though many of these traditional therapies, such as acupuncture and Chinese Medicine, have been around for thousands of years, integrating modern medicine with traditional medicine has not been rapid nor easy for many populated areas in the contemporary world.

A big part of these changes in medicine to accepting traditional options has occurred because the general public wants to have more options to be empowered for their own good health. In the US and other locations worldwide, Integrative Medicine's development has been a critical part of this integrative growth and development.

Pioneering doctors such Dr. Andrew Weil, who is probably one of the most well known in this transformation, has stated in many of his books and lectures that he defines Integrative Medicine as an integration to use "different modalities that utilize best practices from many resources – from both modern and traditional methodologies and treatments."[18]

You may be wondering why I am bringing up this field of Integrative Medicine and its history. The reason is based on a reflection of this progress in medicine towards these integrations and a lack of progress in the fields of architecture. This progress in building and construction can be relative to similar goals that integrative medicine is striving to achieve — best practices towards optimal health.

As medicine has been embracing more traditional therapies for better health, what has been happening in the fields of architecture?

The answer is that there have been some steps to improve architecture to be more ecologically aware and more "green" or energy-efficient. Yet, the healthy component has been slow going and primarily focused on Healthy Hospital Designs. While Healthy Hospital Designs are an excellent step in this progress, it's also a recognition that there is room for improvement for the rest of the built environments – from the average home to the modern commercial building.

A potential to have more rapid development towards these goals is to use this example of Integrative Medicine to show a pathway of development for architecture to take. Embracing healthier approaches to built environments while also utilizing traditional methodologies can help to achieve these goals.

This process can be defined as *Integrative Architecture* to support and work in tandem with the positive developments of Integrative Medicine.

The concept of learning from Integrative Medicine in the field of architecture has many benefits. For one, many people are familiar with the topics of Integrative Medicine and the positive connotation it has to empower the average person. It also can be utilized as a high standard in discovering and using best practices for better health.

The concept of Integrative Architecture is similar to Integrative Medicine in that it strives to utilize best practices while also merging modern approaches with traditional methodologies. It is essentially considering many different methods to achieve the best results, and these "best results" include a process for healthier designs.

We'll go into more details about this topic in chapter 10, Introduction to Integrative Architecture.

Context Is Key

This book covers many various topics, and while over the years, I have been told and taught to focus on a single topic to become proficient at this for a career, it has not been my path to focus on just one subject.

In some ways, I can't argue about this single topic focus, as many people follow this path in life with great success. Some have commented that it takes about 10,000 hours to become an expert at any topic, which can be sourced from Malcolm Gladwell's book *Outliers*. However, this can be questioned or redefined as a focus on the "quality" and not just the "quantity" spent for mastery.

Perhaps this definition of quality includes the many facets and interconnections that a professional will navigate. By recognizing the value of a larger scope of topics, the value of the independent and interdependent connections can be obtained.

While a specific practice of one topic often leads to mastery, the process of gaining mastery of a topic does not reflect on the quality of work relative to other facets of life.

What is meant is that you can be so focused on one thing and become very good at that single topic, yet how does that skill connect with the many other facets of life?

Architectural Medicine integrates many topics into a single focus by merging many various subjects into a scope relative to health in the built environment. It is the integration of many topics that provides the quality of the results and the strength in its approach.

This is not to say that there is less value in the work of a specialist. In fact, it has been the work of many specialists that has provided the increased knowledge and information that has become available to humanity.

In a later chapter, I discuss the subject of the "silo" of work as it is commonly called, where one person becomes so immersed in one topic that they block themselves out from the rest of the world. While I discuss this in more detail later in the book, I want to take this time to discuss a concept that is based on a different approach. It is not a debate of the specialist as is discussed above and not quite the opposite of the generalist approach, but more related to the context relative to integration.

Several decades ago, becoming more knowledgeable was often based on access to information, and this was sometimes hard to find. If you could not find information in the library, bookstore, or know someone as a teacher or friend who knew about a particular subject, it was much more challenging to learn about such topics.

In the modern world in which we live in this 21st century, the opposite has occurred. If you can get online to the internet, you can find almost anything or learn about any topic through some form of online resource.

However, this has added an extra challenge in learning, which is the issue of information overload.

Nowadays, there is so much information that figuring out what to learn and what is relevant to the learning process has become very murky due to the massive number of options.

In this manner, the key to this process is *context*.

With the information age, the context of the information is as important as the information itself. This is perhaps, an appropriate meta-reference during a time when meta topics are plenty.

A big part of the work that I've been doing over the years is in providing context through a systems approach. By taking the big picture overview of how solutions can be provided and then connecting them to the many professionals and groups, the result can support whole systems solutions.

In many ways, this is a fractal relationship, as the microlens of these systems can also be applied to a macro view of the world. This also relates to the scalability of topics from small ideas that can scale as they expand in size and still support the entity in a healthy manner.

This scalability of topics can also be applied to the "DNA of Buildings," which can then become the larger "DNA of Cities" when scaled. This viewpoint of the DNA of the building can help define and support a scalable building approach for the future of architecture focused on health and wellness. This concept is discussed later in this chapter, with more details in Chapter 19.

While this book does span many topics, a focus and goal of this book is to discuss how these various topics relate to each other. This can show the context of how these systems are interrelated and interdependent with each other.

When you discuss the connections between the fields of architecture and the fields of medicine in terms of future solutions, there is a need to understand how these connections can be created and the context of these connections to provide cohesive solutions.

One of the keys of this book is the different processes to creating healthier built environments. There will be discussions on the doctor's and health professionals' evaluation process during these writings, including those involved in the architecture, building, and construction professions. Another facet of the book discusses design topics and how the experience of spaces and places can impact health in terms of physical, emotional, and mental well-being.

This includes the ideas of new systems to implement and support the integration between architecture and medicine and how the designs of built environments can impact overall human health. These topics are discussed in the following chapters.

While the idea of creating systems to support healthy building solutions began for me in the late 1990s, the success of achieving this goal requires many processes to be developed. And this includes the advanced technological capabilities that we now have in this second decade of the 21st century.

When I first began writing this book, a significant focus was on a lack of integration and a lack of systems between these professions.

As I began writing about these topics, there were three key factors involved that drove what I strived to address:

- The lack of integration between Architecture and Medical professionals
- The lack of systems to support cohesive solutions, and
- The lack of technological solutions to support these cohesive systems for each professional

This last point is discussed in more detail in chapter 16, the Architectural Medicine System (AMS), and chapter 18, the Architectural Medicine Software Solution – ARxMD.

Back when I began this work, it was a big surprise to learn how there seemed to be such large gaps and lack of focus on a topic that seemed to me a big deal – the impact of the built environment on health.

In the late 1990s, I began diving deeper into these topics, both figuratively and literally. What surprised me the most was the fact that both of these professions of architecture and medicine were not as focused on these issues.

I could clearly see that each profession focused on many micro levels of issues, from protocols and processes to evaluating pharmaceuticals and building codes. However, this huge topic of built environment impacts on human health often seemed to be ignored or had limited attention. The lack of focus on health in an integrated approach between these professions was a surprise.

The fact that there is still little to no interconnections between these two professions, except the topic of healthy hospital design, is one reason why I kept focused on writing this book through the years.

Another reason is that even today, the doctor hardly includes anything relative to the built environment in evaluating their patient's health. And this is also surprising, knowing that people are spending from 60 up to 90 percent of their lives inside of buildings.

Knowing that people spend all of this time in built environments, how do we do not factor these built environments into the health of the public in any proactive way?

This is confounding, but before I continue on this tirade, let me say that I think I understand "why" there hasn't been a lot of time spent on this topic by doctors and architects.

For me, a big reason is that it requires systems to be in place and complex systems at that. And as we are all probably aware, these two professions of architecture and medicine requires years of tremendously challenging study and training to achieve. Without systems in place for education, training, processes, and protocols in both professionals' daily work, there will be very little chance for these topics to be addressed in each professional's work.

And let me also visit this topic during the current time of 2020, as the world navigates the novel coronavirus pandemic. Perhaps there has been no other time in modern history that has brought to light the importance of the built environment related to health.

If we go back before the pandemic of 1918, another time in recent history that we can look back to was the time of Florence Nightingale's commentary about the importance of the built environment and health. And that was circa 1863!

Over 150 years ago, Florence Nightingale's commentary was based on the importance of a clean interior and building environment to support and regain health.

With my personal experience involved with inspections in buildings and even being around those evaluating health issues, I could see that this topic of health related to buildings was and is a significant issue. When I first began training to do environmental inspections and consulting, my first inclination was to wonder where my training processes would stem from and what guidance would be provided while doing this work.

However, as I soon learned, there were limited support processes. Especially at that time of the late '90s, only a few people who knew about these topics were available for discussions. Once I began working with other professionals, I was able to ask the many questions I had in achieving the goals of this work. Yet, I also realized how hard of a climb it would be to make a difference in helping people have better health in their built environments.

In this manner, there was no chance for these topics to scale up to a larger group of consultants and inspectors to help evaluate these scenarios. And without proper support and systems, the amount of work and education to be done was enormous.

It was at this time during 1998 and 1999 that I began to ask myself the questions, "what would be most helpful to me, and perhaps helpful to support others in their processes of achieving this work?"

At that time, I wrote about these processes and how systems and technology could help achieve these goals. I called this approach the "Electronic Clip Board or the Datalog software approach" and outlined some of these topics that eventually led to Architectural Medicine. These writings formed the basis for the Architectural Medicine System (AMS). It also focused on using technology and software as a solution, which has developed into the topic discussed in chapter 18, The Architectural Medicine Software Solution, as ARxMD.

In terms of building approaches, this context can become significant when viewing the designer and the builder's perspective.

For example, the sustainable builder may often focus on material selections directly from nature with limited processing and manufacturing, thereby reducing the impacts on the ecology from start to finish considering the building's entire life span. This is referred to today as Life Cycle Assessment (LCA).

In comparison, green builders may opt to use a wider variety of materials, both natural and synthetic, to design the structure to save energy in the long run. This would, therefore, increase energy efficiency and reduce the carbon footprint of the building over time.

While both groups may have a similar end goal, the process of achieving these goals can be significantly different. And add to the equation those focused on healthy building, and you have three groups who have different approaches to this goal.

And what makes this even more complex is that these are just three groups with specific building approaches. In reality, there are many other groups with a different approach and design-build philosophy.

These differences become an issue when you view each facet from a single perspective instead of considering all of the different facets as a whole. By having a complete perspective, each of these paths to achieve the goal can factor into the equation and consider all of these important topics.

By considering these different pieces of the puzzle, such as energy efficiency, ecological impact, and the inhabitants' health and wellness, a complete picture can help define the best approaches.

There are many professionals involved in both the building and medical fields, and each profession must view this larger puzzle. By doing so, they can ensure their part of the puzzle fits to create an integrative, cohesive whole.

The Topics of Health in Buildings Related to Each Professional

This brings up the topics related to each professional. Until this point, the issues have been generalized and based on the general public, but what about each professional? What might it look like for each professional to address these topics? And what procedures and processes might be on the horizon for these solutions?

While no one I know has a crystal ball, as mentioned earlier in this book, a critical approach to this integration between fields is to review the history of these developments and view the trajectory of where the pattern is heading.

When you take some time to look at these topics, you will see some common threads among each group. And even if their solutions are different, some of them are striving to create the same outcomes.

When you see all three of these topics of green, sustainable, and healthy building, perhaps a bigger pattern emerges, one that can better show the possible or probable trajectory.

The primary two professions in this book are the architect and the doctor, yet as we continue into later chapters, we'll discuss the importance of the building inspector, which is referred to as a Healthy Building Inspector. We also discuss the importance of the Architectural Doctor in chapter 15.

These are the main groups involved, but the reality is that if many other professionals are not involved, the entire system cannot move forward successfully. The importance of nurses, builders, engineers, electricians, plumbers, caretakers, epidemiologists, and public health professionals are just a few of these essential groups.

The emergence of new professionals such as green chemists and those specializing in biophilia and biomimicry as professionals will likely be critical in the future.

Some of these professions are discussed in more detail later in the book, and there is also a link to these references on the Architectural Medicine website.

As we get into the details of each of these pieces of the puzzle in the following chapters, it will include more information on each professional and how they can function together in these integrative solutions.

Yet right now, the main question might be, why are these three main topics of such importance?

Why Are These Three Main Topics – Green, Sustainable, and Healthy Building Important?

Many people are becoming more aware of their personal health and the impact that their built environments can have on their overall wellness and well-being. And while this individualized experience is critical, there is another perspective to view architecture, which is the built environment relative to planetary health. These topics include climate change and the growing population of humans, which is close to 8 billion people in this year of 2020.

In the year 1900, there were less than 2 billion people[19], and with these growing populations, it means that the resources that we use on the planet become exponentially impactful.

With the planet's finite resources and the increasing negative impacts on the many other creatures and organisms that live on this planet, we have to make some changes to maintain the balance of life. If not, this will impact biological life on this planet and all life, including humans. Humans are part of the integrated network of life that cannot be separated, and if we cause damage to the ecosystems, the results are a negative impact on human life.

The DNA of the Individual Building Becomes the DNA of the City

If we are to make changes, the question might be focused on what changes to make and how to define these changes. One way to do this is to view the built environment as having a specific DNA. Is the DNA of a building supporting the many facets of life on the planet as well as human health?

In a way, the DNA of the individual building becomes the DNA of the city, and if the design or building DNA ignores the basic foundations of the natural ways of the planet, then the city will also fail to live in harmony with these basic tenets. This results in a detriment to society and humanity at large, along with all of Earth's inhabitants.

If this is evaluated in terms of an end goal, then the process becomes that of reverse-engineering the goal and working backward to the world's current state. This process can provide the steps required to achieve this goal and define actions to develop toward these goals.

Many groups have begun working on this process in their specific field, and by working together, they can continue to advance towards this better future that is possible.

In this manner, consistently evaluating the systems and adjusting, improving, and adding to the research, development, and processes can utilize the knowledge learned by each profession. This can be included in the whole process, yielding a synergistic and exponentially beneficial result.

If individuals and professions work on their own development, the collective result is a beneficial result for themselves and the collective whole of society. This is what a collective, cohesive, and whole health approach can achieve. And this is why whole systems thinking, planning, and development become critical to better health and wellness for humanity and the planet.

The DNA of Cities – Epigenetics and the Exposome of Human Health

The topic of the DNA of Cities will be discussed in more depth in chapter 19, which relates to the macro level of architectural development.

This topic of literal human DNA on a micro-level will be discussed in chapters 11 through 13 pertaining to various facets of wellness.

And to add to this DNA discussion, another factor becomes interesting as well, which is the micro-level of DNA topics related to *Epigenetics*.

Epigenetics is the "study of how your behaviors and environment can cause changes that affect the way your genes work."[20]

Your behaviors and environment can impact how your genes are turned on or off, and this can then define how your body literally builds itself. Unlike genetic changes, "epigenetic changes are reversible and do not change your DNA sequence."[21] Turning on or off of certain genes can either be helpful or a hindrance to your health. This is of particular interest with Architectural Medicine in that your built environment can impact the functionality of your DNA. I go into more details on this topic in chapters 11 through 13.

In this segment, what can be stated is there is an essential correlation between the DNA of the individual building and the influence that architecture can have on epigenetics and the DNA of humans.

In the past several years, the term *Exposome* has been another concept that has become more common in the discussions of health and environmental exposures. The CDC defines the exposome as "the measure of all the exposures of an individual in a lifetime and how those exposures relate to health."[22]

What makes this topic different and extremely interesting relative to Architectural Medicine is the fact that it strives to map environmental exposure impacts over a lifetime. This "measuring of the exposures and the effects of exposures" over a lifetime spans from the individual's exposure "before birth and includes insults from environmental and occupational sources."[23]

The Architectural Medicine System (AMS) and the use of big data and bioinformatics can provide an interesting potential for Molecular Epidemiology, which studies the "relationships between occupational exposures and health outcomes." By utilizing biomonitoring and bioinformatics, the issues in the environment, and particularly the pollution in built environments, can yield valuable, usable data for better health.

I will discuss this in later chapters, and go into more details on this topic in chapter 21.

The Term DNA and Architectural Medicine – Two Integrated Twisting Paired Strands

In the previous paragraphs and in later chapters, the use of the term "DNA" is used in a particular format relative to building.

Yet, it should be made clear why and how this term DNA is being utilized.

DNA is defined as the instructions for the development, functioning, growth, and reproduction of all known organisms. It is essential for how organisms grow as "DNA contains the instructions needed for an organism to develop, survive, and reproduce."[24]

In this manner, it can be seen as the *blueprint* of all life.

The term DNA has, in some ways, become synonymous with how a process functions. As humans, DNA is the core of how the body functions and how all cells develop and grow.

In this book, the terms "DNA of Buildings" or "DNA of Cities" is referencing the core blueprint of the development, functioning, growth, and replication of buildings. It refers to the way a structure is built and how it functions as a whole. Whether this is relative to the way it lives with the ecology, how it functions as a system, or the entire impact it has on human and biological health.

A healthy DNA blueprint of a building considers the ecological integrations existing in its environment. It focuses on energy-efficient functionality and ensures its inhabitants' optimal health – physically, mentally, and emotionally.

During the discussions of Architectural Medicine, the word "integration" is used quite a lot. It is discussed due to the importance of the two professions of architecture and medicine working together to create and support health in the built environment.

This integration is discussed in many ways, yet perhaps one of the best analogies is the DNA strand itself.

If DNA is two twisting paired strands, acting in a balance between each other, and yet each supporting its own strand, the combination or integration of these two strands is what allows for life.

And while this may be a very micro level analogy, when you are building a structure or supporting good health, you need to focus on the foundation and core of the issues and then work towards complete solutions that stem from this origin.

As architecture and medicine exist as two separate fields or two strands, in a way, each strand is in a similar fashion to the two strands of DNA. This equation requires that they connect in real ways that are both balanced and yet supportive of each other to have this DNA exist in a healthy format.

The analogy of DNA is both a positive description, an excellent example of what integration is, and the fact that this integration can occur while each strand can maintain its own identity. It is an independent and interdependent example of life at the micro-level. When this is scaled up, it creates cells, organs, and organisms that are literally living together in symbiosis.

And so, the two main fields of architecture and medicine can also remain independent yet interdependent. This can create an integrative approach that, when working together in mutual format, a symbiosis of the built environment can create a healthier environment to live in and within.

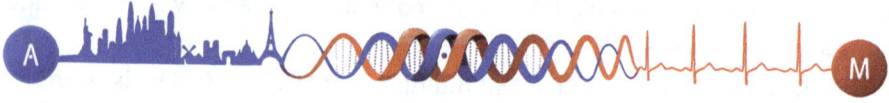

This is why the Architectural Medicine graphic as the "pulse of the healthy built environment" uses the DNA strand to connect the cities' silhouette with the heartbeat of life.

This book will explore both the data-centric views of health and some of the less measurable facets of the built environment regarding how design, shapes, and forms can impact the way we feel. It will also explore how these designs can impact our mental or psychological responses to our environments.

While some of these discussions may be correlated to the soft sciences, meaning those that cannot easily be measured, the fields of Evidence-Based Design have worked hard to measure the metrics in design, along with the above mentioned Epigenetics discoveries.

This also includes the emerging field of Neuroscience of Architecture or NeuroArchitecture. Studying the way the brain responds to the many facets of the exterior environment provides significant insights into how humans are influenced and affected by their built environments in more measured formats.

This book also discusses the topic of healthy building, yet takes this a step further to go beyond just the physical impacts that the built environment has on health. It ventures into the full scope of human life to include the mental and emotional aspects of life and the physical impacts and influences that these built environments have on human health.

It's not just the materials and methods of building. It's how the space affects, impacts, and influences your life – mentally, physically, emotionally, and spiritually.

In this manner, I've chosen the name Architectural Medicine and not just Healthy Building to define these topics. Yet, of course, the field of Healthy Building has made important advancements on these topics and will be addressed accordingly.

To provide the proper framework for the integrations between the fields of architecture and medicine, there needs to be a baseline of understanding of these three main topics within architecture. This will then help to define the concept as Integrative Architecture. These topics can then be combined to better define Architectural Medicine.

And so, before we get into the details on how buildings can affect humans in terms of physical, emotional, and mental or psychological wellness, let's first discuss the three topics of Healthy, Green, and Sustainable Architecture and Building in the next chapter...

"We won't have a society if we destroy the environment."

–Margaret Mead

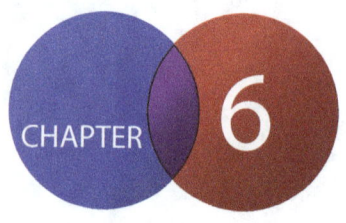

HEALTHY, GREEN, AND SUSTAINABLE BUILDING
A BRIEF HISTORY AND AN OVERVIEW

This chapter is going to jump right into the topics of *Healthy*, *Green*, and *Sustainable Building*. By providing an overview of how these topics are interrelated, I will show the end result first in this chapter. Then reverse engineer the topics in the following chapters as each issue is discussed individually.

The reason why I'm starting with the end goal first is simple. If you have context as to why these topics are important, you can recognize how they need to overlap to support each other.

When each facet is discussed individually, you can get a contextual sense of the importance of the interdependence of them working together.

An essential part of Architectural Medicine is the integration of many different components into a cohesive whole. To start, there is a need to define what these facets are before there can be discussions as to how they can fit together.

So, let's get to these three topics of Healthy, Green, and Sustainable Building.

The following are diagrams that include each of these topics, with overlaps between each segment. This three-part Venn diagram highlights the independent topics, yet interdependent as a whole, with a balanced approach to providing the end goal of health in the built environment.

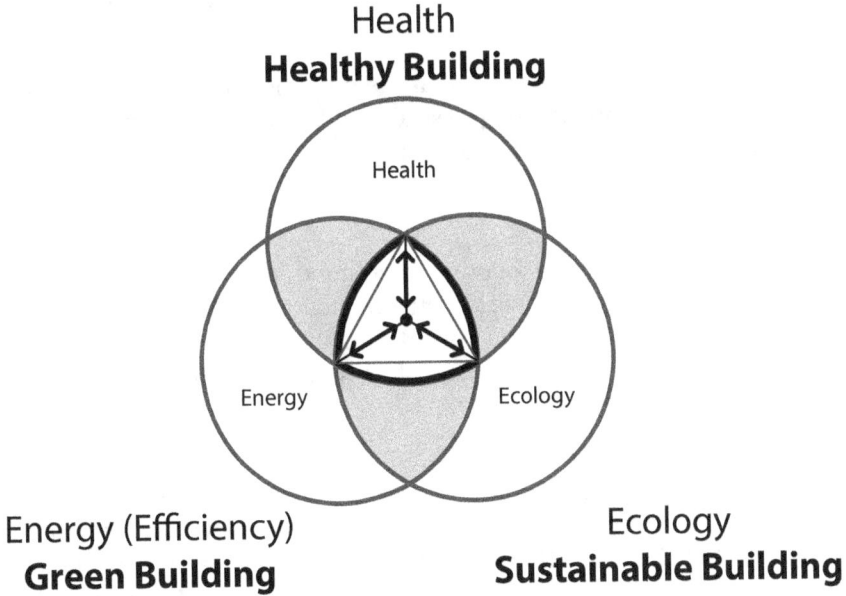

As you can see in the graphic, the overlap between each of these topics is defined as Healthy Building, focusing on Physical Health, Green Building with a focus on Energy-Efficiency, and Sustainable Building with a focus on Environmental or Ecological Design.

For those new to these topics or perhaps not as well versed, it should be stated there are many definitions of these fields depending on who is defining them. To make sure there is no confusion, please note that depending on who is writing the definitions, they will vary from person to person and country to country worldwide.

I discuss why I have chosen these definitions in the following chapters, yet suffice it to say that the main reason I have outlined these definitions is based on my experience in these fields. This, along with the big picture context of why they matter and what goals these topics are striving to solve.

With that said, we can see in the diagram that these three topics are defined as Health, Energy, and Ecology.

These topics are essential because they highlight the main issues critical to providing current and future generations the possibility of supplying and maintaining biological and ecological health and wellness.

Basic Definitions of Healthy, Green, and Sustainable Building

As a quick overview, these three topics will be defined as the following:

Healthy Building: the impact that the building has on the health of the occupants with an emphasis on physical health. This includes topics ranging from Indoor Air Quality (IAQ) to the impacts that materials in buildings can have upon the inhabitants.

Green Building: a main focus of green building is to make the structure energy-efficient, with an emphasis on the reduction of fuel consumption. This includes reducing pollution and considering the energy source in its use as well as its production. Reducing the carbon footprint of the building is also a focus and a goal.

Sustainable Building: a main focus of sustainable building has been to consider the impact that the building will have on the environment and ecology of where it's built. This includes reviewing the overall impact that the building materials, production, and end of use (LCA) - Life Cycle Assessment will have on the local and global biology and ecology.

While some may recognize and be familiar with these three topics, it's also important to note that many other fields are involved in these developments that overlap. While it might seem to make things even more complicated, it is intended to provide the entire scope to evaluate properly. In this manner, all of the facets can be assessed when making decisions.

That said, there are some common attributes that I can pull from many experts in these fields and perhaps sew these together to at least provide a picture of what each is striving to define. I will address all of these topics and then discuss how they may fit together for an integrative approach in the following chapters.

In later chapters, I will comment on some of these other fields and how they are interconnected, from Natural Building and Environmental Design to Organic Architecture and Permaculture.

The first topic of Healthy Building focuses on the impact of physical health parameters in the built environment. This includes topics such as the materials of the building and the potential for these to cause illness, such as lead paint and asbestos. This can also include air quality topics, such as Carbon Monoxide (CO), Carbon Dioxide (CO2), Nitrogen Dioxide (N2O), and such problems as Volatile Organic Compounds or VOCs. This can also include microbial contaminants, such as bacteria and viruses. These can all have a negative impact on health.

The next topic is Energy, and this is grouped with Green Building. As many people are aware, science is showing that humans impact the ecological and biological health of the planet, and our energy use and sources of energy all contribute to these factors. It's also known that up to 50 percent of all energy used worldwide is utilized in building construction and regular building use.[25]

That is a huge percentage, and if we focus on just the energy efficiency of our buildings, it can have tremendous ecological and health benefits. And the reduction in both the use and production of these energy sources means that we can reduce pollution in enormous strides, with outstanding benefits and results.

This brings up the connection to the third topic, which is focused on the Ecology and is highlighted as Sustainable Building. Sustainable architecture and building are often described as striving to increase the ecological connections with the built environment while decreasing harmful impacts on the local and global ecology.

With these energy efficiencies and reductions in pollution, this not only means that the benefits support better environmental and human health, yet the health of the entire biology of the planet.

This includes the many organisms and creatures that we share this planet with, and their good health means that we as humans can also be provided the potential for good health. When we realize that we are in symbiosis with the planet and all of its many sentient beings, it will help provide context for our choices and actions.

There are many definitions of green and sustainable building, but in order to achieve the end goal of comprehending the core topics of these issues, I've outlined these fields and definitions to provide context for the next chapters.

When you begin to uncover the various layers of creating the healthy, green, and sustainable built environment, you might find that these become overwhelming in scope and depth.

A big part of this book is defining some of these issues and providing an overview in a less overwhelming and, hopefully, more empowering format.

In the fields of healthy, green, and sustainable building, each has had its own trajectory, and in the next few chapters, we will discuss some of the similarities and differences. I will also attempt to continue to define these topics in a loose format, as there are no real, concrete definitions of these fields.

The lack of specific definitions can confuse understanding these topics, so while my descriptions may not be an exact standard, I'm doing this to give context to this often overwhelming information.

The big question is, "where to start?" Unfortunately, many people first become aware of these topics when building, renovating, or buying a home or house. People are often unaware of these topics until the deconstruction process has begun on their building projects, creating a rushed time crunch to the already overwhelming amount of changes in their lives.

This becomes a real challenge, as not only are many striving to educate themselves on incredibly complex topics in fields that can often take a lifetime to master, but they now need to learn about all the various components in a condensed amount of time.

To make this more complicated, many of the professionals involved often don't work from commonly integrated standards and definitions. Even if you, as the general public, might have clarity, it doesn't mean that numerous other professionals will have that same clarity and share these specific meanings to discuss these topics.

This is another reason why this book includes the primary professionals of architecture and medicine. It is a hope to bring clarity to all involved or have enough information to know what conversations to have to bring clarity to the table.

You will bring your starting point to this process, yet some basic topics can be discussed to gain a baseline overview.

In my opinion, the lack of context has taken the current age of information to the point of overwhelm. Instead of allowing the information age to empower the general public, it has instead led many to freeze with indecision.

In the following three chapters, we will discuss a brief history and overview of each of the three main fields of healthy building, green building, and sustainable building, and at the end of these three chapters will include a fourth chapter to weave this all together into some form of coherent interconnection called *Integrative Architecture*. While I go into specific details on each topic – as the depth of each of these topics merits a book within itself – it will provide a foundation of these fields. It will give an overview of how they came about and why and for what purpose the pioneers in these fields continued tirelessly to keep the process moving forward towards solutions.

Again, please note that these chapters are summaries, as each topic can themselves be a book. And even many in these building fields would provide varied definitions. That said, there are some patterns in these fields based on their history and the trajectory of goals they strive to achieve.

It's also important to state that the history of these fields plays a vital part in analyzing these three fields, both in how they function by themselves and how they integrate or do not integrate today.

These examples are not defining all of the different professional approaches. However, I'm using these definitions from personal experiences over the past 30 years as a way to highlight some of the main issues discussed.

If you have other ways to define these topics or are personally using these topics in various definitions, please strive to understand what I am trying to convey, as many people are still not aware of these general issues.

The past 50 years shows a rich history in each branch of these three topics and developments. Many people may also be familiar with the fields of natural building, sustainable design, organic architecture, healthy building, ecological design, environmental design, and other fields that began development in the past 20th century to make matters even more complex.

While this entire range of fields will not be discussed in this book, we do have more information on our website where you can read about these specific topics and dive deeper into their definitions and history. By going to our website, you can view these topics by clicking the link "Information on the Various Fields of Architecture and Medicine" from our main book page: https://architecturalmedicine.com/book/

A Quick Overview of These Fields and How They Relate to the Topic of Architectural Medicine

Sustainable building and green building are in many ways striving to create the same or similar solution.

They are both approaches to building intended to reduce the building's energy use and decrease the environmental impacts from the structure. Providing more fuel efficiency and less fuel use, particularly fossil fuels, leads to fewer carbon emissions and less negative impact on the ecology.

From the manufacturing of materials standpoint, the goal in producing these materials is to use less energy and have less negative environmental impact from production to application and, of course, the end use of the product. The result leads to less negative ecological impact, less spending in production, and more cost-effectiveness for a better living environment.

However, each field approaches the solution differently. For instance, in sustainable building, some builders will hold steady in their use of mainly natural materials, meaning materials that come from nature, instead of synthetic materials and products manufactured by humans.

In the last 30 years, many Sustainable Builders have used materials such as timber frame, adobe, and the straw bale building approach. Typically, these builders will source their materials as local as possible to reduce environmental impact. And when sustainable builders are reviewing these environmental impacts, they are often factoring in the entire life cycle of the product, from the cutting down of trees and milling of the wood to the carbon footprint in the transportation of these products. In terms of the whole cycle of use, this includes their use and end of service.

Over the entire cycle of the life of the product or Life Cycle Assessment (LCA), these questions are often factored into the decision making process from the very beginning. And this includes the important factor of where the building is located and what local resources are most appropriate to provide a decreased impact on the environment.

This life cycle of each product or LCA is also referred to by the comment "cradle to grave" of the products. In the past 30 years, there's been an emphasis on sustainability, focusing on the revised version called "cradle to cradle." This philosophy called cradle to cradle was initially coined by Walter R. Stahel[26], yet is most known by the work and writings of architect William McDonough and chemist Michael Braungart in their book *Cradle to Cradle: Remaking the Way We Make Things*.[27]

In this approach, the production, use, and end use of the products mimic the processes of nature. This means that when the product is no longer used, it can be recycled and repurposed back into the natural system, which of course, is how nature functions. Incidentally, this mimicking of nature is the basis of the term *biomimicry*, which is discussed in later chapters.

When plants and organisms die in the natural world, they decompose and return to the soil they came from. And because there is no degradation of the original materials in this process, it can "sustain" the process repeatedly in perpetuity without a decline in the materials' original quality.

In essence, this is what many in the sustainability fields are striving to achieve – the ability for human-created processes and products to follow this way of nature. Everything that is produced and manufactured can eventually be recycled, reused, and repurposed back into its original form without degradation to the original materials.

This allows future generations the opportunities to utilize the materials of the planet in the same manner as previous generations. It provides a return to the original quality of the materials to begin anew.

And to repeat this comment, to say that these three topics are not set in stone as a definition is an understatement. As much as there are writings on defining these three topics, there are as many writings that could be seen as contradictory.

The whole point of discussing these topics is to recognize that the built environment impacts human health and the ecology, including energy efficiency as a goal. Reducing the negative impacts on human and biological health can support healthier ecosystems of the planet, with which human health is integrally connected.

In terms of the definition of healthy building, there are some basic concepts that can provide a baseline of understanding when discussing this topic.

It's quite common sense to think that building should be inherently healthy. After all, a very important part of architecture is to make sure that the building provides shelter and safety for the inhabitants. This would instinctively be defined as the building not falling down and not falling apart. Yet because the building fields have become so sophisticated over the past 50 plus years, it does mean that these issues have to be reviewed. The sick building syndrome (SDS) issues of the 1980s first put this term healthy building onto many people's radar, at least in the US.

Over the past 30 plus years, some important pioneers have been in the healthy building realm and have helped define these issues. They should be given credit for their work to provide healthier solutions and hard work that, for many, has been an uphill battle. I feel fortunate that I have met many of these pioneers and will not hesitate to state that my path and their inspiration planted the seeds to what has become Architectural Medicine. I list their work and books where appropriate during the following chapters. Please be sure to review their work and contributions to gain deeper insights into these subjects.

Their work through the years and my experiences have led to me thinking about these fields and eventually coming up with the concepts of Architectural Medicine.

You might think that I'd begin discussing healthy building in terms of these three main topics, yet I'm going to start with green and sustainable building for a few reasons.

One key reason is the importance of the 1960s and 1970s on these two topics, leading to green and sustainable building developments.

A big reason why many American architects and designers began seeking solutions in their designs to be more energy-efficient and to have less environmental impact was due to the environmental movements at this time. This includes the energy crisis of the 1970s. I was old enough to remember that in the '70s in the US, the energy crisis significantly impacted daily life. It had gotten to the point that there were days when gasoline for vehicles was so sparse that you could only get gas on certain days based on whether your vehicle's license plate ended with an odd or even number.

These were also critical topics on the news, and everyone at that time was immersed in these issues, at least in my life's experiences. The main concerns were the lack of fossil fuel energy sources, which for many, spurred the process of seeking alternative energy solutions. And this, combined with the ecological problems in the 60s and 70s, brought up the fact that buildings have a large impact on the ecology – often a negative and detrimental impact.

And so there were architects and builders at that time who strived to find solutions to these issues. This includes passive solar building solutions, the photovoltaic (PV) solar movement, and the approach of having fewer impacts on the environment that led to terms such as "ecological footprint."[28] This term is meant to describe what happens when you walk on areas of the ecology that are sensitive and, therefore, be aware and cognizant of the detriments to such wear and tear on sites with human involvement.

During this time of energy efficiency and sustainable building, what resulted in many of these design solutions were structures that were tighter and had less energy transfer between the outside and inside. Subsequently, this meant less energy and fuel needed to heat and cool a building, which also reduced fuel use to reduce environmental impacts. So, the goal of reducing fuel and saving money was a twofold improvement.

However, it failed to recognize the impacts on health this would have, particularly in these buildings that had no functioning windows (or *glazing* as it's called in the architecture field[29]). The result was energy-efficient structures, yet the air quality inside became either toxic or reduced oxygen for the inhabitants' health.

In the 1980s, the infamous story of Sick Building Syndrome (SBS) was based on this issue that occurred at the US EPA offices. The office had an upgrade to the building interiors, where the designs had tighter building designs, combined with new synthetic materials installed such as carpets, furniture, and new paint.

This was before the now common topic of VOCs and these upgrades led to people in these office spaces becoming sick. Yet, at first, they did not understand why people were getting sick. It was speculated that these new designs with tighter enclosures for energy efficiency and new materials with high VOC off-gassing created a toxic interior environment to work within.

This influential case of sick building syndrome occurred at the EPA's Waterside Mall headquarters in southwest D.C.[30] While there was controversy in determining if these building issues did cause sickness in those employees working in these offices, it was undoubtedly a milestone in the topic of building health. And it sparked the aspects of fresh air and the questions of health related to these new synthetic chemicals in new building materials.

Another common building health issue was the advent of Legionnaire's disease, which is due to contamination of cooling towers by legionella organisms. Legionella bacteria can cause a serious type of pneumonia.[31] The name derives from the "1976 state convention of the American Legion, a U.S. military veterans' organization, at a Philadelphia hotel where 182 Legionnaires contracted the disease, 29 of them fatally."[32]

Why Designers Should Include the Trifold of Healthy, Green, and Sustainable Building as an Interconnected Whole

There is no doubt that the topics of climate change and health in the built environment have become of greater concern in the past twenty years.

However, I'd say we're about 40 years behind what people in the '60s and '70s were warning us about. In this section, I'm going to talk about the cause-effect relationship of the built environment on both of these topics, as well as the reasons why you can't separate the issues of green, sustainable, and healthy building moving forward into the future.

The main reason you cannot separate these topics is that if we foresee a future that supports better health and wellness for humans and the entire planet we all live on, these topics will all have to be recognized as integrally connected. You cannot separate biological health from ecological health, and each of these topics relates to each other.

In discussing these reasons, I think history can have a role as a learning process and show potential patterns. The trajectory of this history can be utilized to plan for more strategic solutions. With that said, this history is not that far in the past as merely the past 40 to 50 years. In the world of architecture, this is a mere speck on the timeline of history.

However, what's important to note is that never in recorded history have we seen human developments have such a massive impact on the planet's ecosystems and humanity's health.

Since the 1960s and 1970s, there were plenty of warning signs to heed, and perhaps none is as prevalent and epic as the Cuyahoga river spontaneously catching fire. For those unfamiliar with this story, the Cuyahoga river became a dumping location in Ohio's industrial section from the Industrial Revolution onward. It became so toxic from the chemicals being dumped into the river that the river eventually caught fire. And not just once, but multiple times.[33]

For all creatures on this planet, such as humans, who consist of around 70 percent water, the idea that water spontaneously combusts should be terrifying.

This issue of massive industrial pollutants being siphoned into the Cuyahoga river significantly impacted the industry's environmental rules and contributed to creating the Environmental Protection Agency (EPA).[34] It should also show us that these issues should be monitored to prevent such environmental and biological tragedies.

And then, as mentioned previously, in the 1970s, the shortage of oil as the primary energy source brought up a more prominent topic to evaluate, which is the dependency on fossil fuels. In the 1981 Special Edition of National Geographic titled "Energy," this critical topic garnered the attention to such a point that the magazine's entire issue was focused on these topics of fuel, energy, and future options.[35] The magazine issue not only focused on energy but also on the many facets of energy, including human and biological health.

If you have the chance to read this, it can provide meaningful recognition of a pattern emerging from the 1960s into the 80s, which can be traced to pioneers such as Rachel Carson and her book *Silent Spring*. While the mainstream and science community of her time ignored her work and warnings, advocates of environmental concerns in the 60s and 70s brought up these same issues. Even prominent magazines such as National Geographic seemed to be ignored by the masses when they created this special edition for just this topic.

The 1980s in the US were perhaps best summed up by the movie character Gordon Gecko, who stated, "Greed is Good." It was the mantra of many corporations and of the people who benefited from such developments.

However, this spurred many grassroots movements of the time. From the 1990s up until now, many individuals and groups have turned away from the assumption that companies and government would enforce healthy policies and have taken it upon themselves to devote their lives towards solutions.

Those such as Amory Lovins of the Rocky Mountain Institute have been advocates for change and a voice of reason, even previous to his quoted words in the National Geographic magazine from 1981.[36]

As a result of many of these concerns of both energy and ecology, many groups began to seek alternate solutions to the mainstream energy sources of fossil fuels. These "alternative" sources have become more well known today as solar, wind, and geothermal power, to name just a few of these alternative options.

These developments have resulted in this book defining green, sustainable, and healthy building as such.

I'd say based on the trajectory of their developments, they have occurred in the following chronological order – Green Building and Sustainable Building in similar timeframes, followed by the emerging field of Healthy Building.

As mentioned earlier, green building is often focused on the science of researching the energy impacts and the reduction of energy use in buildings. Whether this is focused on the insulation of old and new buildings or the use of higher efficiency heating and cooling systems, the focal point is often "energy-efficiency." And by reducing fossil fuel dependency and increasing the energy efficiency of buildings' electricity demands, this can help decrease the 40 percent of the world's energy expenditure used in building creation and use.

Global Warming and Climate Change – Change the Name, Continue the Progress

Around the same time, sustainable building became a hot topic, quite literally. This is based on one of many topics focused on global warming concerns. Sustainable building is often focused on the environmental considerations or impact that the built environment has on the ecology, both the local and global impacts.

This approach often strives to reduce the use of manufactured materials and reduce the excess materials from the building waste cycle. These design approaches typically range from the initial landscaping in building the structure to the materials and methods of how they impact the environment. And, of course, the long term effects that the building has on the location, the planet, and the building's occupants.

Essentially, many core tenets of sustainable building have the mantra of using fewer materials, having less impact on the environment, and removing the "cradle to grave" concept. This coincides with the common terms today of the *Circular Economy*. This view is often striving to transcend the mindset of how products are made, used, and deposited when they are done being utilized. The common modern perspective is that these products will go to the landfill or be sent away when they are finished being used. As many will state striving to achieve these goals, there is no "away."

The Circular Economy, Sustainability, and the Cyles of Life as Spiracycles

What is meant by this phrase "cradle to grave" is that too often, there is a linear viewpoint of products and the building processes. This linear idea starts with the manufacturing or birth of a product (cradle) to the end use of the product that is discarded and sent to the landfill (grave). From production and use of the product, this linear path becomes garbage or trash after use. This linear mindset is in juxtaposition to how the systems of nature function.

And this term is used in opposition to "cradle to cradle," a term made common by William McDonough and Michael Braungart in their book *Cradle to Cradle*.37 Cradle to cradle denotes a circular process. Circular means that when the product is no longer being used at its end of life, it can then be recycled or repurposed into something else. As opposed to the linear process of cradle to grave, there is a circular process that can continue repeatedly.

If this repurposing of a product can only be done a few times or cycles, then this is referred to as downcycling. This means that each time it is recycled or reused, it degrades or downgrades in quality to the point where eventually it will become waste or garbage.

If it can be upcycled, then each time it is reused, it does not degrade and can be used in perpetuity. This is how nature functions. Each time a living creature is born, from a plant to an animal, it uses the materials of nature to become a living organism. At the end of life, the physical body dies and then returns to its original material components through decomposition. In this process, it returns to the soil as its initial material components. And as nutrients, it then becomes materials for other organisms in which to live and grow.

Each time these natural materials are utilized, they return to nature and do not degrade. In this manner, they can exist as the same components in perpetuity. This life cycle is also referred to as Life Cycle Assessment (LCA).

The concept of a circular economy, or cradle to cradle, is essentially based on a product's end of life to become the beginning of life for another product. Ideally, this occurs without any degradation to the quality of the materials. I use the term spiracycle to define these processes as they circle around and either degrade in quality and spiral downwards or maintain quality and the cycle spirals upwards.

The next topic is that if we focus on human health, especially in preventing illness, we should be looking at the built environment and recognizing that people in the modern-day are spending up to 90 percent of their time indoors.[38] So we might be wondering what types of impacts built environments have on human health.

What new design approaches can be taken to prevent illness and support wellness as a proactive process?

As to the design process, what can be recognized is that the single home or building is critical in addressing these issues. This is because a general blueprint in approaching these building solutions is that the single building often leads to multiple buildings, which eventually leads to our cities.

As mentioned in the previous chapter, the single structure's DNA is actually the blueprint for the entire city or a major influence on cities. If each building is designed in a functionally similar manner, then this single design "DNA" will eventually influence a whole city as the DNA of the city.

So it matters that the individual structure does have a solid blueprint and DNA to address these trifold topics to provide green, sustainable, and healthy buildings. And as such, the focus on all three will impact the individuals who reside in that single building, but the multiplication of such buildings forming a city eventually defines the DNA of the city itself.

And this is part of the reason why I have listed these three topics in this order. It provides a bit of background about how some of these issues came to be, including the motivating factors and some of these resulting processes to find better solutions.

While some of these individual solutions have caused issues, the initial intention of finding and seeking solutions provided a framework for today's energy-efficient and more sustainable designs.

Fortunately for us, in the year 2020, the pioneering research and experimentation have provided many solutions and more in-depth knowledge of these issues for current day solutions.

While sick building syndrome brought great awareness to these topics in the mid to late 80s, it wasn't until the 1990s that healthy building became a topic that more designers and architects began pursuing.

And this brings us to the next chapters with more details on each topic of green, sustainable and healthy building. With these topics discussed and their interconnected importance, we can begin to dive deeper into each subject and how it eventually fits together into Architectural Medicine.

And so, we begin the next chapter with an overview of *Green Building*...

> "What is the use of a house if you haven't got a tolerable planet to put it on?"
>
> – Henry David Thoreau

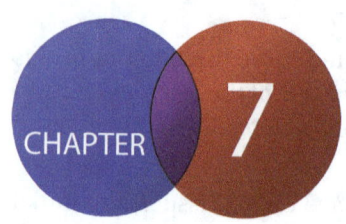

GREEN BUILDING DEFINED AND OVERVIEW

I'm going to start this chapter with a comment about the topics of Green Building and Sustainable Building outlined in this book. It's important to reiterate that there are many different definitions of green and sustainable building locally and globally.

In the US, there are different definitions based on the specific groups that are defining these terms. So, to be clear, there are no set definitions of these terms.

That said, there is an important reason to discuss these terms and define them relative to the ideas of this book. While the definitions used in this book may not be shared everywhere, the important part is to use common terminologies to define these concepts and how they impact the bigger picture of this book's ideas.

Ok, with that said, let's discuss Green Building...

In the late 1960s into the '70s in the US, a big topic in the national news was the energy crisis. The heightened awareness of this issue, brought up by the everyday impact of the lack of energy resources, spurred on a process for many people to seek alternatives to the fossil fuel issues that the energy crisis was focused around. If you look to many of the so-called alternative building developments during this time, many of them were based on striving to find solutions that would replace the dependency on fossil fuels and reduce energy costs.

And these topics did not just start in the US, as there are many other movements around the world that had concerns about energy-efficiency and sustainability.

From my experiences meeting many of these pioneering spirits worldwide, a focal point was to find methodologies to reduce energy consumption and be more energy-efficient. This process of seeking methods to be more energy-efficient as part of this building movement reduces energy use to be resource-efficient. For some, this is defined as "using the Earth's limited resources in a sustainable manner while minimizing environmental impact."[39]

While the definition today may vary and overlap with topics such as sustainability, there are some crucial differences as I've viewed them over the years based on how some architects and builders approach these topics.

For instance, many people involved in green building and *Building Science* are focused on the reduction of fuel consumption to be more energy efficient. While those who are focused on sustainability topics might also strive to be energy efficient, they can approach this in a different way to include the overall ecological impacts that the building imposes on the locale.

Green building can include a wide range of methods to decrease energy use and conserve resources. This can be achieved by several different options, from increasing insulation in a structure for reduced energy costs to using solar photoelectric (PV) panels, wind turbines, and geothermal sources for energy generation. My education and experiences with green building over the past several decades have often been tethered by these forms of technological and mechanical processes to replace conventional energy sources, reduce energy requirements, and improve energy efficiency.

For purposes of this book, I will refer to green building as that which is focused on energy efficiency and the reduction of energy consumption. From my perspective, the purpose of defining it in this way is twofold. One is to make sure that what is striving to be achieved is provided for those who are not as familiar with these concepts. And two, it can provide a baseline of this specific topic for reference.

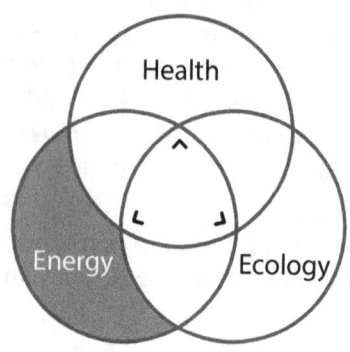

Energy (Efficiency)/ **Green Building**

Energy

Issues related to optimizing Energy use, sourcing more sustainable energy options, striving to reduce pollution, and working to reduce carbon footprint.
Groups and organizations related to this Energy focus include: Architecture 2030 and the
US Green Building Council (USGBC)

It is my belief that once people are more familiar with the issues that are being addressed, then the methods of achieving these goals become more clear moving forward. Eventually, if you spend some time reviewing and analyzing these topics, you will see an overlap of these different naming conventions and segmentations. You can then have your own opinion as to how it should be appropriately defined and approached.

In the next chapter on sustainable building, we'll get into some more of these details and discuss some of the overlap and some of these differences. For purposes of turning some of these abstract concepts into real-world, tangible examples, this naming process can be less jargon and more of getting to the point for discussion.

This jargon includes the word *green* itself. Perhaps the use of the word green, back in the environmental movements of the 60s and 70s, denoted the greenery of nature, symbolizing a healthy ecology and environmental stewardship. When people think of spending time in nature, the imagery of green fields and green trees and mountains can provide a visual representation of a healthy environment to spend time in.

The word green relative to this context can be defined as "of, relating to, or supporting environmentalism" and "a product, service, etc.: designed, produced, or operating in a way that minimizes harm to the natural environment."[40]

In my experiences, the term green was often used by those striving to decrease energy use, and they often approached this by increasing the amount of insulation and providing resource-efficient heating and cooling methods. It will then require less energy and thereby reduce the costs and dependency of the fuel itself. This is often combined with utilizing passive solar energy as heating and cooling methods and using photovoltaics to provide power. Using the benefits of advanced technological materials and processes is often a pathway to attain this goal. Today, many references to this approach can be seen in the "off the grid" movements, where people strive to create more autonomous building and living solutions.

In my perspective, the terms green and sustainable have some district differences. In my experiences, those focused on green building are often very focused on energy efficiency and resource efficiency to the point where modern materials would be a main focal point in decreasing energy use and reducing costs. However, this sometimes can be a different focus than those in sustainable building where the goal is to reduce the negative environmental impacts in the entire construction process, not just energy reduction.

An example of this is the following. Those focused on energy efficiency may choose to use various materials, such as Styrofoam insulation, which will reduce the amount of fuel that has to be used to heat and cool a structure, thereby justifying the use of a petroleum product in order to achieve these goals. In contrast, a sustainable builder might focus on using more natural materials and building smaller structures to create less impact on the environment while also reducing energy use.

Both approaches can decrease the energy required and utilized over the building's lifetime, yet do so with different methods.

This is not to state which is a better approach, yet it is to express a different mindset in achieving these goals.

In the year 2020, many of these goals are approached in a combined format, and the lines between green and sustainable building can often be blurred.

The use of less synthetic materials for both short and long-term benefits can be utilized to both decrease energy use and reduce the negative impact on the environment. This is often approached in a cohesive design approach. In this manner, both goals can be achieved as a beneficial format.

Yet as I've mentioned previously, having some understanding of the history of these approaches can provide some perspective for moving forward that can be of value. And knowing that these two mindsets grew from the energy crisis and the environmental concerns of the 60s and 70s can provide insights into the trajectories of these two paths.

The World Green Building Council defines green building as "a building that, in its design, construction or operation, reduces or eliminates negative impacts, and can create positive impacts, on our climate and natural environment."[41]

If you review the history of the US Green Building Council from the 90s up until today, you can see that they've added and updated these definitions over time with more overlap between energy efficiency and sustainability.

Over the years, my experiences with green building advocates are that they are often focused on technological solutions, such as synthetic insulation and building materials and the use of PV solar panels to achieve these goals. In comparison, those involved with sustainable building are often more focused on connecting to nature and environmental stewardship and using this as a guideline for the designs and selecting building materials.

The overlap in the current day has become much more integrated, yet some design and building approaches emphasize one or the other.

The Pros and Cons of Tight Buildings

As you will see in the chapter on healthy building, one of the issues that can occur from a focus on just one topic in the built environment is that the solution to one problem can cause a number of other issues that didn't exist previously. And as green building is often focused on the use of many different synthetic products, such as using petrochemical products for creating high insulation to reduce energy costs, this single decision-making process can also lead to ecological issues.

A good example of these possible issues is a topic that green building struggled with early on, which was a focus on the idea of making the building "tight."

This idea of making a building "tight" is basically a building constructed to decrease airflow to reduce energy transfer. This leads to the reduction of drafts in buildings. By reducing drafts, it helps to prevent the transfer or loss of energy in the building. It's often achieved by stricter building processes and also achieved by preventing windows from being opened. The approach of a tight building is to reduce the thermal transfer from outside to inside. This example of not allowing the windows to be opened requires that the air filtration and air exchange is done mechanically using the building's ventilation systems.

This example highlights issues that can and have occurred related to creating indoor air quality (IAQ) problems. And while this process may save energy and reduce energy consumption, it can also add another factor to the equation, which is the lack of healthy air quality.

In new construction and renovations where there are many synthetic materials and products used, this can trap high levels of VOCs and reduce the ratio of fresh air. This leaves the inhabitants with toxins to breathe and a possible increase in Carbon Monoxide, Carbon Dioxide, and other gases, including the rise of Volatile Organic Compounds as VOCs that can cause health problems.

This has become a particular issue since around the 1970s forward based on the increase of synthetic materials, paints, and other modern materials. The combination of newer building materials that off-gas these chemicals, combined with these tighter building designs, became a significant health issue for many inhabiting these structures.

When reviewing these green building topics, perhaps the common denominator that has motivated these developments is the amount of energy used and utilized in the fields of construction and building use. The chart below shows that buildings use around 40 percent of all energy worldwide[42] to create and maintain buildings. And with concerns of human impacts on the planet, both in terms of climate change and the negative environmental impacts on the planet, working to reduce this energy use in buildings can have a significant benefit.

Worldwide Energy Use

World total final consumption of 119.8 PWh by sector in 2012:[42]

- Residential (13%)
- Commercial (7%)
- Industrial (54%)
- Transportation (26%)

Architectural Medicine – Building the Bridge to Wellness

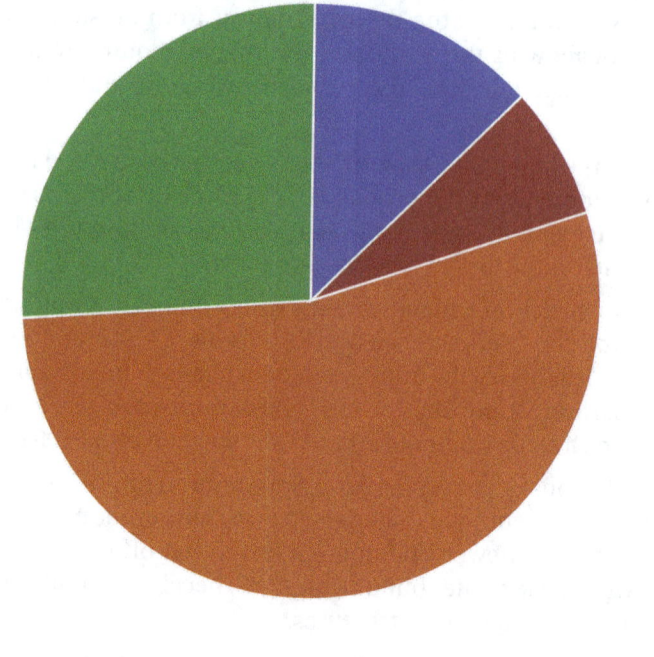

Total World Energy Consumption by Sector

- Residential
- Commercial
- Industrial
- Transportation

As you can see in the diagrams, the charts show that the heating and cooling of buildings, along with artificial lighting, are among the top two culprits of energy use. Reducing the energy needs from heating, cooling, and lighting can help resolve these energy issues the most.

Here's the breakdown of the energy segmentation:

- Residential (heating, lighting, and appliances)
- Commercial (lighting, heating and cooling of commercial buildings, and provision of water and sewer services)
- Industrial users (agriculture, mining, manufacturing, and construction)
- Transportation (passenger, freight, and pipeline)

Chapter: 7 | Green Building Defined and Overview

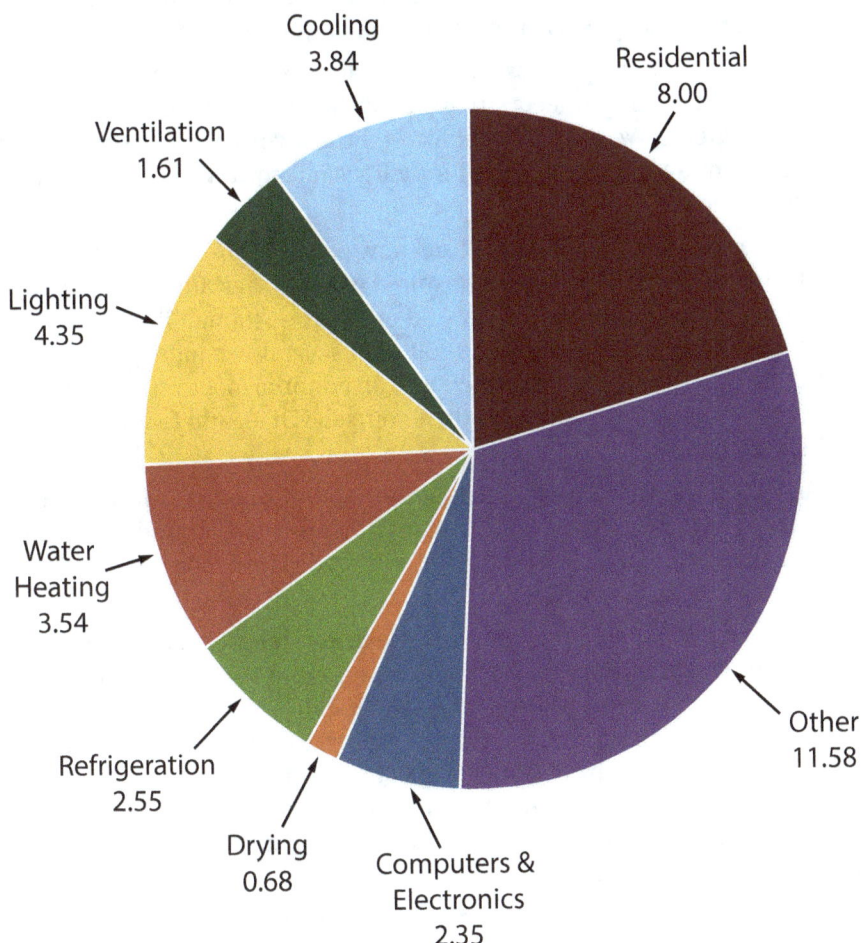

Source: Chapter 5: Increasing Efficiency of Building Systems and Technologies, September 2015 - Figure 5.1 Buildings Use More Than 38% of all U.S. Energy and 76% of U.S. Electricity[43]

Source: International Energy Outlook 2016, Table F1. Total world delivered energy consumption by end-use sector and fuel, 2011–40[44]

And to this end, this is often why green building is often focused on creating these tight buildings to reduce energy losses in terms of heating and cooling expenditures. It's also why a focus on artificial lighting through the years has often been a primary focus. By addressing these two main issues, it can provide a substantial positive impact in reducing energy use.

This green building process has been a large experiment over the past 30 to 40 years, with many pioneers striving to find solutions to reducing these energy requirements. We should be thanking those involved in working towards these solutions and have gratitude for their visions towards finding solutions to these problems.

Another pioneer that should be acknowledged is Steward Brand, whose "Whole Earth Catalog" publication inspired many to seek alternative building and living options to reduce energy and embrace sustainability as a lifestyle and way of life. First published in 1968 with several versions updated until 1972, it provided a catalog of products and an editorial focus on self-sufficiency, ecology, alternative education, do it yourself (DIY), and featured the slogan "access to tools".[45]

I list this publication based on an important information source that was the start of the information age. The magazine provided products and editorials in a similar manner in how the internet today provides information on these topics in today's world.

Brand and many others pioneered these developments and provided a foundation of experimentation. Many seeking these solutions have benefited from their work. In some ways, the fractured processes of these different fields, from green building and ecological design to natural building, sustainable building, and healthy building, began by people focusing on solving one of these many issues. The benefit is that each topic now has more detailed solutions, and the drawback is that these have independently developed, thereby creating other problems.

The good news is that by viewing these developments from a large vantage point, it can become more apparent where the gaps exist and how integrated solutions moving forward can provide more cohesive solutions.

As you will find in other sections of this book, many other resources can provide a deeper dive into these specific topics. Below is a brief list of recommended people and groups to follow and the books and publications that they provide.

Below is a short list of these pioneers, and you can read more information about these fields and these pioneers on our website through the following link:

https://architecturalmedicine.com/book

Highlighting Some Important People and Groups Involved in Green Building

The following is a small list of the great organizations and individuals who have done and are doing great work to achieve these goals of energy efficiency and a reduction of energy use:

Building Science
World Green Building Council
U.S. Green Building Council (USGBC)
Leadership in Energy and Environmental Design (LEED)
Rocky Mountain Institute
Solar Energy International (SEI)
Yestermorrow Design/Build School
Architecture 2030
Living Building Challenge

Amory Lovins
Steward Brand
Joseph Lstiburek
Bruce King
Eric Corey Freed
David Bainbridge
David Eisenberg
Michael Reynolds

With an emphasis on the reduction of energy use, which is obviously an important topic, there can be important lessons gleaned from the focus on only one facet of the building equation.

My direct experiences in the field of green building provided me of a valuable lesson. It showed me that you could often create different problems that you are trying to solve when you view only one facet of the whole picture.

In the early days of green building and even in many scenarios today, making buildings tight to reduce energy transfer from outside to inside can be problematic. It does solve the problems of energy loss and can reduce energy costs to achieve the end goal of being more energy-efficient. Yet, the fact that these buildings are built so tight introduces these other problems such as particulates, VOCs, Carbon Monoxide, and Carbon Dioxide, to name just a few. And so, as the goal of energy efficiency was provided, it added these toxins into the mix, harming those inhabiting these spaces.

Without an integrated knowledge and background of creating these solutions, many are left to follow basic guidelines. This can limit creativity in developing solutions and results in more problems. Don't get me wrong, guidelines, standards, and protocols are critical. As you can see later in this book, there is a list that Architectural Medicine defines as ARxMD processes. More details on this term can be found in chapters 16 and 18.

However, to define these standards without the framework of knowing "why", leaves the context for decisions in a confusing and fractured manner.

Focusing on just one topic of energy efficiency and leaving out the health of the occupants, and ignoring the environmental impact on the location creates a lack of health for both occupants and the planet.

This brings us to the next topic of *Sustainable Building*...

> "Reality must take precedence over public relations, for nature cannot be fooled."
>
> – Richard P. Feynman

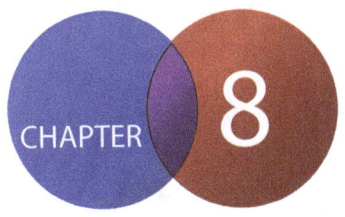

CHAPTER 8

SUSTAINABLE BUILDING DEFINED AND OVERVIEW

As I mentioned in the previous chapter, the Green Building and Sustainable Building topics have many different definitions, depending on who you are talking to and who is writing about these topics.

For purposes of this book, the concept of Sustainable Building is defined as the awareness of the building's environmental impacts, from the materials being used to the building's actual use, and these impacts on the local and global ecology. This, of course, includes the impacts on the environment at the building's end of life.

Ecology

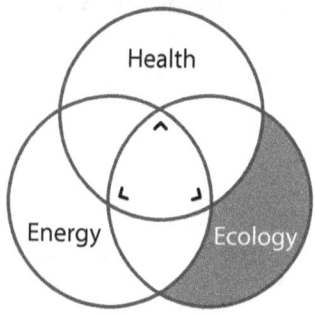

Ecology/**Sustainable Architecture-Building**

Ecology

Recognizing and designing for the Ecology, creating more sustainable solutions with materials and methods. Considering Life Cycle Assessment (LCA) in all designs. Groups and organizations with an Ecological focus in the built environment include: Biophilic Design and the Permaculture Institute

When a building is no longer being used, will the building be destroyed and added to the landfill? Or will the building materials be re-used and re-purposed to become another built object? The latter of which is typically referred to as cradle to cradle, as opposed to cradle to grave.

Sustainable building can be defined as buildings "that are environmentally responsible and resource-efficient throughout a building's life-cycle: from planning to design, construction, operation, maintenance, renovation, and demolition."[46]

An early advocate of this architectural focus is Sim Van der Ryn, whose book *Ecological Design* helped define this field. The book, co-authored by Stuart Cowan, defines ecological design as "any form of design that minimizes environmentally destructive impacts by integrating itself with living processes."[47] There are many overlaps between ecological design and sustainable building, and the definitions are very similar.

And these topics include the question of the carbon footprint of a building in the life span of the building's use. These are part of the discussions that architects and designers have when considering the impact the building will have on the local and the global environment.

This can include many variables, such as the impact it has on the wildlife and topics related to wastewater and water runoff, to the impact that the people have on the balance of the local ecology.

What are the overall impacts the building has on the environment during its lifetime?

Of course, this does include the energy resources impact, which is why green building and sustainable building often have many overlaps when viewing all of the building puzzle pieces.

Part of the reason why I have chosen to discuss these topics in this order is due to my own experiences in these fields, where green building in the 90s was often focused specifically on energy efficiency, sometimes without much attention to the other facets of the building's lifespan and environmental impacts.

The way in which I've experienced these different topics in the real world has been a delineation between the energy efficiency and energy costs and the impacts that building has on the ecology. With this lens, I'm using the term sustainable building to include the energy impacts, which is part of the bigger picture of ecological stewardship. The use of the word sustainable is the focus, which asks the questions, can this type of building and the use of the building processes be "sustained" over time? Can this be achieved without massive degradation to the quality of the ecology and other life on the planet?

In this manner, if it is sustainable, the life of the building and its inhabitants can maintain this process from generation to generation without destroying the ecology in the process.

Many people might refer to this topic in relation to previous environmental issues, such as the Cuyahoga River in the US. This infamous river caught on fire many times in the 1950s and 1960s. It caught on fire due to the many industries on the river that were dumping toxic chemicals into the river.

The river's industrial pollution was so extreme that the river was stated as "oozing as opposed to flowing"[48], to the point that the water, several times, spontaneously caught on fire. This was part of the signaling of a time of environmental concerns and spurred the Environmental Protection Agency (EPA) development in the United States.[49]

This was also happening during the time of the famous book by Rachel Carson, *Silent Spring*, which began signaling that toxins and pollutants were causing health issues for human biology and the entire biology of the planet. It wasn't the first time that industry and nature would be at odds. The clean up of the Cuyahoga River, to this day of 2020, is still an issue after over 150 years of reports of there being these pollution issues. Of course, the Cuyahoga River in Ohio is only one of many examples of these pollution problems.

While many debate the question of how much pollution is allowable or acceptable, the better question might be to ask how these issues can be a design problem to be solved.

These debates and contemplations can also include the Green Chemistry and Biomimicry fields, which view these as design challenges and seek solutions in a larger scope and view of life on this planet. The developments of these two fields, which have been emerging over the past 20 plus years, have resulted from these topics needing solutions to ensure that the ecology is protected while still moving forward in human developments.

And again, in the 1960s into the 1970s, there were many architects, designers, or simply the general public that had concerns about these negative impacts on the environment. Many chose this path seeking better solutions for designs of the future. In the US, if you travel from the east coast to the west coast, and particularly in the American southwest, you will find many examples of these alternative design processes. And some include forgotten building methodologies re-examined, tested, and implemented.

From Adobe buildings, timber frame, and straw building processes to the Earthships in Taos and even hemp used as a building material, many of these alternatives are striving to help solve these energy-efficiency and environmental stewardship issues. Unknown to many, hemp was a typical agricultural material used for many industries across the US before the material became illegal to grow and cultivate in the early to mid-1900s.[50]

Many experimental architectural projects were based on this challenge to find better solutions, and all around the world, you can find examples of such explorations.

If you were to look up a definition of sustainable building, you'd find many different meanings. Yet when you view the term as defined in the Oxford English Dictionary, the following is the actual definition of the word:

sustainable, adj.:

a. Capable of being maintained or continued at a certain rate or level.

b. Designating forms of human activity (esp. of an economic nature) in which environmental degradation is minimized, esp. by avoiding the long-term depletion of natural resources; of or relating to activity of this type. Also: designating a natural resource which is exploited in such a way as to avoid its long-term depletion. Cf. sustainability n. 2b.[51]

sustainability, n.

a. The quality of being sustainable at a certain rate or level.

b. spec. The property of being environmentally sustainable; the degree to which a process or enterprise is able to be maintained or continued while avoiding the long-term depletion of natural resources.[52]

The definition as a noun in the segment above draws attention to the environment, and it is this version of the definition that, in my experience, has had the greatest connection to sustainable building.

The outline of being "environmentally sustainable" where the "process or enterprise is able to be maintained or continued while avoiding the long-term depletion of natural resources" is often at the core of the sustainable building mantra.

Of course, there are still many ways to view this topic, and therefore there can always be many viewpoints. Yet, the essence of Sustainable Building is often focused on the long-term impacts on the natural resources and the ecological consequences.

And the main reason why this is important is based on the fact that a healthy ecosystem allows for healthy biological organisms. And of course, humans are biological organisms, so this includes the health of humanity.

Sustainable building can be viewed as a mindset to reduce the building's impact on the environment by choosing materials, products, and methods that reduce the negative impacts that buildings have on the environment.

This includes the reduction of the production of materials and a design focus that works with nature's systems, striving to have less impact on the local and global ecology. Choosing to design to sustain better ecological health over a long time period in a mutually beneficial way is a common goal.

An example is to use timber if the location where you are building is within forested areas for a timber frame structure. If you are in a desert region, use local materials such as adobe to build thick walls with these earthen materials. For example, if thick walls are created, such as adobe, it will provide both insulative and thermal mass solutions to decrease energy costs and provide less heat transfer. This process reduces the energy use and the subsequent pollution caused by the manufacturing of the materials, yet also reduces energy costs over time in the building's actual use.

As well, when a timber frame structure or an adobe structure is no longer used, the materials can return to nature without degradation to the environment, as nature can recycle these materials back into the ecosystem from which it originally came from.

Nature, after all, is the greatest engineer in terms of reuse, recycling, and sustainability. This is why subjects such as biomimicry have become so common over the past several decades. The lessons of nature's engineering can be studied and applied to human-created designs for a whole systems approach.

Sustainability as a Spiracycle

And when it comes to the topics of cycles and circular patterns, as opposed to the linear start to end process of life, an excellent example of this is the "cradle to cradle" work of William McDonough and Michael Braungart as a transition from the previous "cradle to grave" concepts.

A key here is also to recognize the wisdom of the McDonough/Braungart cycle called cradle to cradle, where in the past, the process was often seen as cradle to grave, meaning that a product was made, bought, consumed, and then thrown away to the landfill. Cradle to Cradle specifies that the "beginning to end" process yields a cycle in itself. A product's life cycle begins from another product's "end waste," leading to a proper breakdown of the materials involved and then utilized to create another group of products.

And this cycle will continue ad infinitum, just as the natural world functions.

This concept of human-created designs, products, and processes was first evaluated in the whole systems approach of John T. Lyle's "regenerative design."[53][54] The Swiss architect Walter R. Stahel defined the "Cradle to Cradle" mantra as part of his work in the 1970s. This helped support the idea of a process that was concerned about the future of products and processes, with the eventual goal of understanding how to design and build products, materials, buildings, and anything human created to have less negative impact on the environment and planet.

For many, the concept of there being garbage or "throwing things away" is a human concept that has become normal, yet nowhere in the natural world is this normal. The natural world exists in a constant cycle of life, death, and a rebirth of life again. Otherwise, the world as we know it would emulate a garbage planet of the Pixar movie WALL-E. And anyone who watched that movie knows that humans had to leave earth to survive, as the planet was dying.

In this manner, there is no garbage. With nature's cycles, nature does not make garbage, as the waste of one product or organism is utilized by another organism or process.

This is a big part of the sustainable definition where a spiracycle is progressing forward beneficially, with iterations providing updates to the process each step along the way.

Chapter: 8   Sustainable Building Defined and Overview

A Key Difference Between Green and Sustainable Building

As you can see in these writings, the differences between Green and Sustainable Building have many overlapping concepts that can make the exact definition confusing or fuzzy. Two concepts that I have seen time and again in these fields might provide some clarity.

Often, the goal of Green Building is to reduce energy and become more energy efficient as the end goal. Whether you achieve this by using natural materials or synthetic materials to increase insulation, as an example, is often not a focus in green building. Using a synthetic material, such as a petroleum product for insulation to provide large R-values to reduce energy use, is often a different approach than the Sustainable Building process.

With Sustainable Building, you may choose to use natural materials or those materials that have less impact on the environment using more natural materials and methods. This allows for the overall lack of impact on the ecology from the use of highly manufactured products. Many sustainable designs have a larger scope of impact in terms of both the energy used and the long term impacts of material choices. This is opposed to just being focused on the reduction of energy use and the energy efficiency goals.

With Sustainable Building, it is typical in my experience that a whole picture of the design process is assessed, including the materials used and the big picture impact the building has on the ecology as part of the decision making process.

In this way, those focused on Green Building may make choices such as using synthetic materials as a good choice to increase the insulation capabilities, thereby decreasing energy costs and being more energy-efficient. And those who are focused on Sustainability are often looking at these energy topics, yet also the bigger picture such as production, manufacturing, extrapolation, and end of use of these petroleum products.

The 1970s energy crisis was a decision-making process that inspired and motivated the long term views of these building topics to provide good ecological stewardship. This becomes important, especially when you scale up the production of such products from their extrapolation and manufacturing. The question of what happens to the materials when they are done being used is often taken into consideration as a sustainability viewpoint.

While there are many debates on these topics, and these will likely continue into the future, perhaps the takeaway from these discussions is to bring awareness to these issues and see them as a design problem to solve. In this manner, current and future designers can focus on these issues for better solutions.

Permaculture – Supporting Sustainable Landscapes and Sustainable Architecture

While sustainable building became a focus for some architects and builders in North American during the 1960s and 70s onward, halfway around the world in Australia, Bill Mollison worked on similar solutions to environmental stewardship that he defined as *Permaculture* or "permanent agriculture."

Permaculture's approach is to recognize the eco-systems of nature and work with nature in more harmony in recognizing nature as living systems.

Mollison defines permaculture as "a philosophy of working with, rather than against nature; of protracted and thoughtful observation rather than protracted and thoughtless labor; and of looking at plants and animals in all their functions, rather than treating any area as a single product system."

When viewing the built environment as a whole system and factoring into this equation the many interdependent facets, it becomes critical to consider the many impacts that a design will have in both its construction and its long term use.

Permaculture includes many different fields as a cohesive whole, from ecological design and integrated water management to support the whole systems design approach of sustainable architecture. It's less formulaic in the design process and instead requires studying natural systems to learn how nature functions and learn from this wisdom.

When the building becomes part of the landscape in both form and function, then these concepts of permaculture in an applied format can support better integration to live with nature instead of designing architecture and landscapes that supersede the natural environment.

A key takeaway from this inclusion of permaculture is the focus on sustainable design, including the landscape and ecology that the building exists with. By recognizing that there are effects on the locale when designing and building architecture, it can support a more vernacular approach that can help the ecology and biological health of the location while providing a framework for the functions of the structure.

Having a better understanding of these many eco-systems can provide a more creative approach to the design of the building as an integrated part of the ecology, instead of the building being a foreign addition.

In this manner, many various fields providing solutions can highlight the value of viewing whole systems solutions. By utilizing the benefits of various fields, from ecological design and natural building to biomimicry and ecological engineering, the systems approach can provide hopeful solutions to these long term environmental problems we are facing in today's world.

These discussions on sustainable building have included a number of other fields such as ecological design, natural building, and vernacular building. If you're asking what the differences are, it can often be complicated, yet some basic comments can be made to differentiate.

Ecological design is defined by Sim Van der Ryn and Stuart Cowan as "any form of design that minimizes environmentally destructive impacts by integrating itself with living processes."[56] It strives to design buildings and products that factor the product's environmental impacts during its whole life cycle, which is referenced earlier as life cycle assessment and the circular economy.

Natural building often focuses on the use of natural materials, as well as using materials that are local for vernacular building. This might include the concept that if you are living in a forested region, then utilizing wood for most of the building, such as timber frame, would be a logical approach. As well, if you are living in a desert type region, then adobe or rammed earth might be a better option to utilize available local materials.

And vernacular building is often the use of local materials and knowledge, using the definition of vernacular as "of, relating to, or being the common building style of a period or place."[57]

The *Encyclopedia of the City* defines vernacular architecture as "representing the majority of buildings and settlements created in pre-industrial societies and includes a very wide range of buildings, building traditions, and methods of construction."[58]

This can essentially include many of the building materials and methods utilized in ecological design, natural building, and sustainable building. In reality, there is more overlap than there are differences.

You can find more information about each of these various fields on our website by going to the link: https://architecturalmedicine.com/book

The work of the pioneers listed below has helped to provide solutions to many of these problems. The future of architecture owes a debt of gratitude for their care, interest, and experimentations to find solutions as we move into the future.

As you will find in other sections of this book, many other resources can dive deeper into these specific topics. Below is a brief list of recommended people and groups to follow and the books and publications that they provide:

Highlighting Some Important People and Groups Involved in Sustainable Building

Biomimicry
Biophilia
Natural Building
Ecological Design
Permaculture

World Green Building Council
Leadership in Energy and Environmental Design (LEED)
Rocky Mountain Institute
Solar Energy International (SEI)
Institute for Baubiologie (IBN)
CalEarth
Architecture 2030
Architecture for Humanity
Living Building Challenge

Sim Van der Ryn
Stewart Brand
Bosco Büeler
James Hubble
William McDonough
Bill Mollison
Athena and Bill Steen
Carol Venolia
Nader Khalili
Linda Smiley and Ianto Evans
Janine Benyus
Cedar Rose Guelberth
Paula Baker-Laporte and Robert Laporte
Rob Roy

Chapter: 8

Sustainable Building Defined and Overview

Neri Oxman

Eric Corey Freed

The big picture view of how these topics impact human health is a main focus of this book. Yet to ignore the health of the ecology or the impacts of pollution, as well as how our buildings impact environmental and biological health, would be to ignore a huge part of what is required to achieve good human health.

This brings us to the next topic and chapter – *Healthy Building...*

"It is no measure of health to be well adjusted to a profoundly sick society."

– Jiddu Krishnamurti

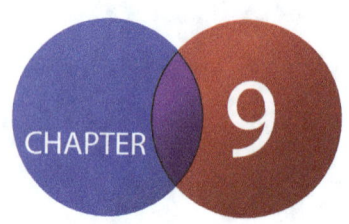

HEALTHY BUILDING DEFINED AND OVERVIEW

HEALTHY BUILDING – A BRIEF HISTORY AND OVERVIEW

With the essence of this book focused on health in the built environment, healthy building is an important focus, yet it has also been the slowest in developing relative to the topics of green and sustainable building. The latter two topics have had more advances in the past 30 years.

I state this as an important aspect of these three developments and it might explain why it's critical to have the medical and public health fields more involved moving forward.

Chapter: 9 — Healthy Building Defined and Overview

As an overview of this topic, I will first paint a big picture view and then discuss how they are currently connected or disconnected.

The fact that there exists a topic of *Healthy Building* infers in some ways that there is unhealthy building. For most people, the subject of sick building syndrome (SBS) might be the primary thought as to what healthy building is, or at least what healthy building might be based upon.

When discussing Healthy Building, as opposed to Physical Wellness in the following chapters, the main difference is that Healthy Building is typically focused on the physical impacts that materials have on the human body, causing illness and disease. This includes lead paint, asbestos, mold, and other topics of pollution in the built environment.

Health

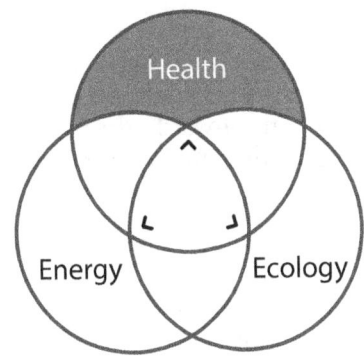

Health/ **Healthy Building**

Health

Issues related to physical health, removing toxic materials and improving occupant health. Groups and organizations with a Health focus in the built environment include: Healthy Building Network, Bau Biologie and Biophilia

If you look into the history of this field, you might recognize that healthy building has been a topic back to the time of Hippocrates. The topics of health in the built environment and ancient places of healing may be referred to as early hospitals.

Many of these ancient greek structures that were built to provide healing environments, in some form or another, were there to remove a form of negative ailment. These early hospital origins called Asclepeions were healing temples located in ancient Greece dedicated to Asclepius, the god of medicine in Greek mythology.[59]

Yet in the eastern parts of the world, or at least in India and Asiatic locations, there's a long history that considers the impacts on health and the built environment. This ranged from vastu shastra and ayurvedic medicine to feng shui and Chinese medicine, all of which closely consider the location and the buildings that the patient is living within.

In both the east and west in ancient times, the powers of place were not just sacred for religious worship but also for the power of healing, health, and wellness.[60] Certain types of mineral waters in Europe, as in other places in the world, became places of healing. The ancient Europeans, such as the greek culture, often built these temples and places specifically for healing, with chambers and places inside of these buildings that they believed brought upon a healing process for the patient.[61]

Yet it probably wasn't until the famous findings of John Snow and epidemiology that more modern ways of recognizing health and "place" in the 19th century became more evidence-based. From that time onwards, the built environment and the various facets of the natural environment became a more significant focus of health and sickness.

Florence Nightingale is also well known for her essential work and her famous quotes referencing the patient's health relative to the building and interior spaces. And Rachel Carson then became most notable in terms of health concerns in modern-day science and chemistry with her book *Silent Spring*. The explorations into the health issues of synthetic chemicals and their impacts on human, biological, and ecological health began due to her work.

Perhaps the most notable timeframe of the healthy building movement was defined by sick buildings or built environments causing sickness from the late 1950s and '60s in Europe. In post-World War II Europe, many of the cities rebuilding after the war used newer methods and materials in construction. These were often built with a new emphasis on saving energy, which resulted in making buildings more "tight," a word that is in common use in the building world today. As mentioned in previous chapters, the term "tight" is often defined as making the building or the building envelope built tightly to reduce the airflow and energy loss. This means that the building's airflow from exterior to interior does not directly impact the thermal transfer in the building space.

For those who have ever lived or stayed in an older building that was built before the mid- 20th century and earlier, these buildings were and often are drafty. This is where you can feel the outside air or temperature differences entering the interior spaces. These drafty structures often let in cold air in the winter and allow hot air to infiltrate the building in the summer. This makes the building less temperature controlled and causes energy losses.

In the past, these drafty buildings would let in the hot summer air and lose the warmth of a fireplace or heating devices in the winter, which led to energy inefficiencies and uncomfortable spaces. Advanced building processes began to make these more recent structures more efficient by making them tight, which meant that they would close off the drafty crevices to prevent the exchange of air and reduce energy losses.

At this same time, the construction fields also began using more synthetic materials, such as synthetic carpets and new paints and plastics that were becoming more commonplace in the built world.

And this combination of making the buildings tighter and adding these newer materials created a kind of perfect storm in these buildings. By making them tighter, it prevented the outside temperatures from impacting the inside temperatures and allowed for more efficient heating and cooling systems, but it also prevented fresh outside air from entering. This, combined with more modern synthetic materials, created a kind of toxicity inside the buildings and then kept these toxins inside without any dilutions with the outside air.

In post-WWII Europe, many people were getting sick, and it befuddled the doctors and general public. A few doctors and groups seeking a solution eventually realized that these tight buildings and newer materials were the culprits. In much the same way as John Snow recognized that one water source affected the entire city population's health where epidemiology began, this new understanding of tight buildings causing sickness began the emphasis on healthy building. These developments were pioneered by those such as Dr. Hubert Palm, who published the book *Das Gesunde Haus* in 1968[62] after discovering that these buildings were making people sick.

Soon after, Dr. Anton Schneider developed the field of Bau Biologie and the Institute of Building Biology (IBN). This Institute has continued onward from the 1970s, expanding to many parts of the world to educate professionals on building issues related to health.

In the US, the 1980s sick building syndrome (SBS) became popular when the newly redesigned EPA building was causing illness to those working there. They didn't know it at first, yet after exploring these reported health issues, they discovered that the combination of the newly created "tighter" building envelope combined with new synthetic carpets, paints, and other materials seemed to be causing the occupants to become ill.

Since that time, many people worldwide have become more educated on the impacts that the built environment has on health. These fields have become more complex as built environments and human progress has become more complex. Today, other fields are becoming more aware of these issues, from Environmental Medicine to the toxicology and epidemiology fields utilizing big data to show patterns of sickness and ailments related to buildings.

Bioinformatics and research in the 21st century have shown medical and health conditions related to chemicals as endocrine disruptors as well as creating nervous system issues.

Several years ago, an article in the NY Times discussed health issues connected to the endocrine system and exposure to chemicals. The author stated there is "significant evidence that several types of chemicals can interfere with the hormones that our bodies use as messengers for everything from sexual maturity and fertility to how we handle appetite and fat storage."[63]

This has certainly been a wake-up call for many. Endocrine disrupting chemicals are now shown as a significant issue related to diabetes, fertility issues, and many other health conditions. The issue of autoimmune problems has also been a red flag for many of these topics. The built environment has become a more common source of substances that are negatively impacting the nervous and immune systems.

This new research and medical knowledge is becoming more helpful in diagnosing public health issues, such as exposure to phthalates and bisphenols. These two chemicals have become popular discussions based on their negative impact on health as hormone-disrupting plastics. With more of these discoveries from the medical research professionals, the expanse of these topics is becoming more common in the public domain for individuals to make lifestyle choices with greater awareness.

After all, it was only recently that the medical community discovered that the brain has a lymphatic system[64] , and with the advent of aluminum being causation for Alzheimer's, there is certainly much more to learn in how these toxicants are impacting health. What might be found in the built environment causing health issues is just emerging.

Yet, most medical professionals are still unaware of these topics in the built environment. What's worse is that even if the average doctor or health professional was aware of these topics, they have very few protocols to navigate such ailments, let alone a lack of accurate workflow as to what to do about these issues.

After all, the doctor already has enough to handle in their profession. How can they be expected to deal with the architecture and built environment fields?

As well, the architect and building professional already have their workload to handle, so how are they supposed to be the ones that will learn more about the medical professions on top of the required knowledge in the design and building profession?

In many ways, these are the gaps that exist that prevent true collaborative efforts to create synchronized solutions for healthier building. At the same time, it will be incredibly challenging for there to be any major change without such integrative and multi-disciplinary development between these professions.

Physical Health and the Impact of the Built Environment

When discussing physical health, a critical analysis is based on the physiological impacts of toxins and chemicals on the body. While there can be a material or pollutant that is toxic for the physical body, physiological issues are based on functions of the body. And this becomes especially important when the body is handling stressors. There is overlap between all of these physical, emotional, and mental or psychological health and wellness topics, yet they do have some specific differences unique to each facet.

As well, Healthy Building has a similar situation to the previous two chapters in discussing Green and Sustainable Building, as it has many definitions according to who you ask and who is writing about the topic.

To be clear, the Healthy Building definition in this chapter and in this book is mainly focused on physical health. This includes the topics of materials that can impact health, such as lead paint, asbestos, VOCs, and mold, but also topics related to materials and methods that can either support good health or issues that can cause illness.

If you read the previous two chapters, you will see a pattern here that defines each of these topics for a big picture view and why they matter. And when it comes to Healthy Building, this is critical to the subject of Architectural Medicine.

In the US, the Healthy Building movement became a more common topic after the US EPA building scenario, yet these issues also included the topics of lead paint, asbestos, and modern synthetic materials, which back in the day had limited VOC regulations.

Another part of the Healthy Building movement was that some people responded to these issues of outgassing and exposure to certain materials in more sensitive formats, such as those with weakened immune systems. Another group of people who were paying attention to these problems were those seeking healthier living, as the health kicks of the late '80s and '90s became a hot topic.

While these issues were often called Sick Building Syndrome (SBS), after the US EPA building issues, in the 1990s, many began to use the term Building Related Illness (BRI) instead. This terminology helped discuss topics that are not always easy to measure. Instead of stating that the building is sick, the BRI acronym states that there are illnesses related to certain building issues, as opposed to the building itself being sick.

Many of these issues were discovered in Europe in the 1960s but did not become common in the US until the 80s and 90s. I was fortunate to have swiss architect Bosco Büeler as a mentor, as well as Helmet Ziehe, who first translated the german Bau Biologie course into English and offered training in the US. Those in Europe had already been studying and learning about these topics since the 1960s and 1970s, so there was a great wealth of knowledge that they shared with the rest of the world.

Today, many researchers are involved in health-related topics in the built environment based in Europe, and there is a growing depth of knowledge worldwide on these building health issues. And this points to the importance of working together on these topics, not just across different professions, yet also inclusive in global collaboration.

Industrial Hygiene Professionals, Environmental Inspections, and the Healthy Building Inspector

Throughout this book, there are references to several professionals with overlap between each field. This segment will reference three groups with such overlap, and I will expand upon this in chapter 17 on Healthy Building Inspectors.

For those familiar with the profession, Industrial Hygienists address issues in the commercial and industrial fields related to safety. Industrial Hygiene is a "science and art devoted to the anticipation, recognition, evaluation, control, and confirmation of protection from those environmental factors or stresses arising in or from the workplace which may cause sickness, impaired health and well being, or significant discomfort among workers or among citizens of the community."[65]

In the US, Industrial Hygienists (IH) are also known as occupational and environmental health and safety professionals (OEHS). The AIHA defines IH professionals as "scientists and engineers who are dedicated to ensuring health and safety in the workplace."

An occupational or industrial hygienist has a wide range of topics that they address in the commercial and industrial setting. This includes topics from the evaluations of physical, chemical, biological, or environmental hazards in the workplace to physical hazards such as noise, temperature extremes, illumination extremes, ionizing or non-ionizing radiation, and ergonomics.[66]

When health issues in buildings are considered, perhaps the numbers that are impacted by such illnesses and deaths are not as widely known. There are some staggering statistics based on occupational diseases, sicknesses, and deaths in the United States alone. According to the American Industrial Hygiene Association (AIHA), approximately 275 people die from occupational injuries and illnesses daily. In 2017 "about 3.5 million workers suffered occupational injuries or illnesses, and approximately 95,000 workers died in 2017 from occupational diseases."[67] And globally, approximately "2.7 million workers die from occupational injuries and illnesses, as one worker dies from occupational causes every 11 seconds."[68]

These topics related to occupational and industrial hygiene are often focused on commercial workplaces, yet what about these evaluations in residences and homes? Shouldn't these evaluations exist for residences and personal spaces? And shouldn't these inspections be provided in tandem for doctors and health professionals to evaluate patient health?

This question and topic is discussed in more depth in chapter 17, which is focused on the Healthy Building Inspector and inspection.

This also becomes an interesting integration potential when added to the discussions earlier in chapter 5 on the exposome, which is defined as the "measure of all the exposures of an individual in a lifetime and how those exposures relate to health."[69]

If the industrial hygienist, the environmental inspector, and the Healthy Building Inspector work to gather these types of exposures over an individual's life, this can be powerful bio-information for health professionals to have insights into personal health metrics. By understanding how the "environment, diet, lifestyle, etc. interact with our own unique characteristics such as genetics, physiology, and epigenetics"[70] impacts our health, this can provide exposome information as a valuable health resource.

Green Chemistry and Solutions to Creating Healthier Buildings

As an aside, in a previous chapter, I commented that there were the two primary professionals of architecture and medicine that are the most prominent two groups in terms of the big picture.

However, I also stated that the integration of these two groups and the collaboration of many other groups would be vital to make sure that the big picture was being considered in terms of a cohesive approach.

In this manner, it seems critical to comment on a group and profession that has become more popular and perhaps will have a huge role in the next stages of green design and healthy design development. This profession is "green chemistry." In her book, *High Tech Trash*, the author Elizabeth Grossman brings to light some of the health issues related to synthetic materials. And in her book *Chasing Molecules*, she follows up with some solutions being developed in this up and coming field of green chemistry.

Green chemists are in many ways functioning as the engineers of materials akin to the biomimicry field. Those such as Janine Benyus in the field of biomimicry are mostly focused on the design and engineering of products and processes. In contrast, green chemistry is focused on the chemical composition of the materials themselves.

In green chemistry, much of the focus is to review how the actual chemistry and microscopic focus of the products are developed and how they impact ecosystems.

Again, there is overlap with many of these new approaches to design and engineering solutions. The more these fields and professions work together, the better the result will become.

What is common between these two fields is that their approach is reviewing the entire process and how the material will impact and integrate with the other facets of biological systems. Green chemistry strives to reduce and remove the significant toxicological and resultant adverse effects of this chemistry, to ensure that a solution can be created without destroying the rest of the environment.

Biomimicry is working similarly. While green chemistry can be viewed as approaching this in the micro-level of material creation, biomimicry is often approaching this in the macro or design process. With each field, you will see much overlap between the two, and this, in my opinion, is a great overlap to see happening.

As I will iterate again in the following chapters, this thread of overlap and goal-oriented processes for green chemistry and biomimicry to achieve whole systems solutions is becoming common when you view these fields' trajectories. Essentially, this means that a provided solution does not negatively disrupt or destroy the collective health of the environment.

In the past, the solution might have been to save energy or reduce fuel and fossil fuel consumption or create a healthier building to reduce carbon footprint. These may have all been individual goals in the past. Yet, they are quickly becoming less individualistic goals and more of a set of goals combined as one overall goal to be healthier, greener, and more sustainable, all in one design solution.

The Coronavirus Pandemic and the Built Environment

Right now, as I am finishing the writing and editing of this book, the pandemic of the novel coronavirus is impacting the health of humanity around the world. And as this continues to be a major health issue, it's also signaling the importance of health related to the economy and the global interconnectivity between humanity.

The more these topics evolve, the more we can see and hopefully recognize the interdependency of all living creatures on this planet. And the more we can build our architecture – from the individual structure to our large cities with these principles in place for health and wellness – the more we can achieve these goals. As soon as we forget or design against these principles, the more disasters will occur around the world as the scaling of issues means the scaling of problems.

As we take more time to evaluate these topics, we can begin to see that the DNA of the single structure in a rural development can become the DNA of the suburb — eventually, the DNA of the city scales from this single building to extensive urban city developments.

The DNA of the single structure can define the DNA of an entire city. And in this manner, it behooves humans as designers and architects to think this through on a scalability factor to ensure that the single dwelling can scale to a huge city and not destroy the very land and natural resources needed for a healthy life and living. The DNA of these designs can directly impact the outcome of the quality of life for millions of people who inhabit these cities.

In this manner, you might begin to see why the topic of health in buildings is not separate from the discussions of energy efficiency as Green Building, and the impacts that our structures have on the ecology as Sustainable Building. All three of these topics are tied together, and the more overlap there is with a focus on providing solutions to all three topics, the more cohesive these solutions can provide for global health.

To add to the discussions of these topics, the social determinants of health have become more common in the medical and health professional fields for many years now. And many of these topics include the built environment. We get into this discussion later in the book, as these topics are critical for implementing and defining issues of limited systems in place for best practices between the architecture and medicine fields. This is discussed specifically in chapter 16 with the Architectural Medicine System (AMS).

As I mentioned earlier, I'm not getting too far into the details of these topics for an important reason. And the reason is for the purpose of context.

Providing a brief but hopefully sufficient overview of these topics can provide the foundation for the contextual understanding of how these various factors relate to each other.

In this manner, the gist of the topics are provided to allow the context of the subjects to be discussed appropriately. There is a wide range of subjects discussed in this book, so to provide an overview, these basic principles are provided for the best context.

And as this topic is being discussed, it might be a good segue into the questions of Healthy Building and the differences between that of Architectural Medicine. As mentioned, a significant difference is the inclusion of emotional and mental or psychological impacts that the built environment has on health and wellness.

The Differences Between Healthy Building and Architectural Medicine

While there are similarities and overlap between Healthy Building and Architectural Medicine, one of the key differences is the scope that is typically involved with both topics. For the past several decades, Healthy Building has mainly focused on the building materials and the physical health of the inhabitants.

And while this is critical to discuss and address, Architectural Medicine also includes the impact that the built environment has on physical health as well as emotional and mental or psychological well being. This addition to Architectural Medicine has some differences that add to the scope of these topics.

And when these facets of the built environment are added into the equation for doctors and health professionals, there might be questions such as "what should doctors and the medical professionals be looking at? What should they be aware of?"

Some of these questions, focused on defining processes to support doctors to include the built environment in evaluations, are discussed in chapter 16 on the Architectural Medicine System (AMS).

Many groups and individuals have developed the field of healthy building over the past 30 to 50 years. Please note the list of pioneers below, where you can find more information on their past and current work, as well as more in-depth information from their books and publications.

Highlighting Some Important People and Groups Involved in Healthy Building

As you will find in other sections of this book, there are many resources that can provide a deeper dive into these specific topics. Below is a brief list of recommended people and groups to follow:

Architecture for Humanity
Biophilia
Environmental Inspections
Evidence-Based Design
Healthy Building Network
Industrial Hygienists
Institute of Building Biology + Sustainability (IBN)

Bosco Büeler
Diana Anderson, MD @dochitect
Cedar Rose Guelberth
Carol Venolia
Christi Graham
Paula Baker-Laporte and Robert Laporte
Dr. Esther Sternberg
Eve Edelstein, MArch, Ph.D. (Neuroscience)
Mary Cordaro
Richard Scarborough
Bill Walsh
Peter Sierck
Dr. Richard J. Jackson
Dr. Andrew L. Dannenberg
Howard Frumkin
Dr. Shelley Miller
Joseph Allen
Helmet Ziehe

In the following chapters, these topics of physical, emotional, and psychological wellness will be outlined, and then in chapter 14, these pieces of the puzzle will be factored into the whole equation.

Before we go into these details of physical, emotional, and psychological wellness, let's first discuss these previous three chapters as an integrated whole, which leads us to the following chapter on *Integrative Architecture*...

"What I do is the opposite of building walls. I build bridges. A bridge is something that connects instead of separating."

– Santiago Calatrava

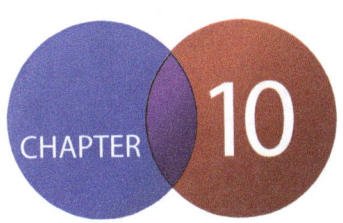

INTRODUCTION TO INTEGRATIVE ARCHITECTURE
HEALTHY, GREEN, AND SUSTAINABLE ARCHITECTURE

By now, you might begin to see a pattern emerge of an integrated necessity for excellent health and wellness in our lives in the built environment. And this brings us to the concept of *Integrative Architecture*.

As a method to provide the necessary overlap between *Green, Sustainable*, and *Healthy Building* approaches, this is being defined in this book and within Architectural Medicine as Integrative Architecture.

You might be asking how this differs from Architectural Medicine – and this is a good question.

The main difference is that Integrative Architecture is integrating the many facets of the built environment to provide green, sustainable, and healthy building solutions.

Yet Architectural Medicine includes the other facets of human health and wellness related to medicine and the medical fields, including physical, emotional, and mental or psychological wellness.

For many, the concept of architecture impacting your emotional and mental health may sound abstract. Yet, the more time you spend reflecting on how your environment influences your health in these realms, the easier it is to see how much the built environment impacts your overall health. We'll get into those details in later chapters.

The ideal focus of Integrative Architecture is to combine the best of many approaches, materials, and methods for best practices in a similar format that Integrative Medicine achieves this combination of medical modalities for best practices. I originally came up with Integrative Architecture as I was inspired by Dr. Andrew Weil's processes and those who have championed Integrative Medicine.

In a similar manner in how Integrative Medicine takes the best ideas and puts them together for the best health, Integrative Architecture takes this same approach.

An Introduction to Integrative Architecture

The history of medicine has seen great changes in the past 50 to 100 years in the contemporary world. In the past few decades, these changes have begun to embrace traditional therapies. This has been differentiated in relation to Complementary Medicine's (CM) growing developments – also known as modern medicine. Even though many of these traditional therapies, such as acupuncture and Chinese Medicine, have been around thousands of years, integrating these modern medicine changes with traditional medicine has not been rapid or easy for many areas in the modern world.

A big part of these changes in medicine accepting traditional options has occurred because the general public wants to have more options and be empowered in their good health. In the US and other places globally, the development of Integrative Medicine has been a critical part of this growth and development.

Pioneering doctors such as Dr. Andrew Weil, who is probably one of the most well known in this transformation, has stated in many of his books and lectures that he defines Integrative Medicine as integration by using different modalities that utilize best practices from many resources – from both modern and traditional methodologies and treatments.[71]

You may be wondering why I am bringing up this field of Integrative Medicine and its history. The reason is based on a reflection of this progress in medicine towards these integrations and a lack of progress in the field of architecture relative to similar goals that medicine is striving to achieve — best practices towards optimal health.

As Medicine has been embracing more traditional therapies for better health, what has been happening in the field of Architecture?

The answer is that while there have been some steps to improve architecture to be more ecologically aware and more green or energy-efficient, the healthy component has been slow going and mostly focused on Healthy Hospital Designs.

While Healthy Hospital Designs are an excellent step in this progress, it's also a recognition that there is room for improvement for the rest of the built environments – from the average home to the modern commercial building.

A potential to have more rapid development towards these goals is to use this example of Integrative Medicine to show a pathway of development for architecture in which to take. By embracing healthier approaches to built environments while also considering traditional methodologies, many of these goals can be achieved.

This process can be defined as *Integrative Architecture* to support and work in tandem with the positive developments of Integrative Medicine.

The concept of learning from Integrative Medicine in the field of architecture has many benefits. For one, many people are familiar with the topics of Integrative Medicine and the positive connotation it has to empower the average person. It also can be utilized as a high standard in discovering and using best practices for better health.

The concept of Integrative Architecture is similar to Integrative Medicine in that it strives to utilize best practices while also merging modern approaches with traditional methodologies. Essentially, it is considering many different approaches to achieve the best results, and these "best results" include a healthier approach for healthier designs.

Why Exactly Is Integrative Architecture Important?

My first job in the working world in my early teens was working as a bricklayer and construction laborer for a mason. During my childhood summers spent at my grandmother's house growing up, I had met this wonderful man named Joe Pitelli. For many years, he raised and rebuilt his home to prevent any flooding issues as the house was next to an area of water. And being that I had wanted to be an architect since a kid – and let people know this – I would visit him often. I spent many days visiting him as he worked, as I was young enough to bug him with tons of questions. He was semi-retired and a good enough person to oblige me and encourage me with his answers.

As he was semi-retired, he was still working, and in my early teens, he offered me a job to work with him and his son, who had taken over his business. It was very hard work, yet hauling bricks and learning the construction specifics were all part of the learning curve for my construction knowledge. The first building I worked on was a medium-sized business structure, which was clad in brick.

One afternoon, during lunchtime, as we were all sitting together, Mr. Pitelli Sr. began talking to his son, Mr. Pitelli Jr., about an issue that they were dealing with in the building process. The situation was that the largest of the exterior walls had a dimension problem that required them to cut bricks at each of the rows in staggered layers due to the length of the wall.

After discussing the topic between him and his son, Joe Sr. then turned to me and said, "you see, as you are planning to be an architect, you must understand what we are discussing. Because the architect did not plan for the proper length for bricks, this main wall will require each row to have a significant cutting of bricks to ensure that it looks correct. If the architect had construction experience, they would have known to adjust the wall length to an appropriate size for the brick type specified. This would have ensured that the wall would look as good as possible and to support the brick installation process."

Basically, he was saying that the aesthetics of the wall would have improved, and the extra work could have easily been avoided if the architect had designed the size of the wall accordingly.

And this was a key factor for my beginning experience in construction and building. My understanding of how buildings are constructed began, and I've used this knowledge throughout my life to understand the importance of big picture, integrative planning in any design process.

Unfortunately, most architects, especially back several decades ago, didn't have any experience with construction. This was later echoed when I attended the Yestermorrow Design/Build School in Vermont in the US. Several architects created the Yestermorrow school in 1980 who graduated architecture school with no building experience and have been working ever since to help provide hands-on education for architects and designers in the building fields.[72]

This story and experience have followed me in my life, and the core of this teaching was that there needs to be an understanding of the many systems involved to plan accordingly.

This experience highlighted the importance of integrated systems, which is essentially what Integrative Architecture is all about. Being aware of the many systems involved helps create designs that either anticipate or plan for the multitude of components involved in the design-build process in architecture. And if not factored into the design process, the result can lead to short and long-term problems.

The concept of Integrative Architecture is akin to Integrative Medicine, which strives to see the whole picture and to consider the many facets involved for the best solutions.

Integrative Medicine, at least in the US and in other places worldwide, has become more than just a buzzword for better health care. It has become a symbol of how integrating different approaches for the goal of best practices can embrace a wide range of modalities to achieve better health and wellness.

As defined by the Arizona Center for Integrative Medicine:

"Integrative Medicine (IM) is healing-oriented medicine that takes account of the whole person, including all aspects of lifestyle. It emphasizes the therapeutic relationship between practitioner and patient, is informed by evidence, and makes use of all appropriate therapies."[73]

And Dr. Weil, who is often seen as the father of and one of the strongest supporters of Integrative Medicine, defines Integrative Medicine as:

"a healing-oriented medicine that takes account of the whole person (body, mind, and spirit), including all aspects of lifestyle. It emphasizes the therapeutic relationship and makes use of all appropriate therapies, both conventional and alternative."[74]

The Defining Principles of Integrative Medicine

The following is a list of principles from the Andrew Weil Center for Integrative Medicine at The University of Arizona.

The principles of Integrative Medicine:[75]

- A partnership between patient and practitioner in the healing process
- Appropriate use of conventional and alternative methods to facilitate the body's innate healing response
- Consideration of all factors that influence health, wellness and disease, including mind, spirit and community as well as body
- A philosophy that neither rejects conventional medicine nor accepts alternative therapies uncritically
- Recognition that good medicine should be based in good science, be inquiry driven, and be open to new paradigms
- Use of natural, effective, less-invasive interventions whenever possible
- Use of the broader concepts of promotion of health and the prevention of illness as well as the treatment of disease
- Training of practitioners to be models of health and healing, committed to the process of self-exploration and self-development.

There is an interview with Dr. Weil from February of 2010 that is a very concise overview of what Integrative Medicine is and is not, and how its focus is on health and the healing of the patient.

Below are some comments from this interview, as he begins with stating the following when asked about Integrative Medicine's definition, "The short answer is it is the intelligent combination of conventional and alternative medicine, but that doesn't capture this movement".[76]

And he goes on to say, "I think Integrative Medicine is a real movement, and in essence, it is trying to restore the focus of medicine on health and healing away from disease symptom management. It emphasizes whole-person medicine meaning that we are more than just physical bodies – we are minds, spirits, and community members."

While the interview is a bit longer than two minutes, he follows up with the interviewer providing this description in more detail. Dr. Weil states, "It looks at all aspects of lifestyle; it emphasizes the importance of the practitioner-patient relationship to the healing practice."

And finally, this quote can be applied to the fundamental approach of Integrative Architecture in a similar manner to his statements on Integrative

Medicine, "and then it's willing to look at all methods from whatever tradition they come from that may be of value in treating disease – that is the alternative piece."[77]

Suppose these same approaches to Integrative Medicine are applied to the concept of Integrative Architecture. In that case, a few key points can be redefined in terms of how it is applied to architecture.

So you may be asking, why have Integrative Architecture? Why not just focus on Architectural Medicine?

The ideal in architecture is that all of the crucial factors in the built environment, including healthy built environments, green building for energy efficiency, and sustainable architecture, are appropriately defined to ensure proper shelter, the preservation of the ecology, and inspiring surroundings to live within. These are factors that all biological life depends upon, and it should automatically be a given.

Sadly, these are not always seen as actively essential and the main focus in today's modern world. And in medicine, some modalities do not embrace the best patient health and healing, which then requires integrative medicine. In this manner, integrative architecture is necessary if the path towards green, sustainable, and healthy architecture are goals to achieve.

It can help achieve optimal health and wellness goals if there is a process for the architecture world to embrace and utilize integrative architecture and the developments of integrative medicine for best practices of both professions. In essence, the combination of these two can become integrative architectural medicine or, said in a more straightforward term, Architectural Medicine.

The key to Architectural Medicine is that it can provide a bridge between these two professions. This can provide integrations between each of these professions to help guide and support these initiatives.

Both of these two professions will require the openness to recognize that there are issues and problems and are also open enough to explore various modalities to achieve better results.

When both of these professions are open enough to embrace and explore these options, the result can allow integration and interconnectivity between these two groups. The result of this integrative, multi-disciplinary focus is Architectural Medicine.

Integrative Medicine and Integrative Architecture require an open-minded approach for best practices in their fields, which, when applied together between architecture and medicine, yields health benefits in the built environment.

So, in moving forward, how can Integrative Architecture be defined?

Taking the lead from the already successful Integrative Medicine processes, perhaps these principles can be redefined with a focus on the field of architecture in the following formats.

The Defining Principles of Integrative Architecture

Integrative Architecture can be defined using the following principles:
- Client and architect/designer are partners in the creation of green, sustainable, and healing environments
- All building factors that influence human, biological, and ecological health are taken into consideration
- Appropriate use of both conventional and alternative methods and materials facilitates green, sustainable, and healthy buildings
- Effective design solutions that are natural and less invasive should be used whenever possible
- Integrative Architecture neither rejects conventional architecture nor accepts alternative building approaches uncritically
- Good architecture is based on good science. It is inquiry-driven and open to new paradigms
- Alongside the concept of design solutions, the broader concepts of green, sustainable, and health promotion for human, biological, and ecological health are paramount
- Architects and designers of Integrative Architecture should exemplify its principles and commit themselves to self-exploration and self-development

Yes, these are the verbatim eight principles of Integrative Medicine reworded to fit the field of architecture. Why start from scratch when many, such as Dr. Weil, have already created a solid path and put into practice years of work to achieve approaches and definitions to guide the way?

Taking this one step further, the definition of Integrative Medicine can also be applied to Integrative Architecture in setting a framework of this approach with similar beneficial goals. As such, the following statement can be referenced:

"Integrative Medicine is healing-oriented medicine that takes account of the whole person (body, mind, and spirit), including all aspects of lifestyle. It emphasizes the therapeutic relationship and makes use of all appropriate therapies, both conventional and alternative."[78]

And applying this to the field of architecture, we may have this wording to work from:

"Integrative Architecture is an energy-efficient, sustainability-focused, health-oriented approach to architecture that considers human, biological, and ecological health, including all aspects of the built environment and lifestyle. It emphasizes the therapeutic relationship between occupant and the built environment and makes use of all appropriate building materials and methods, both conventional and alternative."

In many of Dr. Weil's talks and writings, he has encouraged and has been a proponent and believer of places and spaces that promote wellness. Courses at the Andrew Weil Center for Integrative Medicine, such as Environmental Health,[79] recognize the importance of the natural and built environments as places where healing can be either supported or unsupported. This also provides the recognition that medicine is not just a general Rx modality of drugs or food, but includes your surroundings and all facets of your life and lifestyle.

This includes the built environments that you live and work within. Therefore if you are to achieve this form of optimal health that is advocated, then the architecture that you live and work within must embrace and support this health and wellness as well.

For the past two to three decades, the introduction of Integrative Medicine has been an evolving process. From its origins to the current recognition of this topic as a serious and vital part of medicine – at least many whose interests in providing the best health solutions to patients are pivotal. Integrative Medicine is known as using the wisdom of traditional medicine in combination with modern medicine for best practices.

In this same way, the concept of Integrative Architecture utilizes the wisdom of traditional building materials and methods, along with modern materials and methodologies. This combination is striving for a result of best practices in architecture and building for best biological and ecological health. It is also working to support climate change issues and better environmental stewardship on this planet.

While these best practices are still being defined in many ways, this book's approach and focus on Architectural Medicine strives to support these three fields of healthy building, green building, and sustainable building to merge in defining a better built environment. With more focus on a greener and more energy-efficient building process, and a more sustainable and ecological built environment, the future of buildings will encompass more of these topics over time.

Therefore, how they integrate will be essential to have these solutions work together instead of causing more issues. This concept of Integrative Architecture can be seen as a merging of these three topics and can help integrate the many facets of these approaches into a cohesive whole.

But the reason why Integrative Architecture alone is not a complete system solution is that health in buildings requires the medical fields to become more integrated to provide better health for occupants in the built environment. An emerging focus of social determinants of health, for example, requires that the architecture and medical fields work together.

Therefore, there must be a group of best practices defined for both architecture and medicine to combine in creating built environments in support of health, wellness, and well-being. It will be a process of combining this approach of Integrative Architecture with the benefits of Integrative Medicine for a whole systems solution between the architecture and medical professions.

As an example of this critical overlap, many have become aware of the current interest in decreasing dangerous plastics in products, such as BPA and phthalates, which is often being driven by toxicologists and epidemiologists, not architects and designers. So this is a new age and day where those in medicine are overlapping with the fields of product manufacturing and the building fields, and these emerging interests in health are creating new paths.

And these new paths include the built environment as part of their evaluations of patient health. This is akin to the past, where doctors who provided house calls may have gathered information on the patient's place of living and factored this into their analysis. While some doctors in parts of the world visit people at their homes, this has not been a common practice for many decades, if not a half-century and longer in most parts of the world practicing modern medicine.

The advent of telemedicine can provide a window into a patient's living spaces, yet the inclusion of an evaluation process of their patient's location is still uncommon at this time.

I revisit this topic in the Architectural Medicine System (AMS) in chapter 16 and discuss future processes that can utilize telemedicine to evaluate the built environment later in the book.

So perhaps now, revisiting the concept of a doctor visiting and viewing the patient's built environments to help provide more information and data about building conditions is not so far-fetched.

Introduction to Integrative Architecture

Integrations and the Wisdom of Nature

The previous chapters described an example of the differences between sustainable building and green building. It becomes evident that there can be many examples defined that can open the debate of the differences between the fields.

In the current day, it would take a small encyclopedia to achieve all of these differences and definitions, and I'm not quite sure this would be fair to these fields. I can state that the purpose of this book is not to define or describe each difference, but instead to highlight some of the differences and some of the similarities. In this manner, it can provide a large paintbrush picture of these topics so there can be some overall big picture understandings about these fields.

There are resources on our website that can provide more in-depth details of these different fields. You can visit these resources at this link: https://architecturalmedicine.com/book/

After all, the purpose of this book is to be broad enough for the general public, yet with information to provide details relevant for the professionals. However, it's also important to note that the purpose of doing this is twofold.

One is to give the general public an overview of why they may want to have such solutions. Secondly, to hopefully encourage the general public to demand these changes for healthier built environments for people to live within.

Dr. Andrew Weil once stated that the real reason the medical professionals changed in support of Integrative Medicine was the public's demand.[80]

To be fair, many architecture and medical professionals may not be able to change these on their own, even if they wanted to. These fields are often so highly regulated and controlled and are already tightly configured that it requires outside demand from the public to make sufficient changes.

So, change has to come from both the outside and inside of these professions, which means that the general public must demand such changes. In turn, the architecture and medical fields can then provide a supply to this demand with solutions.

And it is the latter comment where it becomes evident these professionals also need to be aware of these topics. If they are to provide solutions, these topics will need to be defined and delivered accordingly.

This supply and demand will not work with the current building-related processes. There will be a need for new and more updated solutions to be provided, and it will also require these two professions of architecture and

Architectural Medicine – Building the Bridge to Wellness

medicine to work together in ways they never have, at least in recorded history that we know of.

As we go forward on this topic, by visiting the word origins of "integrate," we can build upon why this word can be seen as important and what exactly is meant in the use of this term:

integrate (v.)

1630s, "to render (something) whole, bring together the parts of," from Latin integratus, past participle of integrare "make whole," from integer "whole, complete,"[81]

As can be seen in each of these word origins, the key to this phrasing is to "bring together the parts to make whole." And these "parts" are a significant portion of this book, which is to strive to "bring together" the many facets of the built environment topics – physically, mentally, and emotionally – for health and wellness.

In this way, this integration is bridging these various facets into a cohesive whole. And this interconnectivity can bridge together the many pieces to achieve this goal.

However, to achieve this goal in the material world, there are the topics of both personal health and the concept of global health. As the world becomes smaller and smaller in terms of the impacts we have on the planet, you cannot separate your health from planetary health.

And as I'm finishing up the writing and editing of this book during the time of the coronavirus global pandemic, this topic is even more critical than when I began writing this book many years ago.

And this means that we must factor personal and global health into the architecture equation, along with the components of energy efficiency and sustainability.

The current system of building is in many ways sick, and therefore a new system and model must be created that is focused on wellness.

This includes the well-being of the ecological system that we depend upon for life. When these systems are analyzed, one can find that pollution created inside the house does not allow high performance and functioning for the occupants, just as pollution outside of the house or on the planet does not allow well-being for this system we call nature.

This does not mean that we need to go back in time and live in the way that our ancestors lived. Yet, it does mean that we need to relearn the systems of nature and design and build using the rules of natural systems. This way, we can design to sustain healthy life – generation after generation.

Our current abilities to create technological advancements are a modern-day progression that has served humans well on many levels. Yet, there is also a time when the same technology used for benefit becomes a hindrance to our human progress. If technology is created to live a better, more realized, and beneficial life, then at what point does this very technology hinder our health and well-being from enjoying this better life?

Technology is a tool. It is a human characteristic to want to create, to design, to build, and to solve problems. And while nature is often seen as primitive and lacking sophistication, have you ever considered the complex technology required to design and build a flower? What about a tree?

Is this not advanced technology? Nature is not primitive; nature is the most advanced technology on this planet.

Let me state that again — *Nature is the Most Advanced Technology on this Planet.*

Yes, humans have created and are creating fantastic technology, yet most of this, if not all, was inspired in some way by nature's amazing technological designs. And this includes how nature has solved the many issues that humans are striving to solve.

When contemplating nature's incredible sophistication, from DNA to the colors of a rose, one can begin to see that it is indeed the most advanced technology that exists.

This is not to put humans down nor to be overly critical. It is to create the opposite. It is to inspire what we can create and do so with the great teachings that nature offers, with lessons learned over millions of years, and mind-boggling solutions.

For instance, have you ever looked at a plant or tree from the perspective of how it lives?

Have you ever realized that this incredible creation began with the blueprint in a seed? It then grew to create its power by photosynthesis, converting sunlight into sugars as its energy source, and then builds itself using only the raw materials of soil, sunlight, and water to create itself? Ponder that for a while.

It then perpetuates its design as offspring by creating a very complex flowering seed, which has been designed with fantastic beauty and engineering in its materials and methods.

And then, after it has lived, it returns to the soil where it grew and then decomposes back into the materials required for more plants to grow.

And this cycle can last an infinite amount of times, allowing for the "sustaining" of this species without destroying the surroundings in which it has existed. It has the inherent blueprints to build itself and grow and propagate using the most advanced technological processes known to humans.

Nature is the most advanced technology on the planet, and the systems of nature are the most complex.

Humans can learn much from these systems, and we can choose to change and update our current models of building and living, whether it be the buildings we live and work in, the vehicles that we travel in, the products that we use in our daily lives, or even the clothes that we wear.

All of these materials and methods can be created to work with nature and coexist with the planet we live on and depend upon. It is a system that is very intelligent and very advanced, and the more we recognize and appreciate this, the more we can have reverence and appreciation for this system. This will allow us to respect and learn from nature, like an elderly grandparent who we cherish, care for, and learn from.

Guess what, the grandparent is the planet, and our ancestors' bones are not only particles from distant stars and galaxies, they are also the materials that make up your bones, organs, and skin to create you as an organism.

You are cosmic, in a very practical format.

New systems require a big picture viewpoint with practical nuts and bolts solutions and a connection in between. Einstein searched his whole life to find a relationship between the micro and the macro worlds of physics, and this he called the "unified field theory." That which connects the micro-universe with the macro universe.

Nature has already done this. The answers are there. Find the answers without destroying that which you are exploring, and you will have found the solutions.

While Integrative Architecture encompasses the fields of healthy building, with a focus on physical health, energy efficiency, and sustainable architecture – Architectural Medicine adds physical, emotional, and mental or psychological wellness into the built environment equation.

And now that we've discussed the more physical components of architecture, the following chapters include these other facets in combining the topics of wellness. Including the facets of physical, emotional, and mental or psychological wellness in this equation forms the all-inclusive definition of Architectural Medicine.

To discuss this in more detail, the next three chapters will focus on these facets of wellness relative to the built environment.

And we begin with *Physical Wellness* in the next chapter...

"The good physician treats the disease; the great physician treats the patient who has the disease."

– William Osler

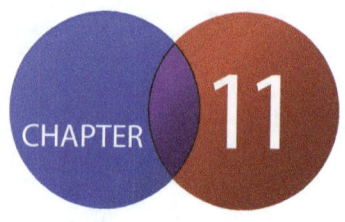

HOW DO BUILDINGS AFFECT PHYSICAL WELLNESS?

In the next few chapters, we will venture into these three facets of *Physical*, *Mental* or *Psychological*, and *Emotional Wellness*. These three topics are critical to creating architecture that supports health and well being, and are as important to Architectural Medicine as green, sustainable, and healthy building.

The topic of *physical wellness* may sound similar to the concepts of *healthy building*, but there are some distinct differences.

Chapter: 11 — How Do Buildings Affect Physical Wellness

In chapter 9 on healthy building, I discussed the issues of disease and illnesses related to the factors in the built environment impacting the physical body. In this chapter and the following chapters on wellness, the focus is on thriving and not just the absence of illness.

Physical Wellness

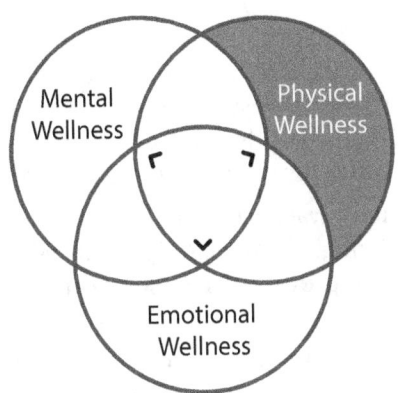

Physical Wellness

Physical Wellness

Are you surrounded by stagnant, polluted air? Are there chemicals and chemical smells in your space all day? Is your body getting enough sunlight? Is your body being cared for and allowing for topics such as ergonomic functionality? Are you around constant stress? What is this impact on your physical wellness and your immune system?

Wellness and health are similar, but not exactly the same. To be clear, these definitions often have overlap depending on the source. Many dictionaries include both health and wellness in similar formats.[82]

Yet, I will refer to "health" as the physical body being free from disease for our discussions.

And I will refer to "wellness" as the focus of well-being and striving towards a life that is not just lacking disease but flourishing.

An interesting part of the definitions of wellness includes "an actively pursued goal."[83] There are also references to wellness as a lifestyle. The National Wellness Institute defines wellness as "multidimensional and holistic, encompassing lifestyle, mental and spiritual well-being, and the environment."[84] Just because you do not have an illness and have good health does not mean that you are thriving, and this is a good reference point to note moving forward.

In the next three chapters discussing physical, mental, and emotional wellness, this concept of thriving in life is critical to factor into the equation. Many topics in healthy building are striving to ensure there are no issues causing illness. This chapter on physical wellness is focused on going beyond the removal of illness to achieve a life of flourishing and a better quality of life.

There are many overlaps, and in many ways, you cannot separate the physical, mental, and emotional state of being. The recognition of these overlaps and a focus on providing solutions can provide synergistic results when considering all components.

What might be interesting for many people to observe on this topic of physical wellness, is how places and spaces impact our physiological health, which is often a new concept.

The idea that a building space can have a physiological impact on our bodies, causing us to experience well-being or biological illness, is quite abstract for many. Yet, these topics have become more common in research in the past few decades, and the findings are fascinating.

This research can go back to the early 1980s to the study by Dr. Ulrich showing that post-surgery hospital patients who had a view of nature healed faster than those whose view was a brick wall.[85] It began the field often referred to as *Evidence-Based Design*.

In the past several decades, the advent of neuroscience has provided insights into the physiological responses to shapes and objects. Objects that are sharp with harder textures and materials have been shown to stimulate the amygdala, promoting stress hormones in the body.[86] And while many people might not be consciously aware that they are under this stress, the body does know.

And so, in this chapter, we begin to recognize that there are physical responses to the designs of the built environment that can support physical calm and relaxation or can cause physiological stress.

Chapter: 11   How Do Buildings Affect Physical Wellness

The Impact of Stress on Human Health

60% to 80% of primary care doctor visits are related to stress
– JAMA Intern Med. 2013;173(1):76-77

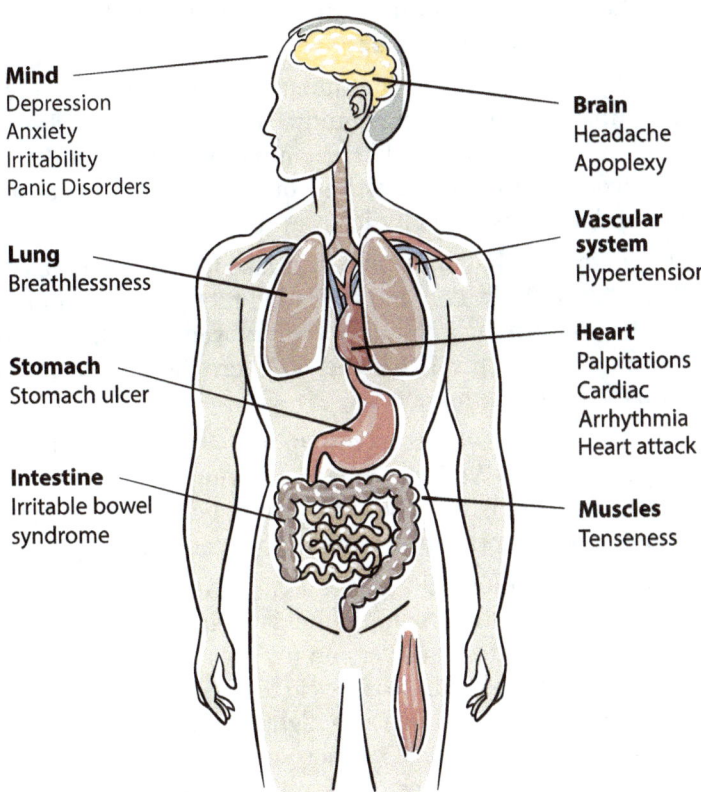

With all that I discussed in the previous chapter about physical health, we can review those topics and discuss a few more items that should be included in this realm.

To begin with, one of the interesting factors on the physical health spectrum is that, at least currently, very few doctors or health professionals consider the built environment in evaluating their patient's health. While healthy building professionals have become more focused on material selections that reduce the negative impacts on health and strive to design solutions that support better health, the medical fields are often not involved with these topics and issues.

And so we'll talk about a few issues that are based on physical health in buildings. I will also talk about the lack of interconnections between these two fields.

Let's begin with some common building issues that many might be familiar with. And that is the issues with lead paint, asbestos, mold, and in general, bad air quality in homes and buildings.

In the 1970s, the issues of lead became a large topic because of the medical research showing a decline in cognitive abilities from children exposed to lead ingestion.[87] It doesn't help that lead has a sweet taste, and as we know from history, lead in drinking water and other sources of ingestion led to many stories of sicknesses both physically and mentally.[88][89]

Many forget that, at that time, there was also lead in gasoline, as the options in those days were leaded and unleaded fuel. And so lead paint, lead in fuels, and lead in products began to be removed over the next decades. Around the same time of the 1970s and 80s were the issues of asbestos in buildings and the abatement process.

This was particularly evident in my upbringing from childhood to my young adult experiences. While in college studying architecture in the late 80s, when I asked my professors about options to learn about ecological and healthy building, I was referred to an asbestos abatement and planning class.

Of course, this was not what I meant at all in terms of my interest, yet it was this lack of common thought in the fields of architecture and construction that led me to seek these answers on my own. However, I still took the course and learned a lot about these issues in terms of the asbestos inspection and abatement process. This course also highlighted the actual health issues of asbestosis and the physiological impacts on the body. Perhaps this could be seen as one of the first courses I took related to Architectural Medicine, and as such, it served as an introduction to the health issues and these types of impacts on human biological systems.

Air quality and mold issues became popular building health topics in the 1990s, and mold abatement started as a small procedure and eventually led to very large companies requiring proper abatement. What many don't realize is that these mold issues have substantial impacts on both the occupant's health, yet also the structural health of the building. The increase in water infiltration over time can break down many building materials, so it is not just a health issue, it's also a structural integrity issue.

Indoor air quality is also a high priority for good health, and there are many buildings in the US and worldwide with forced heating that can often create indoor air quality issues. This is because the filters that many people are familiar with replacing in their heating units are not meant for human health. They are there to protect the machinery of the heating, ventilation, and air conditioning (HVAC) systems. This can bring up many questions about these forced air systems and why there are not better filtration standards for human health.

Environmental Health and Environmental Medicine

Environmental Medicine, Integrative Medicine, and Architectural Medicine...what are the differences and why have different names for each?

When I first began this project, I thought about the issues of creating another name for topics that already had several different names and a history of developments in building health.

Yet each time I worked on these concepts to define them in cohesive terms, both the words "Architecture" and "Medicine" included a centric view of whole person health. It also had the big picture view of the many facets and fields involved in the built environment. When viewing the many facets of human health and wellness, as well as how the human being is impacted and influenced by the built environment – physically, mentally, and emotionally, I kept coming back to the two words "Architecture" and "Medicine" as ways to define and discuss this large group of topics.

I should make it very clear that Architectural Medicine does not intend to make things more confusing and unnecessarily complicated, as these subjects are already extremely complex.

The real reason I've used this name is that in my experience and concerns for a wide range of topics related to health and the built environment, Architectural Medicine is at the core of these two topics and serves as an umbrella in discussing the many other fields involved.

As Integrative Medicine has become more common in certain parts of the world, providing a more "healing-oriented medicine taking account of the whole person"[90] is inherently more open to include the built environment in terms of health. Because the process is informed by evidence and uses all appropriate therapies, it can include topics such as social determinants of health when evaluating health factors.

However, in chapter 10, discussing Integrative Architecture, I addressed the issue that Integrative Medicine does not currently have the connections between the building fields to properly evaluate and include the built environment into their patient's health equation. And so Architectural Medicine strives to help bridge these gaps between these fields to highlight and support the great work that has already been developed.

Some of these other fields that can be included in evaluating environmental impacts related to physical health and wellness are Environmental Medicine and Environmental Health.

Environmental Medicine is defined by The American Academy of Environmental Medicine (AAEM) as the following:

"Environmental Medicine is concerned with the interaction between mankind and the environment. More specifically, Environmental Medicine involves the adverse reactions experienced by an individual on exposure to an environmental excitant. Excitants to which individual susceptibility exists are found in air, food, water, and drugs, and are frequently found in the home, work, school, and play environments."[91]

The topics of Environmental Medicine and Environmental Health are defined by the World Health Organization (WHO) as a field of study that "addresses all the physical, chemical, and biological factors external to a person, and all the related factors impacting behaviors. It encompasses the assessment and control of those environmental factors that can potentially affect health. It is targeted towards preventing disease and creating health-supportive environments. This definition excludes behavior not related to environment, as well as behavior related to the social and cultural environment, and genetics."[92]

A goal of the WHO in terms of Environmental Health is towards "preventing disease and creating health-supportive environments."[93]

The Andrew Weil Center for Integrative Medicine at The University of Arizona offers a course for personal and professional education on the topics of Environmental Health. The course describes Environmental Health as "a broad, complex, rapidly evolving field of medicine. It is not necessarily a new type of medicine, but is new to many health care providers, and practitioners may be pushed out of their comfort zones when incorporating environmental medicine into their work."[94]

The course helps to educate professionals and strives to help the healthcare professional be more informed on environmental impacts on health and to "raise awareness about diseases related to environmental toxicants in patient population."[95]

This focus is terrific and increases awareness and action for doctors and health professionals in dealing with diseases.

Architectural Medicine and Environmental Health

The challenge for someone like myself in using environmental medicine and health to define the many facets in this book as a field is that these other fields don't always encompass the psychological and emotional characteristics of how the built environment impacts human health.

The field of Healthy Building has had a huge positive impact on the promotion and awareness of health and the built environment. Yet if one were to bring into the equation the topics of Environmental Medicine and Architectural Phenomenology, as merely two examples, then it can get tricky to determine where exactly this might fit into the discussions of Healthy Building. We will discuss the topic of Architectural Phenomenology in the next chapter.

As someone who has been directly involved with Healthy Building, I felt that the scope is often focused on topics related to decreasing toxicants and contaminants from the built environment. As much as this is critical, I didn't always feel that it addressed emotional well-being and the design topics of shapes and forms relative to the whole experience of architecture.

Organizations such as the Healthy Building Network and the Institute of Bau Biologie (IBN) in Germany have been great leaders in the fields of environmental health, toxicology, and building material safety for human health. So this is also not meant at all to state a lack of focus on these topics.

In fact, I would state the opposite, in that a major purpose of Architectural Medicine is to highlight these fields and the work they have done and are doing. And to this end, there are many fields and many people who are doing tremendous work related to health in the built environment.

Architectural Medicine is focused on the foundation of this work, yet also striving to be inclusive and help support these interconnections as a multi-disciplinary approach that can be a powerfully beneficial team effort when working together.

Integrative Medicine, Biophilia, and Fields Focused on Physical Wellness

The Architectural Medicine website has a list of fields that relate to health and the built environment, from topics such as Environmental Medicine, Evidence-Based Design, and Medical Sociology to Environmental Psychology, Neuroscience in Architecture, Biophilic Design, and Salutogenesis.

The latter terms Biophilic Design or Biophilia and Salutogenesis are good examples of how there are many different fields that are focused on this beneficial viewpoint of architecture and the built environment supporting wellness.

The term "biophilia" means "love of life or living systems."[96] It was first used by Erich Fromm to describe a psychological orientation of being attracted to all that is alive and vital. The biophilia hypothesis, also called BET, suggests that "humans possess an innate tendency to seek connections with nature and other forms of life."[97]

Edward O. Wilson popularized this in his book, *Biophilia*, where he defines this as "the urge to affiliate with other forms of life."[98] Wilson uses the term in the same sense when he suggests that biophilia describes "the connections that human beings subconsciously seek with the rest of life."[99]

And another topic related to how humans connect or relate to their natural and built environments is Salutogenesis. This term was coined by the professor of medical sociology Aaron Antonovsky.[100] It describes an approach focusing on factors that support human health and well being, rather than on factors that cause disease. More specifically, the "salutogenic model" is "concerned with the relationship between health, stress, and coping."[101]

In terms of stress, this becomes particularly interesting when considering the latest neuroscience findings related to architecture, mainly that angular and sharp shapes can cause increased activity in the amygdala. This, in turn, causes fear and an increase in stress levels.[102] Whether recognized consciously or simply an underlying physiological constant, this increase in stress can cause the reverse of salutogenesis and a general lack of ease. The term salutogenesis is better defined in contrast to pathogenesis and disease.

Antonovsky's theories reject the "traditional medical-model dichotomy separating health and illness." He described the relationship as a continuous variable, which he described as the "health-ease versus dis-ease continuum."[103]

In just a few different selections of these professions and fields, you might see one focused on a specific nuance, and another group that seems to have similar viewpoints yet may have a different approach.

What might be important to recognize is that some of these fields, such as healthy building, are striving to remove pollutants and toxicants from the building. In contrast, others, such as Biophilia, are focused on providing experiences of well being, and connecting to nature for physical wellness. Each has its strengths and positives, which is vital to recognize when it comes to integrations between professions.

So as to not make things more complex or having to decide specifically on one field or another, the term "Architectural Medicine" came to be.

My viewpoint on Architectural Medicine is that using the core words of each of these big fields, it sets both a foundation of a model and an umbrella to connect and highlight the many other fields that work towards the goals of health and wellness.

It is this reason why I use the motto of "Building the Bridge to Wellness" as part of the mantra in building bridges between various modalities, fields, and facets of life into a hopeful cohesive whole. This can result in wholeness in the built environment for each person for better health, healing, and wellness. As mentioned in a previous chapter, the term "heal" has its word origins as:

"restoration to health," Old English hæling, verbal noun from heal (v.). Figurative sense of "restoration of wholeness"[104]

And this work is to help integrate and connect many of these fields and topics, in realizing that while you cannot separate health from the built environment, you also cannot separate the many people who create the fabric of society in achieving these goals.

In mentioning healthy building, a few examples that differentiate healthy building from physical wellness consist of designs that increase natural light, decrease noises, and provide improvements of ergonomic functionality of chairs, desks, and other objects in the building.

These design strategies focus less on removing the negatives and harmful toxins and focus more on the improvements that can be made for better well being and quality of life – especially physical wellness.

In the long run, these design efficiencies can better support health by reducing stressors, and therefore decrease the potential chances for adverse health impacts.

Both architects and doctors play a massive role in working together to achieve better health in the built environment. And of course, these are just two professions out of a large and growing group of professionals that can work together to achieve a better outcome for wellness in the world.

As the world continues to become increasingly complex, the many facets of professionals involved must work together if solutions are to be created that solve one problem, yet don't create more problems in this process.

And this becomes even more important to recognize as population health becomes more focused on going beyond survival and striving to thrive. This wellness and quality of life may not be an exact science, yet there are science-based facets in life that can support better health.

And it is this mindset that can transcend survival through architecture and medicine in all facets of human life. The physiological benefits of connecting to nature, improving designs to soothe the senses, and improving designs that support physical wellness can provide synergistic benefits when combined with mental and emotional well being.

And this brings us to the next chapter discussing *Mental* or *Psychological Wellness*...

"We shape our buildings; thereafter they shape us."

– Winston Churchill

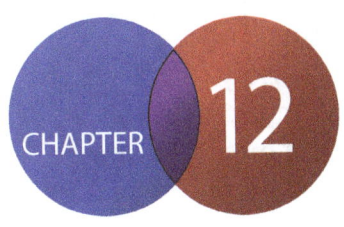

HOW DO BUILDINGS AFFECT MENTAL WELLNESS?

Have you ever tried to focus on your studies, your work, or topics you are striving to understand, and the environment you are in is causing it difficult to concentrate? Perhaps there are loud sounds, or the room you're in has busy patterns and bright colors, and all of this is distracting.

While these scenarios in the built environments and spaces you are in may impact your experiences in a physical and physiological format, via sight, sounds, smell, touch and even taste, the resulting impact prevents your ability to stay focused and maintain concentration.

Mental Wellness

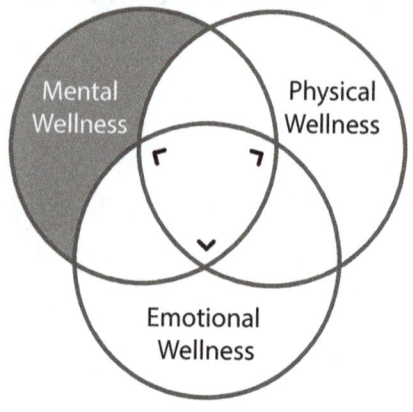

Mental Wellness

Mental Wellness

Do you have the ability to think clearly?
Is the space you're in comforting for your mind or chaotic in sights, sounds, and thinking as well as sensory stress? How does this affect your mindset? What impact does this have on your ability to concentrate, on your mental wellness and on your immune system?

And this is where buildings can impact how you are thinking and feeling. The shapes and the textures of your surroundings can have a positive or a negative impact on your well-being, such as your capacity to stay focused or to concentrate on topics that require your cognitive functions to work at a high level.

This can provide a difference between cognitive functions in either a survival mode or a thriving mode.

Clarity of Thought and the Ability to Concentrate

Buildings and rooms that have busy patterns, loud sounds, undesirable smells, and excessively bright colors, textures, and shapes can create a disruption in focus. While your response to such scenarios can be healthy to ensure that you are aware of potentially dangerous or disadvantageous scenarios to navigate, it does mean that your mind is focusing on something other than your main interest.

There are reasons why there are quiet rooms in libraries at universities and why libraries are places that respect this quiet. The connection between these locations that are quiet to allow you to think clearly is not a mistake. Oftentimes, people chose to work in places that are quieter so they can be more relaxed and removed from outside distractions. This can enhance the capacity to have such cognitive capabilities during times of learning or focused work.

And places that promote contemplation also offer these quiet zones, where your mind can focus on specific topics instead of being distracted by sounds, smells, and designs that reduce your ability to stay focused. The mindfulness movement developing over the past several decades has promoted this time of focus and contemplation. Often, these events are done in quiet rooms, with fewer distractions in the room itself.

Of course, these experiences can be subjective, and some thrive in quiet environments, while others may not find this ideal for their concentration. Yet physiologically, the reduction of exterior stimulus can provide less stress and allow for an ideal environment in which to remain focused.

Architectural Phenomenology & Environmental Psychology

The fields of Architectural Phenomenology and Environmental Psychology are two such examples that study these capabilities that better understand how humans are impacted by the spaces and places that they spend time within.

Architectural Phenomenology can be defined in one way as, "the environment defined as 'the place,' it is this atmosphere which allows certain spaces, with similar or even identical functions, to embody very different properties, in accord with the unique cultural and environmental conditions of the place which they exist."[105]

The architect Juhani Pallasmaa in his book *The Eyes of the Skin*, provides more in-depth discussions on these architectural experiences. He brings attention to the idea that buildings are more than just the visual experience, and great architectural spaces include all five senses in these experiences. This concept can provide "multi-sensory architecture which facilitates a sense of belonging and integration."[106]

While Pallasmaa's work can be classified as phenomenology, it's perhaps more important to recognize the fact that the experiential connection that one has with architecture can be a profound and vital part of human life.

With Architectural Phenomenology's focus on an experiential perspective, the sensory and experiential connection is related more to the personal experience of architecture on the individual in a subjective manner. This contrasts with the more common evaluation of architecture based on a more intellectual "form and function" approach. As such, a focus on the sensory experience can provide a more human approach to the designs of the built environment.

This can become particularly important for wellness, as this can often be defined in terms of sensory experiences. And while the experience of spaces and places through the senses can be defined as a physical aspect, the idea that these topics are all-inclusive in the emotional, mental, and physiological experience can better explain these as an interconnected, nodal experience.

If the term *nodal* is abstract relative to "hierarchical" developments, this differentiation is discussed in more detail in chapter 15 in the section "the tree analogy – from silos to nodal integrators".

Another field that researches the impacts of the exterior world on mental well being is that of Environmental Psychology. This is defined as "an interdisciplinary field that focuses on the interplay between individuals and their surroundings."[107]

This becomes particularly interesting to include psychology in exploring environment-behavior studies into the mesh of the architectural experience. This perspective on human behavior and the impacts of natural and built environments, can provide deeper insights into human health and quality of life. These evaluations that the built environment has on human behavior "examines the way in which the natural environment and our built environments shape us as individuals."[108]

The field defines the term environment broadly, encompassing natural environments, social settings, built environments, learning environments, and informational environments.

Dr. Daniel Stokols at the University of California at Irvine provided an online course open to the public in 2012 that is still accessible and a valuable overview of this subject.[109]

Both of these topics of Architectural Phenomenology and Environmental Psychology show how the tenets of healthy building might not include these other facets of life beyond physical health. To include the complexities of design in terms of mental health, it better describes the relevance to Architectural Medicine as a multi-faceted spectrum of fields in a cohesive format for well being.

Neuroscience and Buildings – NeuroArchitecture

Neuroscience in Architecture or NeuroArchitecture, is a relatively recent development in neuroscience that studies the physiological responses to spaces and places.

The book *Mind in Architecture*, by Sarah Robinson, which includes the above-mentioned architect Juhani Pallasmaa, highlights the work of neuroscientists and architects in how the built environment "affects behavior, thoughts, emotions, and well-being."[110]

While the amount of time spent indoors by the average person is increasing, with up to ninety percent of life spent inside buildings, the book goes on to state that "we understand very little about how the built environment affects our behavior, thoughts, emotions, and well-being."[111]

The authors state that "it stands to reason that research in the life sciences, particularly neuroscience, can offer compelling insights into the ways our buildings shape our interactions with the world."[112]

In the neuroscience research paper titled "Visual elements of subjective preference modulate amygdala activation," Moshe Bar and Maital Neta summarize their research by concluding that "people generally like objects with a curved contour compared with objects that have pointed features and a sharp-angled contour. Using human neuroimaging to test this hypothesis, we report that the amygdala, a brain structure that is involved in fear processing and has been shown to exhibit activation level that is proportional to arousal in general, is significantly more active for everyday sharp objects (e.g., a sofa with sharp corners) compared with their curved contour counterparts."[113]

Their research indicated a "preference bias towards a visual object can be induced by low-level perceptual properties, independent of semantic meaning, via visual elements that on some level could be associated with threat."

This low-level threat can elevate stress levels, thereby causing long-term stressors that many may not even be aware of due to their physiological reactions to such design objects.

Their research shows the behavioral results to "provide initial support for the link between the sharpness of the contour and threat perception. Our brains might be organized to extract these basic contour elements rapidly for deriving an early warning signal in the presence of potential danger." [114]

Certain shapes and designs, such as the curving forms in parametric architecture, can provide a less stressful response for those experiencing these designs, especially over time. This topic of parametric architecture is discussed in chapter 13, with an in-depth discussion in chapter 19.

In her book *Welcome to Your World: How the Built Environment Shapes Our Lives*, Sarah Williams Goldhagen discusses recent research in "cognitive neuroscience and psychology to demonstrate how people's experiences of the places they build are central to their well-being."[115] This wellness can stem from the community and social life, as she states, "the world needs better-designed, healthier environments that address the complex range of human individual and social needs."[116]

Evidence Based Design and Social Determinants of Health – (SDoH)

As mentioned previously, Evidence-Based Design is another important facet in the design world focused on science and the benefits that designs can have on health. Starting with Dr. Ulrich's study in the 1980s showing the benefits of viewing nature to speed up healing, this study is often seen as the origins of these scientific evaluations, which today supports design decisions in hospitals across the world for healthier hospital outcomes.

The World Health Organization (WHO) defines the social determinants of health as "the conditions in which people are born, grow, live, work and age."[117] The Centers for Disease Control and Prevention (CDC) include in their definition the "aspects of the social environment, the physical environment (e.g., place of residence, crowding conditions, built environment [i.e., buildings, spaces, transportation systems, and products that are created or modified by people]), and health services."[118]

This connection between the built environment and wellness can be seen in the places and spaces where people live and work, and the group Healthy People 2030 organizes the social determinants of health around five key domains: " Economic Stability, Education, Health and Health Care, Neighborhood and Built Environment, and Social and Community Context."[119]

An essential facet of this definition is in reference to the built environment. This includes the social experience of architecture. Whether or not someone is surviving or thriving can often be connected to the built environments that they live, work in, and spend most of their time in and around.

The power of architecture and the ability for buildings to either enhance human existence for thriving or to prevent this development and leave people in survival mode, can make a significant difference in the lives of millions and even billions of people.

This impact on mental wellness can be extremely important for many, and ensuring that designs can support this well being and quality of life is essential. In this manner, the importance of architecture should not be reduced to simple aesthetic grandiosity. Instead, it can uplift the spirit for good mental health in both practical and esoteric ways.

And a key factor to Architectural Medicine is striving to take these important ideas, concepts, and theories and apply them in practical formats. After all, if these individual organizations are not implementing these processes into the common day workflow of doctors, architects, and many other building and health professions, then the benefits of this research cannot provide positive societal change.

Epigenetics and the Built Environment

And speaking of change and the positives of societal change, one of the more interesting developments over the past few decades has been the topics of Genomics and Epigenetics.

According to the National Human Genome Research Institute (NHGRI) at the National Institutes of Health (NIH) in the US, Genomics is the "study of all of a person's genes (the genome), including interactions of those genes with each other and with the person's environment."[120]

Since the discoveries of DNA and the double helix designs from the mid-1800s into the 1950s, nature versus nurture questions were mostly philosophical, with little scientific evidence to provide any details on this question. While many recognize Watson and Crick for discovering the helical nature of DNA[121], there had been a long string of events that had led to this knowledge. And as such, the ongoing research since that time has provided an even deeper understanding of these fascinating insights of biology and life.

In the 1990s, the topic of epigenetics became more common, with a more defined description provided at an epigenetic conference in 2008.[122] Over the past thirty years, this topic has become critical in these questions of nature or nurture – what impacts do life experiences have on a person's life?

The Centers for Disease Control and Prevention (CDC) defines Epigenetics as "the study of how your behaviors and environment can cause changes that affect the way your genes work."[123]

In essence, it studies how certain environments and lifestyles can turn genes on or off. And of particular interest is that epigenetics defines this process as changeable. Where genomics is the DNA that you were born with, epigenetics is the process of specific genes turning on or off, impacting one's health in many different realms.

When applied to topics of the social determinants of health (SDoH), as an example, it can show potential for changes in one's life towards the positive, as opposed to viewing many challenges people have in life as being set in stone.

This direct correlation between one's environment and epigenetics can have an impact on human physiology. Whether it is the natural environment or the built environment, these can profoundly affect human health and long-term effects on life quality.

With many people suffering from depression and other mental and emotional challenges in their lives, evaluating their environments, either built or natural, can provide potential solutions to help them towards healing and wellness.

Even if people have been struggling with epigenetic changes from a young age onward, if the causes are based on epigenetic alterations of their DNA, then there is hope that these issues can be resolved when providing healthier environments and lifestyles.

And this brings us directly to the topic of this chapter as to how buildings affect mental wellness. While wellness is a multi-faceted and complex topic, there is a hopefulness that the examples of epigenetics, social determinants of health, and neuroarchitecture can all be included in design decisions that can support well being.

This topic also applies to the previous chapter on physical wellness and the next chapter on emotional wellness. There is an overlap between physical, mental, and emotional wellness that, in many ways, cannot be separated. Due to behavior being closely related to mental well being, I chose to discuss epigenetics in this chapter. Yet, upon further research, this subject can span all of the facets of human wellness.

There are still many questions on epigenetics and genomics and how this new knowledge can be applied in a constructive format. With insights into behavior through neuroscience and evidence-based design, the future of understanding how the built environment impacts human health can provide more wisdom to apply to designs of the future.

As research into the topics in this chapter provides more insights into how environments impact health and wellness, this knowledge can inform future architects and designers to build for better health.

It can also offer psychologists and doctors more insights into what might be at the core of a patient's ailments. It can then allow these professionals to include their patients' buildings that they work and live in as potential sources of disorders.

However, for these to become beneficial processes, there needs to be better systems and integrations to enable these professions and professionals to work together to achieve such goals. We will discuss some possible solutions to this situation in chapters 14 and 16, yet right now, we'll continue these discussions on wellness.

As mentioned, this topic of wellness includes emotional illness or wellness, and this discussion continues in the next chapter focused on *Emotional Wellness*...

"Well-being is not just a mere pleasurable sensation. It is a deep sense of serenity and fulfillment. A state that actually pervades and underlies all emotional states."

– Matthieu Ricard

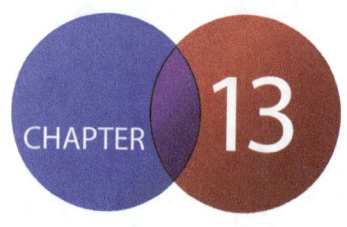

HOW DO BUILDINGS AFFECT EMOTIONAL WELLNESS?

In this chapter, as the built environment's emotional impact is discussed, it's important to acknowledge this as subjective and challenging to define. Different people indeed have different experiences in the buildings where they live and work.

This is where the progress in neuroscience is helping to provide a window into the physiological impacts of these experiences.

Emotional Wellness

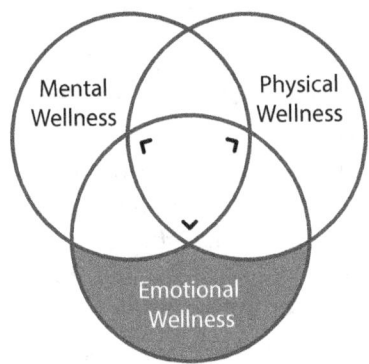

Emotional Wellness

Emotional Wellness

Are you surrounded by loud noises and a chaotic emotional environment? How does this affect your nervous system? Are the sights, sounds, smells, and sensory inputs impacting your emotional wellness? What impact does this have on your stress levels, your emotional wellness, and on your immune system?

This can be particularly interesting when discussing the quality of life and the current popularity of wellness movements. In the previous chapter discussing mental wellness, there were many overlaps between mental and emotional wellness that can be observed.

There can be arguments that a vital learning process in the 21st century is to comprehend the interconnectivity between the many facets of life and cause-effect relationships. And indeed, I propose this to be an important realization. As Matthieu Ricard states, "well-being is not just a mere pleasurable sensation. It is a deep sense of serenity and fulfillment. A state that actually pervades and underlies all emotional states."[124]

While a deep sense of serenity and fulfillment is created differently for each person, perhaps this is an excellent example of how the built environment can affect overall wellness. And in viewing the complete picture of designs, recognizing the overlap and interconnectivity between the physical, mental, and emotional responses might become more notable.

In the previous chapter, we discussed how the built environment could impact your senses and affect your ability to concentrate. And this included a sense of relaxation to thrive, as opposed to being affected negatively, which triggers a more survival-based experience.

And this survival or thriving response has a significant impact on your nervous system, which in turn can impact your emotional well being.

If you are in an environment where your brain center or your amygdala is triggered in response to the discomfort of loud noises, upsetting visuals, smells, or other negative sensory scenarios, it can create underlying stress. As a stress response, the body reacts to fear in either fight, flight, or freeze modes. Many do not realize that the stress impact of small stressors can actually impact your physiology in similar manners as large stressors.

And if you are in an environment with continuous stressors, the impact on your nervous system can increase stress hormones and reduce a sense of relaxation.

This becomes particularly challenging over time, where your body responding to constant stressors can add to major health issues in the long term.

And this becomes relevant in the built environment, especially when there are designs that you are not necessarily aware of or are not paying attention to how you are responding to such impacts.

While a certain amount of stress can actually be positive in life, the experience of daily stressors, such as those incurred by the environments that you work and live within, can build up over time and cause long-term health problems.

As stress is often cited as the number one contributing factor related to death in the modern world,[125] it should be a high priority on the list to pay attention to if wellness and quality of life are meaningful values.

From Pathogenesis to Salutogenesis: The Salutogenic Model

Salutogenesis is a word coined by the medical sociologist Aaron Antonovsky, who stated that the "salutogenic model" is concerned with the relationship between health, stress, and coping.[126]

Antonovsky was more focused on factors to support human health rather than focusing on pathogenesis – the mechanism that leads to a diseased state. Hence the word "salutogenesis" from the latin word origin salus – from salùt-, salùs "safety, well-being, health."[127] In his 1979 book *Health, Stress and Coping*, he discussed the issues of a "health-ease versus dis-ease continuum." This focus on health generation, as opposed to disease generation, has steadily become a profound mindset change in the US over the past few decades.

In his book *Salutogenic Architecture in Healthcare Settings*, Dr. Jan Golembiewski states, "architecture can be psychologically manipulative, for better or for worse. Architecture does this by providing a narrative context that affects a person's behaviour, neural and endocrine systems, and through its influence on the brain and the body, architecture can directly influence health."[128]

This is a powerful statement, and other fields, such as the neuroscience of architecture research, are also showing the physiological impacts of architecture on mental, emotional, and physical health. Golembiewski goes on to state that "Antonovsky's salutogenic theory provides an accessible overarching logic for determining these effects in design."[129]

This topic of salutogenesis, along with evidence-based design, leads to questions of how to create designs and environments to support better health. And in the next section, we briefly discuss this topic and discuss more details in chapter 19.

Evidence-Based Design and Emotional Well-Being

With a focus on exercise and diet to yoga and meditation activities, many have become more interested in these modalities to improve wellness. This has correlated in the medical fields with Integrative Medicine and has gone from an abstract and alternative field to a more fully comprehensive view on health and medicine.

The design world has started to embrace more of this mindset, yet it has been a slower process. An example of this is Dr. Roger S. Ulrich's study, referenced in earlier chapters from the early 1980s with the now famous research "view through a window may influence recovery from surgery".[130]

This study by Dr. Ulrich began a design movement focusing on the positive impacts that the built environment and views of nature can have on health and healing.

It is commonly referred to today as Evidence-Based Design.

In both of these movements, Salutogenesis and Evidence-Based Design, there is a health-focused viewpoint instead of a pathogenesis viewpoint. And this process can create a positive design approach towards supporting health and well being, as opposed to focusing on the disease.

Perhaps these new design approaches can be viewed as more preventive approaches to illness as a pro-active process for better wellness.

Epigenetics and Emotional Well Being

Design topics can always be subjective, as each person responds to shapes, forms, colors, textures, sounds, and lighting in many different formats.

However, the inclusion of neuroscience in understanding the physiological responses to these shapes and forms as architecture can also be added to another facet in how humans respond to the exterior world. And that includes the recent science of epigenetics.

As discussed in the previous chapter, the topic of Epigenetics is a fairly new field, and as such, is still providing insights as potential solutions when talking about overall wellness. Yet, the topics of mental and emotional well being can have profound results with this new knowledge. The knowledge that a change in behaviors can be impacted by one's environments, for better or worse, can provide new possibilities for health.

These discoveries show that certain genes can be turned on and off, resulting in different physiological responses. And another important factor in these equations for health is based on stress. I discussed earlier that neuroscience studies have shown that particular objects that are sharp or objects of harder materials can induce a stress response to the brain center. This produces a fear response, where the amygdala is stimulated, and the fight, flight, or freeze response is triggered. As studies have shown in these stress responses, there is no difference physiologically to how the body responds to a minor stressor or a significant stressor. It is stressful either way, and during these exposures to stressors, stress hormones are released into the body.

So over time, these small stressors can add up in the health equation, even if the person is not fully aware of the stress. Perhaps the person has become used to the stress, and they consciously ignore this. Yet, the stress response and the chemical cascade that ensues still exists.

While stress is not always negative, to have enduring, continuous stressors in one's life based on the objects, shapes, and forms that one lives around and within adds unnecessary suffering with significant impacts on health.

Over time, this can also have a major impact on quality of life.

The potential for lifestyle changes and environmental changes to help make significant health improvements should be good news in a world that isn't often so positive. In places where social determinants of health have substantial negative impacts on wellness, the recognition of design and architecture as a salve for better health should be enough to pay attention to these developments.

Parametric, Curving Architecture and Wellness

There is a type of design that is often labeled parametric design in architecture. Although some may use other terms such as curvilinear, organic, and other adjectives, many of these terms are referencing the same type of designs.

The essence of these design styles is that the shapes and forms are curving. Over the past centuries, architectural styles have been many, yet most designs have had a standard set of principles at the foundation or core of these forms. And this common thread of design standard has been shapes and forms as rectilinear shapes, or basically a box-type design.

Excepting the pyramids and dome-shaped buildings worldwide, most architecture has similar characteristics that most people expect when purchasing a house or experiencing a building. The walls are flat or planar in form, meaning they are identical to the sides of boxes as flat walls – ninety degrees from the floor to the ceilings. These walls are also typically ninety degrees when connecting to other walls, with a flat roof, like a box top, or having two or more angled flat panels that merge at a certain angle, as in the ubiquitous gable roof.

Obviously, there are many variations of these shapes and roof angles, yet the typical house or building around the world is in the form of these box-like shapes.

In the past three decades, architecture has literally taken another shape – that of parametric design. In chapter 19, we'll get into more details about these designs and why they have deeper meanings. Yet, for now, these curving shapes and forms can open up the discussion to different designs that can support health.

As discussed previously, the latest research in neuroscience shows that sharp objects and materials with more rigid characteristics can trigger the amygdala, thereby increasing stress levels and causing more fear. With this new information, the benefit of this knowledge is that shapes and forms that are more curving and less sharp have the potential to create less stress. This, combined with materials that have softer characteristics, can create built environments that can support better wellness.

When views of nature are added and designs that are more curving and less harsh with less sharp angles, there is the opportunity for the body to be less reactive and, therefore, under less stress.

Over time, these designs can provide more uplifting architectural experiences that support better physiological health. The results can lead to less emotional stress and provide better overall health.

Perhaps after reading these chapters, the concept of a building impacting one's physical, mental, and emotional wellness can be more tangible.

Whether spaces and places are directly and consciously experienced or indirectly impacting a person in the periphery, natural and built environments can profoundly change human lives.

The many fields supporting solutions for emotional wellness continue to work towards these beneficial goals. There have been exciting developments in the past several decades on this topic of emotional health supported by the fields of environmental psychology, neuroscience of architecture, evidence-based design, and architectural phenomenology, to name a few.

The broader scope of wellness connected to the fields of public health, epidemiology, and even sociology has been slowly providing more data about the physiological health impacts of environments. And the topic of social determinants of health is beginning to include the effects that different settings can have on mental and emotional states. As well, insights into the beneficial facets of design that can nurture and support good health are being discussed in more mainstream design platforms.

Designers have been creating nurturing spaces for eons. Yet, it has only been in the previous 20th century that technological developments have availed this level of focus beyond survival towards emotional wellness and thriving on a larger scale.

This, of course, varies significantly worldwide from location to location, as there is still a considerable level of economic and technological differences on the planet in achieving these building goals.

With a better sense of the numerous building puzzle pieces that need to be navigated in providing cohesive solutions, it's a good place for us to discuss how they all fit together. And this is exactly what we delve into in the next chapter...

> "An investment in knowledge pays the best interest."
>
> – Benjamin Franklin

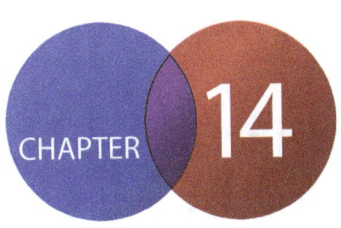

ARCHITECTURAL MEDICINE – PART 2

HOW DO ALL OF THESE TOPICS FIT TOGETHER?

Now that we've outlined the many building puzzle pieces, in this chapter, we'll talk about how all of these pieces can be put together for cohesive solutions.

In the previous chapters, I discussed two triads of the building puzzle. These pieces are green, sustainable, and healthy building, which are listed in the diagram below as Energy, Ecology, and Health, respectively.

And then, I discussed the triad of Physical, Emotional, and Mental or Psychological Wellness.

The Intersection of Energy, Ecology, and Health in the Built Environment

Health

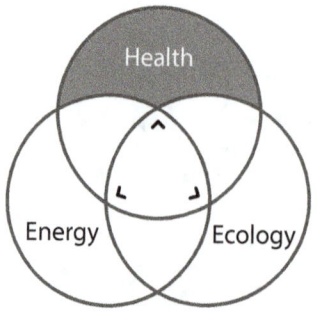

Health/**Healthy Building**

Energy

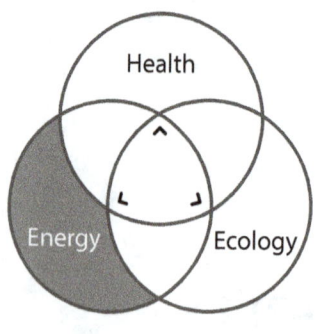

Energy (Efficiency)/**Green Building**

Ecology

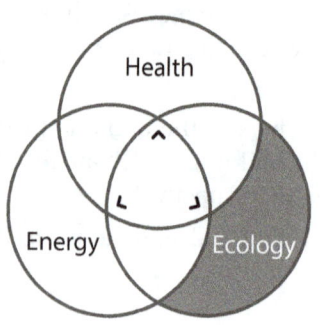

Ecology/**Sustainable Architecture-Building**

The Intersection of Mental, Physical, and Emotional Wellness in the Built Environment

Physical Wellness

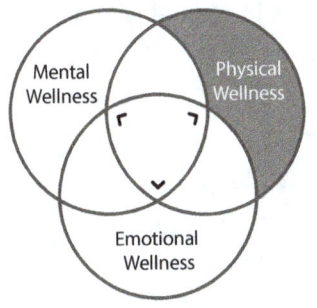

Physical Wellness

Mental Wellness

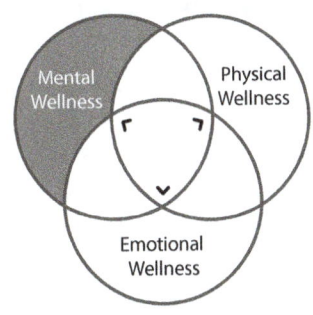

Mental Wellness

Emotional Wellness

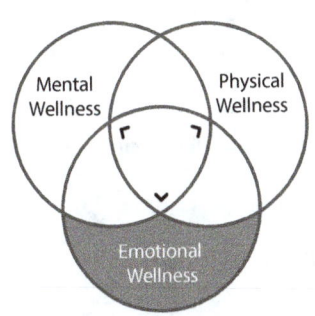

Emotional Wellness

Architectural Medicine – Building the Bridge to Wellness

The double triad of "Energy, Ecology, and Health" and "Mental, Physical, and Emotional Wellness" are interconnected to support the vitality of human thriving. This is what can define a strong foundation of a building – rooted in recognition of having Ecological respect for the planet's systems, the optimal creation and use of Energy, and the focus on ensuring the Health of all occupants. These roots of supporting life can then create a strong base to allow and support the foundation of the branches of mental, physical, and emotional wellness and well being.

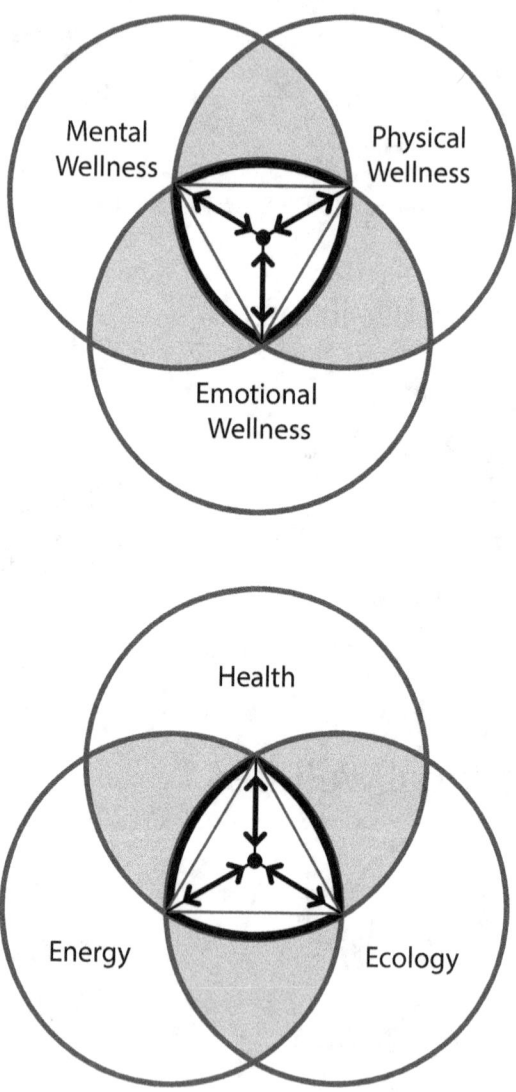

This group of graphics can show the progression of topics, connected as triads, and then each triad placed together to form an integrative, cohesive whole.

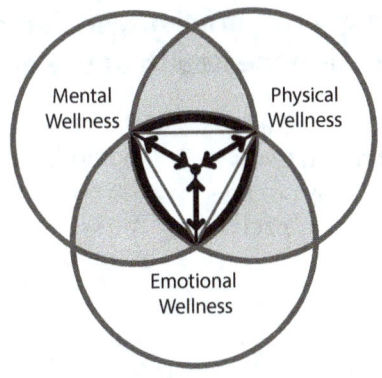

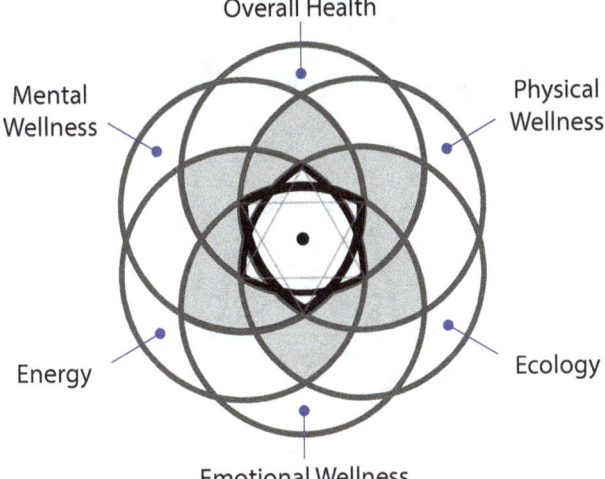

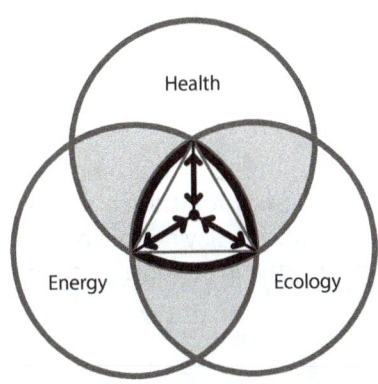

Is the building performing to its optimal potential?
Is the structure energy-efficient, ecologically friendly, and supporting the health of the occupants?

The Result: Healthy materials and methods that are optimal in terms of energy-efficiency, yet may not be focused on the ecological impacts.

The Result: Healthy materials and methods with consideration for the ecological footprint, yet may not be ideal or optimal in terms of energy-efficiency.

Issues related to Health, removing toxic materials and improving occupant health.

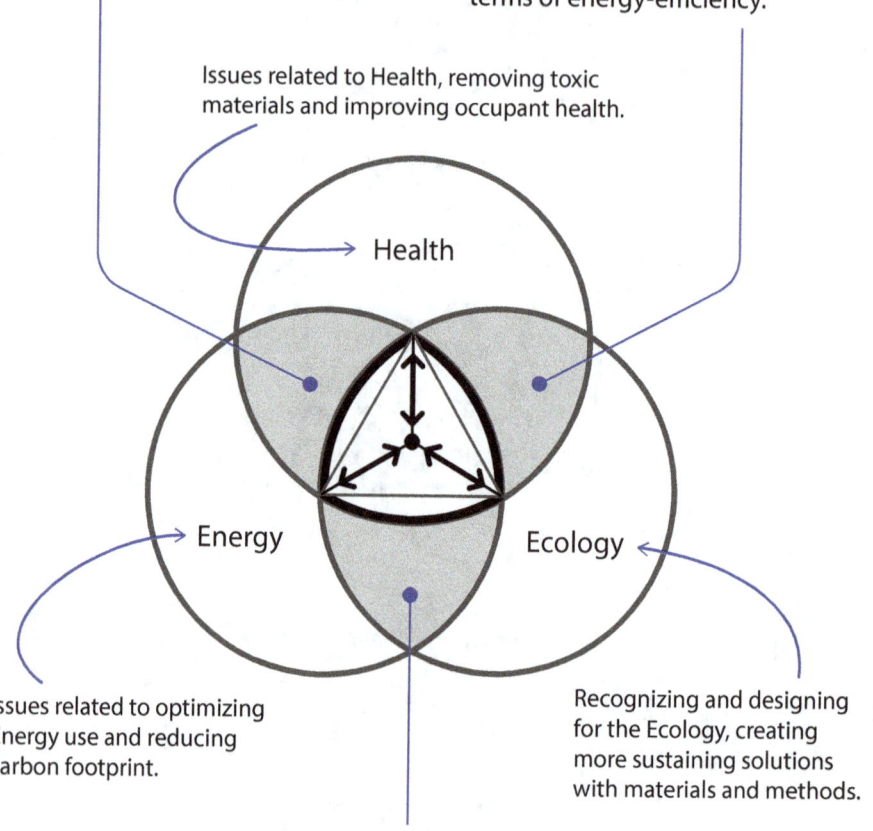

Issues related to optimizing Energy use and reducing carbon footprint.

Recognizing and designing for the Ecology, creating more sustaining solutions with materials and methods.

The Result: Energy-efficiency with consideration for the ecological footprint, yet may not be focused on human and biological health.

Are you performing at your optimal potential?
Or are you feeling gray, foggy, and lacking energy?

The Result: Spaces that are geared towards the mental development and utilization, yet also considering the physical health and wellness of the occupants.

How is the space affecting how you think?

How is the space affecting your body?

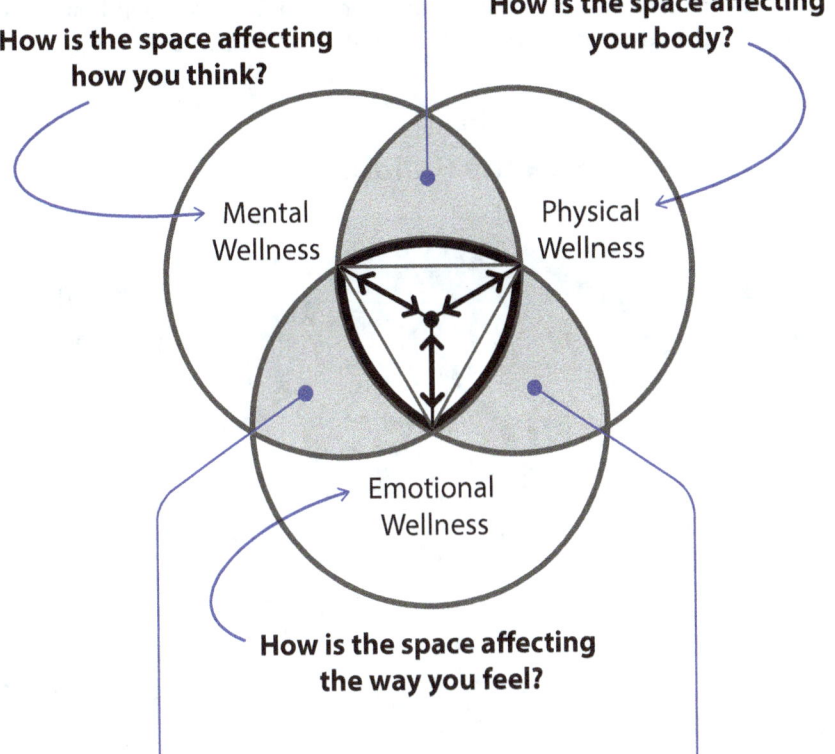

How is the space affecting the way you feel?

The Result: Spaces that are geared towards the mental development and utilization, while also considering the emotional well being of the person.

The Result: Spaces that are geared towards the physical health and wellness of the occupants, while also attending to the emotional needs of the occupants.

In each of the previous chapters, the discussion focused on these topics independently. Yet, a key focus of Architectural Medicine is to ensure that all of these topics are considered together. By considering all of these topics together, it ensures that each subject is integrated into the future of architecture and the built environment. In this manner, the many facets of the puzzle pieces for optimal living can be factored into this big equation.

By putting all of these pieces together in the jigsaw puzzle of the built environment, *architecture* can become *medicine* for preventive health and provide nurturing environments for human health and wellness.

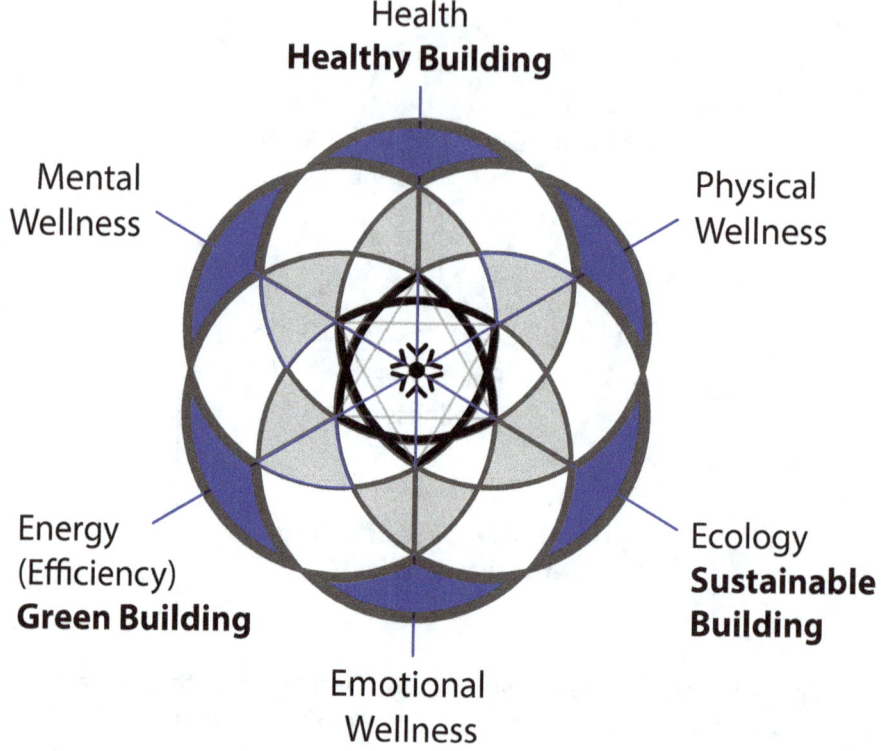

These models of integrated designs can provide a pathway towards wellness, similar to an Rx for health or a blueprint for wellness.

When all of the facets are considered and included in design solutions, it can be akin to how a tree functions as a whole between the root systems, the trunk, and the branches. A tree has an integrated support system, where the roots support the trunk and the branches with stability and nutrients. In contrast, the branches convert sunlight into energy through photosynthesis and distribute this back to the roots and the rest of the tree for health. The trunk provides a functional transportation system to bring the nutrients from the roots to the branches and the energy of photosynthesis to the roots.

This model of symbiosis, where the interdependency of the many facets can support the whole of the organism, can be a model for integration, whether this is an individual human or the entire planet's health.

The roots of a tree can support the branches for vitality, health, and optimal performance, which is then returned to the root systems for ongoing nutrition for the entire tree's health.

This dynamic is comparable to the high-level athlete who can perform at their optimal by having the support for their mental, physical, and emotional health. And a common format in creating the potential of these goals is to have several diagnostic features customized for each athlete.

A customized training plan is required to reach the athlete's end goal of blossoming and reaching their potential to flourish. This requires a strong foundation of support, a solid base to achieve this health and well-being, and a support team to help them achieve this goal.

While this may not be a common analogy in the world of architecture, design, and building, such support can be provided through the architecture and buildings themselves, in which one spends most of their time within. And a game plan to achieve this goal is a similar blueprint in format, simply applied differently by all professionals working together. Instead of the goal being an athlete attaining their goals, the end goal for the built environment is for the inhabitants to flourish in their lives.

Creating a strong support system in the form of the built environment allows for the space in which people work, play, and live to provide the foundation of support to achieve these goals – whether a trained athlete or someone striving to reach their potential in any modality.

Just as the athlete has the support in the form of coaches, diagnostics, and personalized information to provide the best methods for them to succeed, this can be designed into one's life through the architecture they spend time within.

And like the solid roots that provide strength and vitality for a tree, this can provide a foundation of support in a healthy manner in the same way a building's foundation provides support for the entire structure.

Like the branches that provide energy through photosynthesis to support these roots and the entire tree, the building's design and functionality can ensure that the foundation is kept solid and strong. And all of these systems in place can then support the structure's inhabitants to ensure that they are supported, protected, and nurtured for good health.

In this approach, it's not just the materials and the methodologies of the structure. It's how the space effects, impacts, and influences your life — mentally, physically, emotionally, and spiritually.

Architecture and the built environment have a considerable impact and influence in one's everyday life, so much so that it may be unrecognized and even ignored. For many, it has become so commonplace to go to a place for work, and to become so accustomed to their own built environment as their home, that these concepts may be overlooked.

This does not infer that these aspects of life need to be analyzed all the time, yet if one is seeking improvement, good health, and striving to achieve goals, these are factors that one's life is built upon.

Not paying attention to such matters would be akin to a contractor building on a foundation that has not been appropriately analyzed for structural integrity. And to simply build without considering how this foundation will support and hold the rest of the building is a recipe for disaster.

In the process of achieving a goal in which one is striving to succeed, you would not ignore these essential foundations to achieve high-performance goals.

And so why would these fundamentals of the built environment be ignored in one's everyday life?

To not examine this foundation would be to build on grounds that could not support the building. It would therefore create a circumstance where, later on, as the building is developed and more floors are added, the scaling up would not be supported, and all could come crashing down.

Our human health and wellness require a strong foundation to be built upon to grow and to stay healthy.

WHEALTH

Everyone, at some point in their lives, has become sick. Whether it's an acute or chronic condition, the feeling of being sick is horrible, and often when people are sick, their only focus is to get better. They are usually not thinking about thriving, as their illness has taken complete focus to continue in their survival.

And during this time, many people recognize the value of health. It can change behaviors when people get better, as they never wish to suffer in pain or be struggling in survival again.

These scenarios can often be reminders of the value of health, to the point where their wealth in their life is their health. And this term "Whealth" is where a focus of Architectural Medicine can find a home for itself, striving to provide a healthier solution for thriving and wellness as personal whealth.

To be clear, this is not to state that financial wealth is irrelevant, yet instead, to say that to enjoy the benefits of other facets of life, good health and wellness are critical.

Obviously, everyone may have their own definition of this wellness as whealth, yet the common denominator can often be physical, emotional, and mental wellness.

And this is where the previous three chapters on wellness become pivotal. And that's because achieving this overall wellness requires all of these pieces of the built environment puzzle to be in place if seeking the benefits of physical, mental, and emotional well being as a goal.

I had once read the quote, "medicine is the providing of health and healing for wellbeing to the patient, not just to give medicine for the purpose of medicine or drugs." It was listed as a Hippocrates quote, yet I have not found an appropriate citation to name him as the author. However, even if this statement is not from Hippocrates, the sentiment remains relevant and has value. The idea that health is a complex process of evaluations and solutions, and not just a single drug or prescription, is in itself powerful medicine.

The architects and doctors of tomorrow will have to have more integration between the fields to diagnose some of the issues related to health in the built environment. And they will have the ability to collaborate on solutions in the process. The concept that a single drug or a simple design solution will fix all ailments is unrealistic and also antithetical to the processes of nature and life.

As modern materials become more complex and common, there will be even more of these products that may have health impacts. It will require even better integration between these fields to provide analysis and solutions when issues arise.

As mentioned earlier, sick building syndrome was one instance where the medical fields were involved in diagnosing patients whose health seemed to be affected by a mysterious cause. The cause of these issues was often found in the places where people worked and lived. These sick buildings are often found where "tight buildings" are developed, and by tight buildings, this definition is meant to describe a building envelope. A "building envelope" is the definition used to describe the building in terms of the exterior walls, ceilings, and floors as the "envelope." It is that which envelopes the rest of the rooms inside of the structure.

And when these building interiors do not have fresh air circulation, and instead these envelopes tightly contain the air to have better energy conservation and insulating properties to save energy for heating and cooling, it does not mean that this air is healthy for humans. This is a perfect example of how green and sustainable building initiatives have sometimes left out the health of the occupants when not factoring all of the pieces into the equation.

Over time, this sick building syndrome has become a design and engineering issue. While more often reviewed now than it has in the past, it's still a topic with much room for improvement. Even the term Sick Building Syndrome (SBS), since its popularity in the '80s and '90s, has become more critically evaluated and often replaced with another term Building Related Illness (BRI).

Essentially, the main issue with tight buildings to decrease the energy loss or decrease the exchange of interior air with the outside air temperatures can sometimes leave the exchange of fresh interior air out of the equation.

If it is hot outside and desired to be cooler inside, preventing the outside exchange of temperature from getting inside helps decrease energy costs. Of course, this makes sense and logic as the decrease fuel use means less energy used, less degradation to the environment, and an increase in savings. This makes sense for the green of the environment as well as the green in the bank.

This is an excellent example of making the structure tight, reducing the air exchange, increasing insulation, and closing up any areas in the building where there are drafts, which means less heat exchange between the outside and inside air. This is great for saving energy.

The problem with this approach is that these buildings often don't have functioning windows to open and close, which would defeat the purpose of making the building tight to decrease airflow exchange. Yet when there is no fresh air in the building, it can cause health issues, such as reduced oxygen, increased carbon dioxide, and carbon monoxide. As well, many modern materials out gas, known as VOCs, can also cause health issues.

In this example, you can see that one attempt to solve one issue has created another problem. While it's good to save money and be energy efficient for both the environment and the wallet, there can be a lack of recognition of the health issues and problems it can create.

This is a perfect example of why the whole building system should be examined and evaluated to prevent and not cause more problems than solved.

And this is also a perfect reason why these various topics are discussed in this book.

If you only evaluate and factor into the design process one facet, you can create other issues and cause new problems. This is a repeating topic throughout this book and underlines the importance of a cohesive systems approach to these issues.

This is not to say that synthetic materials are all bad and natural materials are all good – there isn't a perfect solution. As many know, many natural materials are harmful when used in buildings, such as lead paint and asbestos. Another example, not as a building material, but as a result of building issues, is the natural process of molds growing inside of buildings. While mold is natural, it has become one of the most significant issues in health-related building topics as a Building Related Illness (BRI) in the USA and other world regions in the past 20 plus years.

Even certain natural paint options such as those with tannins can cause some people to react negatively and have health issues. So it's not to say that all natural materials are good and all synthetics are bad. Instead, it would be more logical to review this in terms of how materials impact human, biological, and ecological health in both the long and short term and how they all react when multiple materials are present in an environment.

After all, reviewing just one product in vitro to determine its impact on human health would be akin to reviewing just sodium or just chloride by itself. Alone these two chemicals are very toxic, yet ironically when placed together, which we call table salt (NaCl), they are not just ok for health, but needed in proper amounts for good health.

This is to state that it is not enough to view one facet of these issues and make broad statements on their impacts and effects. It will require teams of various professionals to evaluate and provide deeper insights in a collaborative process to help guide the future of these materials and methods to find healthy or healthier solutions.

That said, there can be benefits to keeping things more simple and natural, such as natural fresh air, local natural materials, and natural lighting that can keep people connected to the planet's natural cycles. This, in turn, can help people stay in better balance and to become less stressed.

This process requires a nodal system of people, groups, and organizations working together as an integrated whole so that the many pieces can be viewed together. This nodal system reflects the biotensegrity of the human body itself and all living organisms.[131]

Here again, we can see the macro of the world reflected in the micro-processes of a healthy organism and a healthy society – for they are one and the same as systems.

Re-Evaluating the Built Environment and the Many Facets of Health and Wellness

It's important to note that while these comments can be viewed as criticisms in evaluating these issues in the built environment that are causing health issues, it's not to state that it's the fault of those professions and professionals involved in designing, building, and constructing these built environments.

Many are simply not aware of these issues, and in other ways, some problems are created by the eventual breakdown of materials or the use of chemicals and biocides that have found their way inside of these buildings.

Or perhaps there is a lack of awareness of the issues that certain materials and methods can cause related to health, which is an essential part of the writing of this book.

It is to bring awareness to these very complicated systems that we call buildings, which have gone from very simple structures to extremely complicated systems over the past fifty to a hundred years.

In my opinion, in the next several decades, buildings will be seen similarly to airplanes and vehicles as complex, integrated systems. This recalibration in viewing the built environment as complex systems requires a technological and functionally cohesive approach to designing, building, and maintaining these structures.

Towards the end of the book, I'll discuss some thoughts on the future of architecture, particularly concerning health and wellness. And one of these topics includes the idea that, moving forward, buildings will likely be viewed and more aligned with advanced technological designs. They will be seen analogous to an airplane or a sophisticated nautical design, and less so the old version of a building as an advanced shed.

The fact is these modern buildings as systems are multi-faceted and require many parts and pieces to fit and work together as a whole. This is often why many of these issues go unnoticed, as, over time, they've morphed from basic buildings into sophisticated technological structures. And many people do not understand the sophistication of the modern building until that is, an issue is impacting those occupying these structures.

Two takeaways can be gleaned from these comments moving forward. One, the recognition that buildings are complex systems that need to be evaluated on these terms. Professionals involved in designing and building these structures need to work together, have some forward-thinking as to potential issues, and work to resolve them before they become health hazards.

The second is to have more data collected, evaluated, and acknowledged for iterations of current practices. This can evolve into knowledge bases that each profession can utilize and update their facet for their profession.

In this manner, large groups of people involved in building these structures can iterate before there are significant issues, instead of an afterthought or the need to fix something later in the building's life.

After all, buildings have a life as well, and if the building is healthy in terms of the structural integrity of its functions, then it is likely that this building's health will reflect in the occupants inhabiting the building.

Again, this is not to state that those involved are to blame for the lack of a current focus on building health, but instead a factor of the building's materials, methods, and systems changing so much over the past fifty years.

In fact, many of these changes have occurred in the past thirty years in most of the world. Some of the world's most significant changes are areas where newer technologies in building materials have been implemented.

These more contemporary building materials and methods have been utilized without much understanding of these materials' impacts on human health in the short and the long term.

Many architects and doctors have never worked together or considered the overlap between their professions and the importance of working together. This is another reason why the focus of health and wellness in the built environment has been so elusive within these professions.

However, the time has come for the overlap between these professions to become more congruous. With goals of more significant overlap and the sharing of knowledge and best practices between each professional, the future can better support human thriving and well being.

An active working together between these professions of architecture and medicine, setting new protocols, processes, standards, and helpful systems to provide integrative solutions for better health in buildings, is ripe for change.

The advent of the novel coronavirus as the pandemic of 2020 has also shown the importance and need for more focus on health in buildings — and is reason enough for this topic to flourish.

Many building and health professionals, along with the general public, are struggling to navigate this pandemic.

The need to work together to find solutions is more appropriate than ever and has not been as paramount as perhaps the Spanish flu of the 1918 pandemic.

Putting It All Together – Integrative Medicine Plus Integrative Architecture Equals Architectural Medicine

When there is the openness of both the architecture and the medical professionals, who utilize best practices in each of their respective fields, their focus can be on their patient and client's best and optimal health. And when there are professionals who have this mindset and approach, they will seek ideal solutions for their patients and clients.

When it comes to medicine and health, the doctor may begin to recognize that external factors such as the built environment, where the average person is spending up to ninety percent of their time each day, may significantly impact their health and well being.

When the architect begins to recognize the impact of architecture and their designs on health and wellness, they may conclude that their approach to health-focused designs stems from the knowledge of the health and medical fields.

Each of these professionals may be wise enough to realize that they cannot achieve these goals alone and, therefore, may conclude that they can work together to accomplish these large goals. This can be achieved by combining the knowledge, wisdom, and best practices of the many other fields involved, from building inspectors, nurses, and epidemiologists to those in the areas of green chemistry, evidence-based design, biophilia, and environmental psychology.

This workflow can be constructed of toxicologists, epidemiologists, and public health professionals utilizing big data and medical research to define issues. This knowledge can then be resolved by working together with the fields of green chemists, material manufacturers, and product designers to explore new solutions. And then, when these products are developed and implemented into the building material world, the resulting impacts can be evaluated over time using the same process of data retrieval and analysis in an iterative format.

To extend the range of these professionals does not necessarily mean that they have to be well versed in all of these facets, yet to know how they can all work together and have these connections is perhaps the key.

In practical terms, this means that both the sharing of knowledge and the ability to work together in various ways, which may be new and unprecedented, can yield synergistic and beneficial results.

New systems can be introduced to support these integrated processes, and along the way, these new integrations can lead to more robust systems that provide better solutions over time. In chapter 16, the Architectural Medicine System (AMS) is discussed with more feedback on how these systems may function together.

As we've discussed in previous chapters, there are many pieces of this puzzle of health and wellness in the built environment that can be placed together for better solutions.

The following diagrams revisit these topics and visually show how these fields can be connected with better communication and overlap for cohesive solutions.

Current Building Model – Limited Integrations

Limited Communication and often no direct review of building health related issues between the building fields, the health fields, and the occupants (general public).

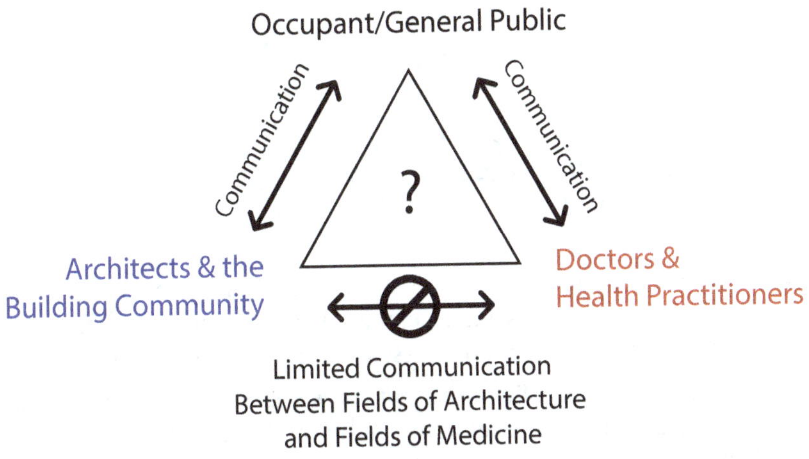

Occupant/General Public

Communication ↔ Communication

?

Architects & the Building Community

Doctors & Health Practitioners

Limited Communication Between Fields of Architecture and Fields of Medicine

As you can see in the graphic above, the communication status between the fields of architecture and medicine is limited. There can be better integrations and new systems created to support these integrations resulting in better health and wellness in the built environment.

The following diagrams show these new integrations with the support of the Architectural Doctor. We'll discuss the details of the Architectural Doctor in the next chapter.

New Integration Between the Occupant, the Building Fields, and the Doctors and Health Professionals

Direct Communication and review of building health related issues with the building fields, the health fields, and the occupants (general public) through interconnections among all groups and the Consultant-Architectural Doctor.

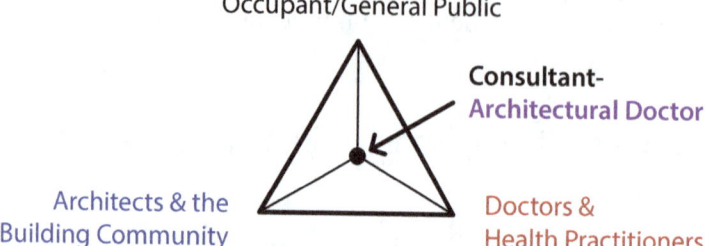

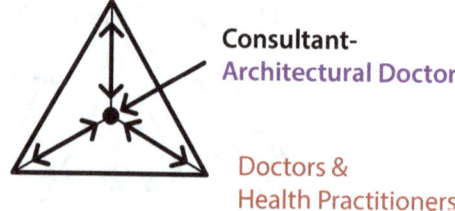

We'll also get into the details of the Architectural Medicine System (AMS), which shows how these professionals can work together in more cohesive formats, providing procedures and processes to achieve these healthier goals.

As we revisit the initial diagrams that show a lack of integration between the fields of architecture and medicine, including the general public, the following diagrams show the progressive movement in the direction of integration.

Starting with the first triangle diagram, we have the general public at the top, then the architecture field in the lower left and the lower right is the medical field. Building upon this integration, with the Architectural Doctor's support, we begin to add these connections into the diagrams where the fields start working with each other.

This communication also includes the general public as the occupant and leads to more clarity about the built environment's health for all involved.

Chapter: 14 — Architectural Medicine – Part 2

New and Revised Building Model for Health and Wellness

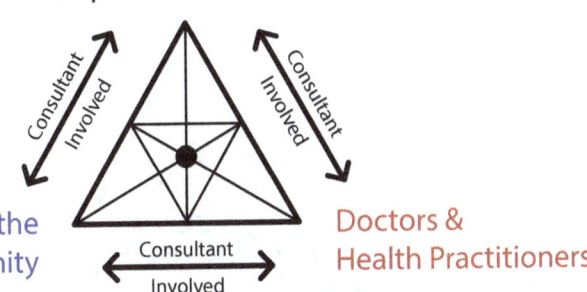

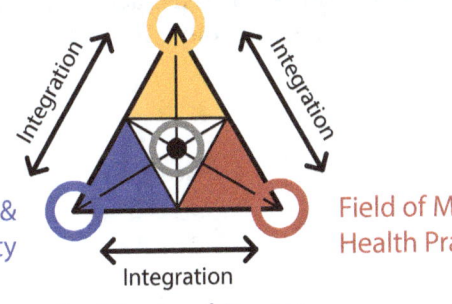

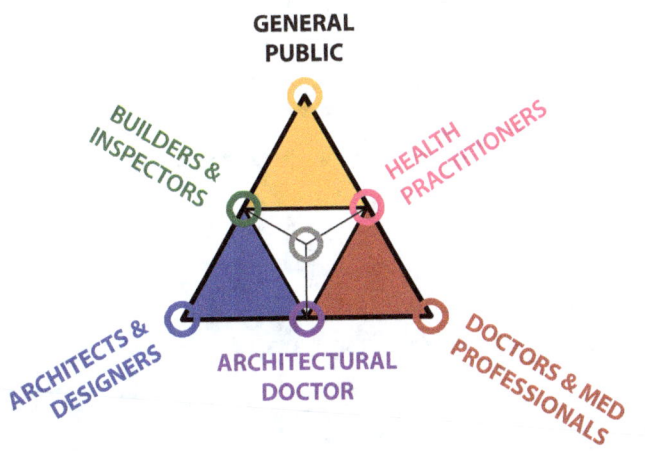

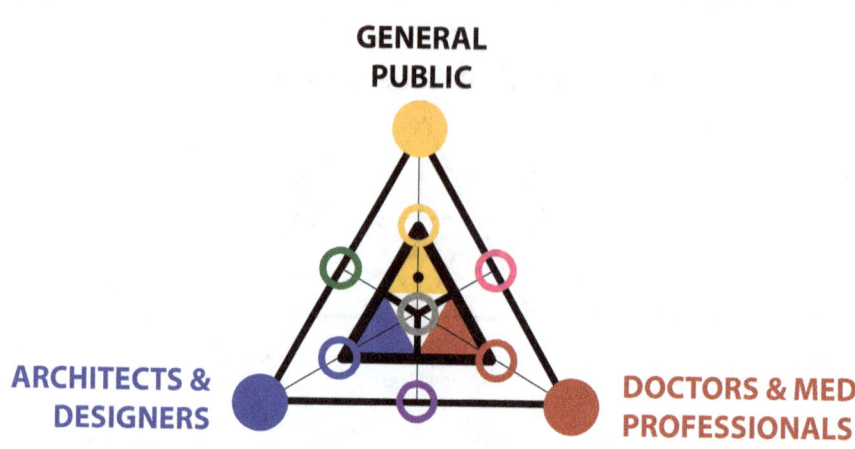

The next step is to include the Healthy Building Inspector and the building professionals, along with the health practitioners. This can consist of nurses and psychologists and the many other professionals involved in health care and caretaking.

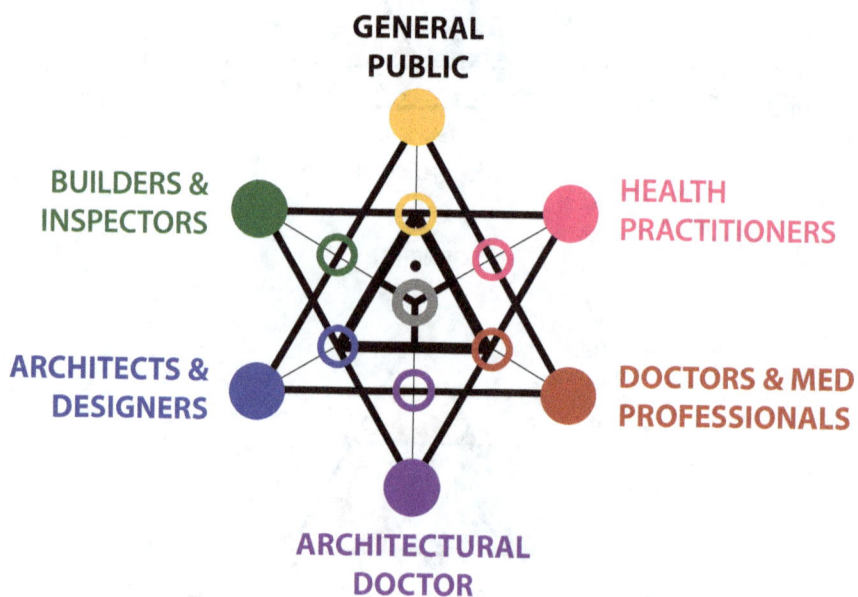

Once we have these integrations in place, there can be better support systems to achieve integrative solutions between all groups to benefit the patient and the general public.

As shown in the graphics, the process consists of connections growing between each field and all of the many parts. As discussed in chapter 5, "Reviewing the Many Pieces of the Puzzle," these diagrams outline the many pieces and the processes to connect them.

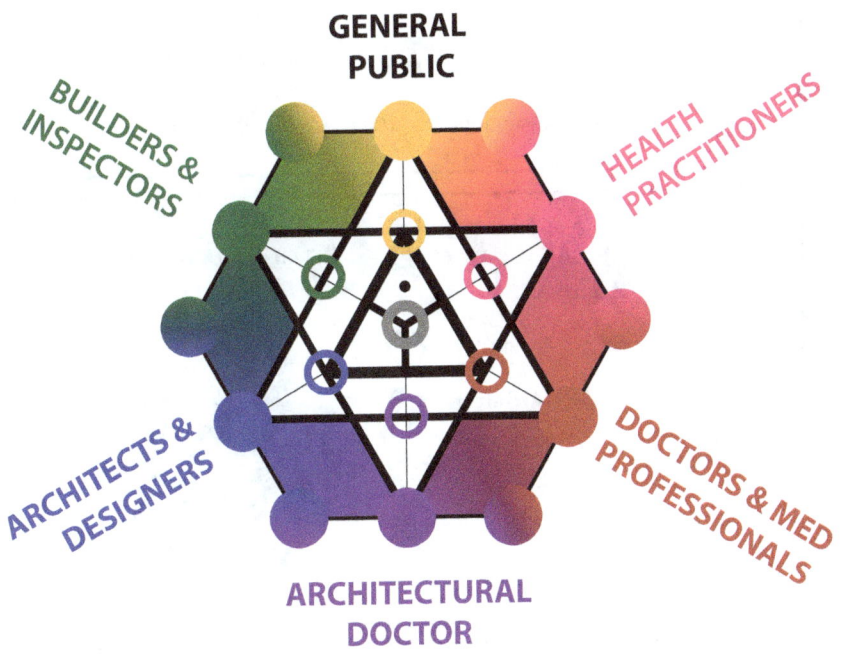

Having these integrations can provide pathways for various fields to work together and provide more cohesive solutions by viewing the many parts of the puzzle together.

With a view of all of the different facets, there can be planning and considerations to provide whole system solutions. Instead of piecemeal solutions that can create more problems, these connections can ensure all aspects are factored into the equation.

The following diagrams show more details along with a key for each of the diagrams. The final diagram shows all of the facets of these topics as a cohesive whole.

Key to Diagrams

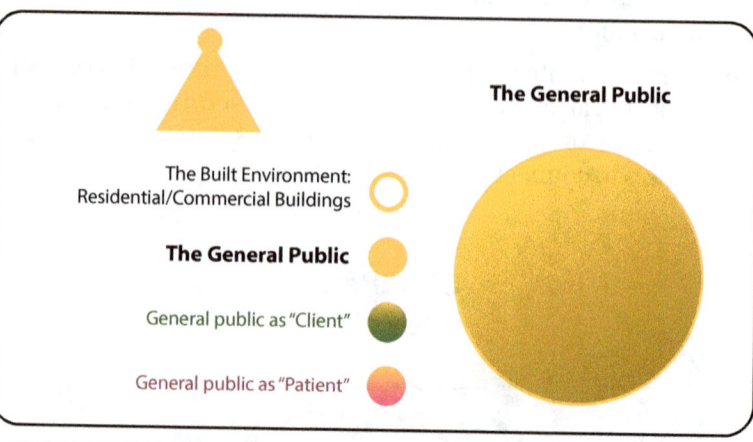

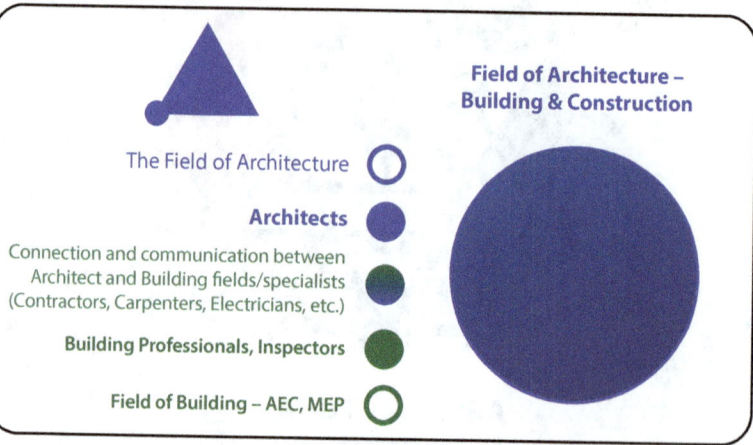

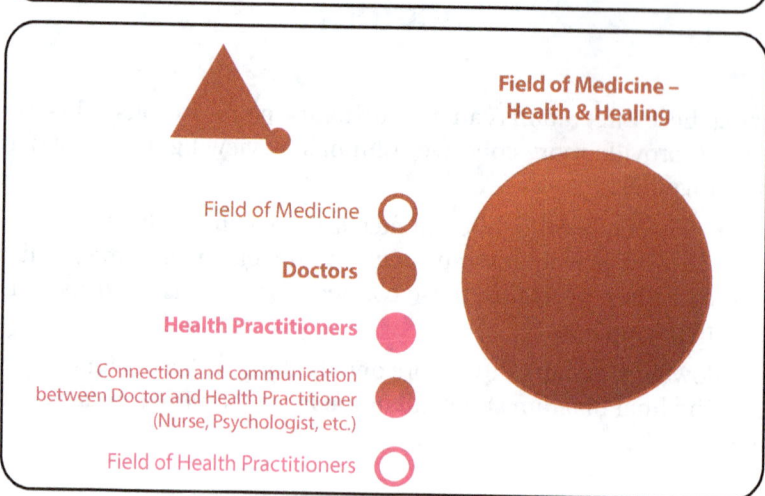

Chapter: 14 — Architectural Medicine – Part 2

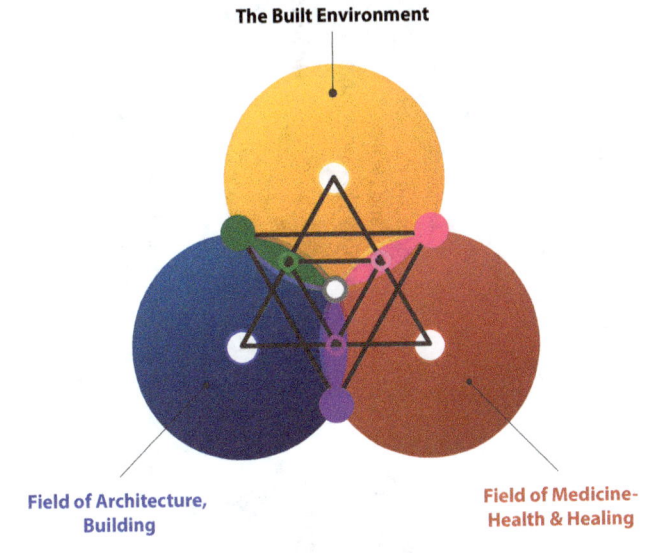

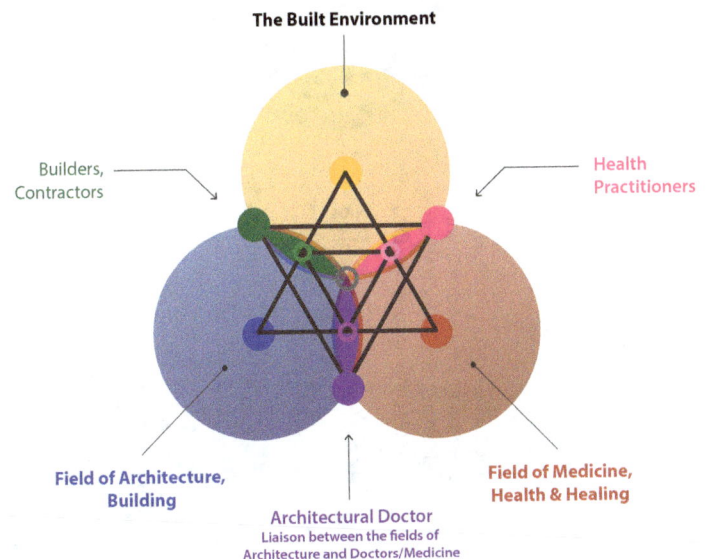

Architectural Medicine – Building the Bridge to Wellness

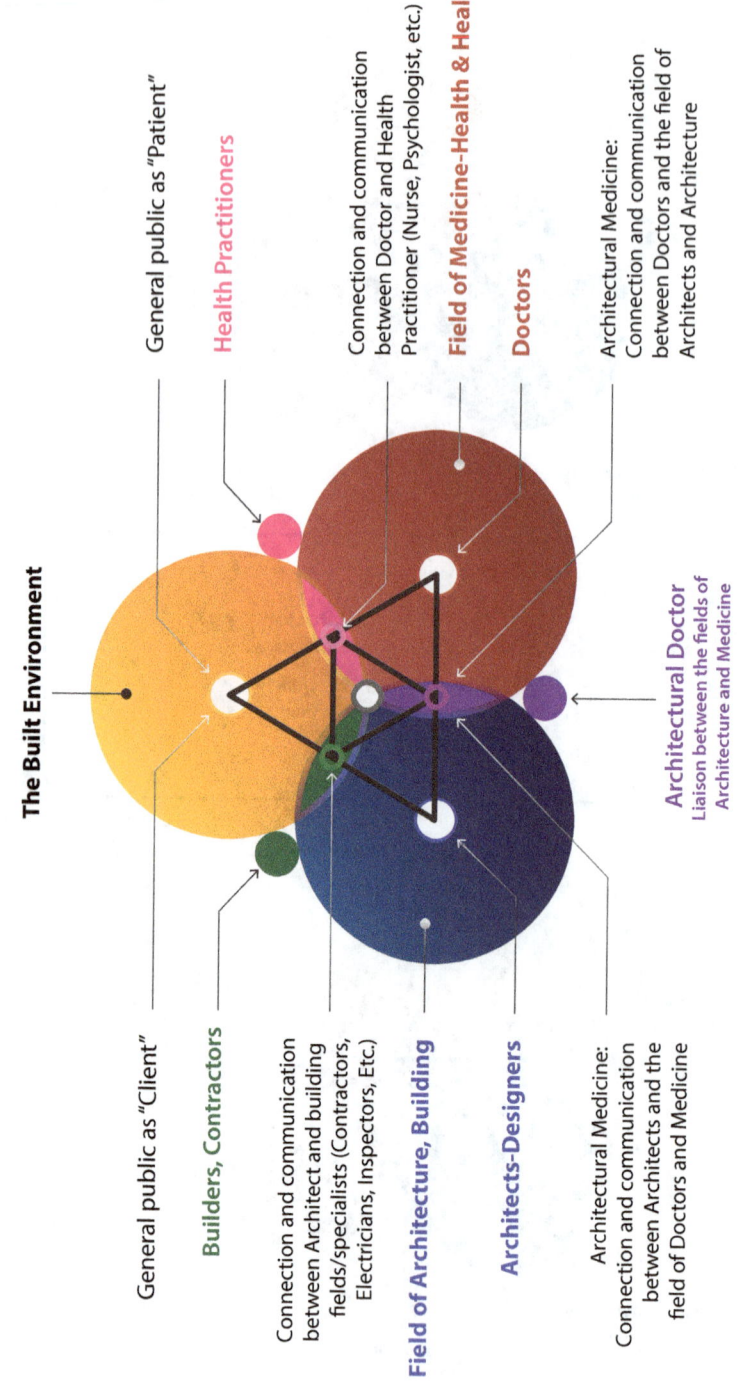

Chapter: 14 — Architectural Medicine – Part 2

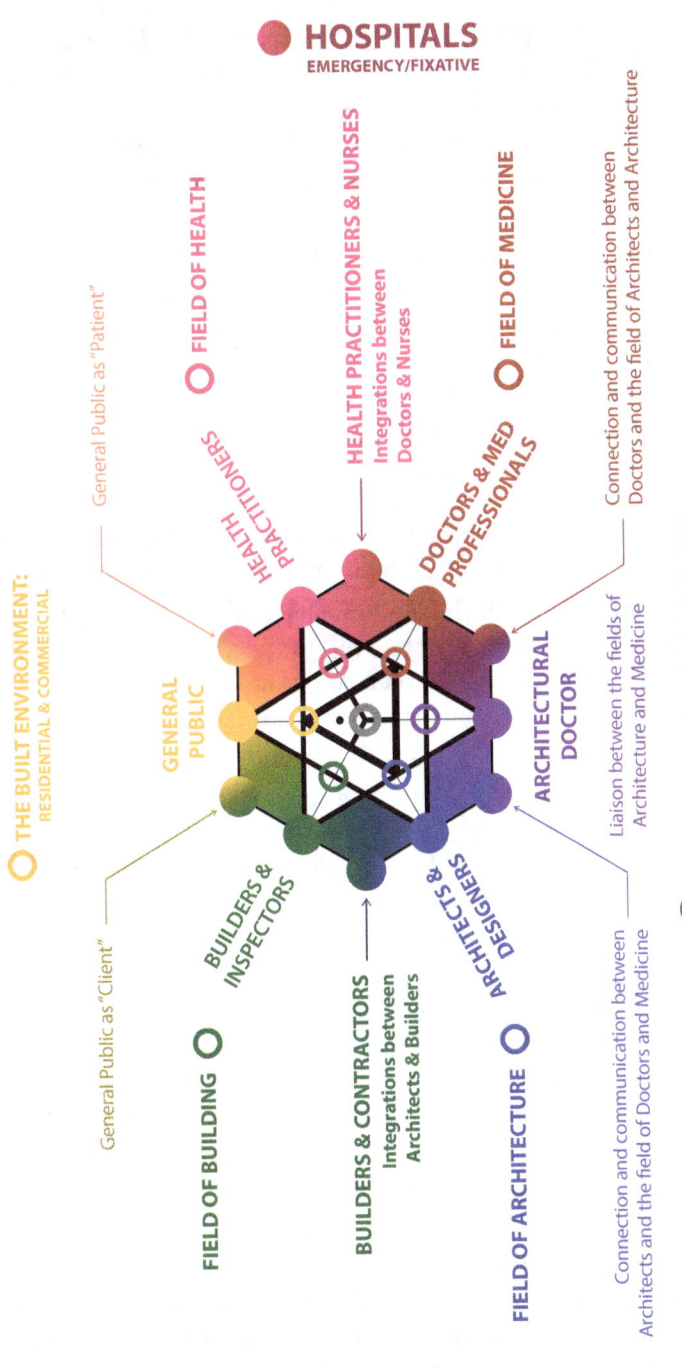

In the following chapters involving the Architectural Doctor and the Architectural Medicine System (AMS), I will discuss these integrations in more detail and explain how these fields can work together in providing solutions.

Right now, in this time of the second decade of the 2000s, we are still in the infancy of these developments – even if they have been evolving for the past forty to fifty years.

The reality is that these developments have existed in smaller pockets of professional approaches yet often have not been embraced and accepted by the masses and larger groups of professionals. When it comes to architecture and the built environment, there is a need for group efforts in co-creating cities on this level for integrative solutions.

Some people reading this may tremor at the thought of the scenario in the book *The Fountainhead* of a Howard Roark moment of group design colloquiums supporting mediocrity. However, the process and end goal does not have to be one of group designing, yet should be inclusive of the various components to achieve healthier, greener, and more sustainable architecture.

This goal cannot be achieved if all involved are not on board to accomplish these goals, and so there must be overlap and a "working together" mantra to accomplish these goals. These can still produce beautiful, amazing, and unique architecture to inspire and soothe the soul.

As the field of architecture already works with many different professionals, it is a matter of how these groups work together, not whether they do at all. Architects such as Santiago Calatrava and Zaha Hadid have already shown that beauty and functionality in design approaches can be achieved using new methodologies.

Of course, many previous designers and architects from history, from Leonardo da Vinci to Buckminster Fuller, have shown that the integration of design and engineering focused on human-centric benefit have not only worked, but they've also lasted for generations.

The approaches of medicine to support the individual's health and well-being by including the built environment in their equation for best health, have endured from Hippocrates to Florence Nightingale.

The wisdom of best practices, in many ways, has not changed. The facets that have changed are the more modern ways of life and the complexities of materials, methods, technologies, and the scale of architecture and cities.

This, along with the faster pace of life and larger populations, has led to more complex processes. Yet, the overall approach and goals of better living and more well-being remain to be, as Dr. Weil states, focused on "optimum health."[132]

And this is where the many fields can work together to achieve integrated goals in providing optimal health and wellness in the built environment from the single building to cities. This collaboration can occur from the fields of Environmental Psychology, Architectural Phenomenology, Green Building, and Environmental Medicine to Integrative Medicine, Green Chemistry, Epidemiology, Biomimicry, and Biophilia, along with many others.

The collaboration of sharing and evaluating data and processes can help in placing the many puzzle pieces together to provide these whole systems solutions.

Parametric and Curving Forms and Designs to Support Health and Wellness

In this book, up until this point, actual design solutions have not been discussed very much. Except for the earlier comments about the International Design style, the focus of design solutions has been limited. And that's due to a few critical reasons.

One of the main reasons is based on the idea that there is no design "style" that altogether provides green, healthy, and sustainable designs. Many of these designs encourage a vernacular aesthetic based on the definitions provided by the materials and the methods. Yet, as you will recognize when researching green, healthy, and sustainable designs, you will find a vast range of design styles.

That said, there are specific designs as forms and shapes, as mentioned in the previous chapters discussing the neuroscience of architecture, which have shown that curving and less sharp designs can reduce stress on a physiological level.

What can be learned from these studies is that these newer forms of curving designs, commonly known as parametric design, can offer a built environment that can nurture human beings and reduce stress. I go into more details about parametric architecture in chapter 19. Yet, for now, it's important to state this in reference to these newer design styles and the topic of putting the many pieces of the puzzle together.

After all, the built environment's actual designs will be important to include in these health discussions, not just the materials and methods of construction. And this topic requires a segment to itself. I will state this now as an important component and provide more details about this design approach in chapter 19.

A Systems Approach

As I mentioned earlier in this book, a key facet of Architectural Medicine is the fact that, while there have been great strides in the emerging fields of health in the built environment, a big part of what makes this book a bit different is the focus on systems.

In the previous chapters, I outlined the many facets of these topics relating to health in the built environment, and in this chapter, I've been outlining these pieces and how they can fit together.

In my honest opinion, a cohesive systems approach in a multi-disciplinary format is key to providing healthier built environments for current and future architecture.

And by systems, I am specifically referring to the fact that there is very little integration with the world of building and architecture in today's world of medicine and health.

With people spending from 60 to 90 percent of their lives inside architecture, the fact that we are rarely factoring building health into the equation of wellness, is to me, strange.

The fact that so much time is spent indoors with so many potential pollutants and impacts that buildings can have on health is often a perplexing scenario for me to understand why there are no better systems to evaluate these topics. The fact that there are few standard processes that consider the built environment in evaluating health in diagnosing ailments seems odd.

I am both perplexed and not surprised because of my personal experience working in construction and the architecture fields for so many years. In particular, striving to find solutions for these issues and wondering why these do not exist has led me to question and contemplate this over many years.

What I've learned over the years is that it's often not a lack of interest or concern. It's usually a matter of how to achieve these goals.

How are doctors and health professionals supposed to include the built environment in their evaluations? They aren't trained to go into buildings to inspect and find potential health culprits. And even if they did find these issues, perhaps akin to the previous doctor's home visit, what would a doctor do about a possible health issue they have seen? Would they write a prescription for a healthier building solution?

The answer to this is an obvious, no, yet a follow up is another question "why not?"

My answer to why these solutions do not yet exist is that there have been no systems for these two professionals to work together to provide such evaluations and follow up on health issues in buildings.

An Rx for better built environment health does not yet exist, yet perhaps moving forward, it should and, hint, this is a topic we discuss later in the book defined as ARxMD.

To revisit this comment about systems, these two professions of architecture and medicine are also arguably two of the most demanding careers in terms of training and education. They already have tremendously complex systems to achieve their high level of capabilities, so adding some form of additional steps into their already systemized processes is not exactly fair to these professions and professionals.

When you begin to think about all of the steps and procedures required for this process to happen as outlined in this book, you will soon find many processes that do not currently exist, along with integrations needed between professions that also do not exist.

This process also requires at least two new types of professionals – the Architectural Doctor and the Healthy Building Inspector. The Architectural Doctor, which in many ways can help to build these bridges between professions to support the multi-disciplinary process required, is a central focus and an important part of Architectural Medicine.

And while that may sound like a lot, it is also critical to consider it an investment towards human health. Taking steps to provide this integrated process can offer better health and wellness for humanity at large.

As we discuss the Architectural Medicine System (AMS) in chapter 16, a part of this process will be to create integrated solutions to achieve these goals.

What is meant by system solutions? To begin, if we review the comments above about the doctor needing to evaluate one's built environment to gain insights into potential health issues that can be resolved, that is step one – a prescription for a healthy building inspection.

And this alone requires a few steps. The first is to include evaluations of ailments into the doctor's analysis so that they are aware of health issues related to the built environment.

Once that is achieved, there is a need for connections between the doctor and these healthy building inspectors so a proper evaluation can be reviewed. This is akin to a doctor ordering lab testing for blood work or an X-ray or MRI to provide analysis and insights.

This may sound strange right now, yet 100 years ago, a doctor requesting an MRI or blood test would have also sounded strange.

This process would also require a Healthy Building Inspector trained on such evaluations of buildings related to health issues.

Currently, the typical building inspector does not look for health type issues unless they are related to some building issues in an indirect manner. The discovery of lead paint and asbestos can flag issues that are related to health. For example, mold problems might trigger water infiltration issues related to the integrity of the building materials. However, the average building inspector would not be reviewing most of the building for problems related to health. And they would need to be trained on these protocols and trained in working directly with doctors and health professionals.

So, what can be seen in the above sentences are more systems are required to make this happen.

Then, of course, if there are issues found, the architecture and building professionals would need to help provide the required building solutions.

This would mean that architects and the construction fields would need to be trained on these issues, in both preventing them from occurring in the future and resolving them when they are found.

And there is also another facet of training and education and the integrations required to help connect the inspectors to the builders to the doctors.

Ideally, this is where the Architectural Doctor can help bridge these different fields and act as a liaison between the many professionals involved along the way. And of course, the patient as the client is also essential to keep in the loop, and the role of the Architectural Doctor can assist with this as well.

And so, the process of creating healthier built environments requires systems to be in place, including training and education. This includes working with other professionals, who are often outside of the scope in which each professional is typically working with.

Novel Coronavirus and COVID-19 Teachings

While I've been writing this book for years, the process of putting together and finalizing these writings into a book during the year 2020 seems fitting, as the world is experiencing the novel coronavirus and the COVID-19 pandemic.

One of the crucial lessons to be gleaned from this pandemic is the importance of health in the built environment. While previously there were topics that most of the population had an awareness of, such as lead paint, asbestos, and the more current issues of mold, the current pandemic has heightened the built environment issues and brought this to another level.

And what becomes glaringly apparent, as the populations strive to return to business buildings and schools, are the topics of health and well being in these environments.

For me, a specific facet of this topic is not being discussed, which is the inclusion of new systems and new processes to address these issues. Many have discussed the problems, yet I've heard few conversations that focus on systems approaches with these topics.

In the following chapters, the introduction of the Architectural Doctor and the Healthy Building Inspector are particularly relevant to these issues – including the Architectural Medicine System (AMS).

The coronavirus pandemic highlights these issues and raises questions that many people involved in healthy building research and solutions have been paying attention to for years.

However, it's taken a pandemic to view the importance of these issues, and as such, the solutions will also take time to review and resolve.

That said, one of the essential parts of these solutions is "systems." This includes the importance of systems that provide on-site testing and lab testing for buildings. The importance of systems implemented and integrated between these professions and the general public is critical for safe, built environments.

Many of these solutions are entirely achievable, yet they require multi-disciplinary work in an integrated format. And due to the complexities of these issues, it also entails new methods and a "working together" mindset.

The pandemic has caused a massive amount of casualties, and many lives have been lost. If we can view these as serious issues and work together, I think a positive solution to prevent future health-related issues can honor those whose lives have been lost.

The pandemic has brought about the awareness of one topic – the importance of health on a local and global scale. To ignore these lessons and go back to life as it was may end up creating more harm than good. However, if we can learn from these issues and then develop new solutions and implement new systems, we can recognize the situation to utilize human ingenuity and creativity for a better future.

And this segues nicely into the topic of the next chapter with the introduction of the *Architectural Doctor*...

"The art of healing comes from nature, not from the physician. Therefore the physician must start from nature, with an open mind."

– Paracelsus

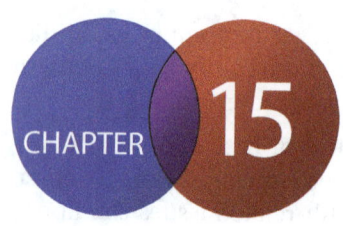

THE ARCHITECTURAL DOCTOR

The importance of recognizing that both professions of architecture and medicine are extremely demanding is of great importance. To master either profession is a massive enough proposition, and to add more complexity to each discipline without proper support is asking too much.

Architects and doctors deserve to be supported to help their clients and patients achieve better health and wellness. And being that the modern-day world spends up to 90 percent of their time indoors, the Architectural Doctor can help bridge these two professions and professionals. With an increasing number of populations living in cities each year, the Architectural Doctor can support the interconnection between fields as a liaison. This new professional can support this integration, so the nomenclature and the general overview of each profession are comprehended.

What Is an Architectural Doctor and What Is the Architectural Doctor's Purpose?

The Architectural Doctor is well versed in each profession and can also help support the many facets of these connections, from the inspection process to evaluating the building scenario for both consideration and planning for required solutions.

The Architectural Doctor can also communicate with the patient or client and support their needs for information when there are fixes that are needed. And the Architectural Doctor can also confer with the doctors and can be there to work with the architects to support the steps towards education, information, and planning.

Vital facets of the Architectural Doctor are twofold. The first is to support the process of bridging these two fields of architecture and medicine through information and education. The bridging is the actual connection of the two fields to help patients, whose health is negatively affected by their built environments.

The second is to support and develop new processes and protocols for these interconnections between professions to occur. As the current method of a doctor's evaluation is to analyze and utilize various lab tests to gain insights into conditions and ailments, this extension of lab tests can go beyond the typical blood sample, for example, and expand to the patient's built environments for testing.

These tests will require Healthy Building Inspections, provided by inspectors – Healthy Building Inspectors – to evaluate the built environment in a more advanced format than the typical evaluations with current building inspections. Topics such as lead and mold have become more common in the past several decades for the inspector to include in their building inspections. The addition of other testing related to potential health issues for preventive measures and proper evaluations will become more commonplace for this building inspector in the Healthy Building Inspector role.

And for this to become a reality, there are many moving parts involved, including procedures and processes required for the Architectural Doctor to orchestrate and support.

These types of inspections can be provided as a single evaluation, such as a specific blood test, or more inclusive, offering a broader scope of information to eventually be evaluated by the doctor. As such, there is a need for a process, a system of protocols for the specific inspection, and the recording and submitting of reports to all involved for proper evaluation.

As discussed in chapter 18, the Architectural Medicine Software Solution –ARxMD – is another option that has been created to fill such a need. Use of other recording processes and procedures can be utilized as well. The purpose of the inspection is to provide more information and insights into how the patient's built environment may negatively impact the patient's health, which is the focus of this entire process.

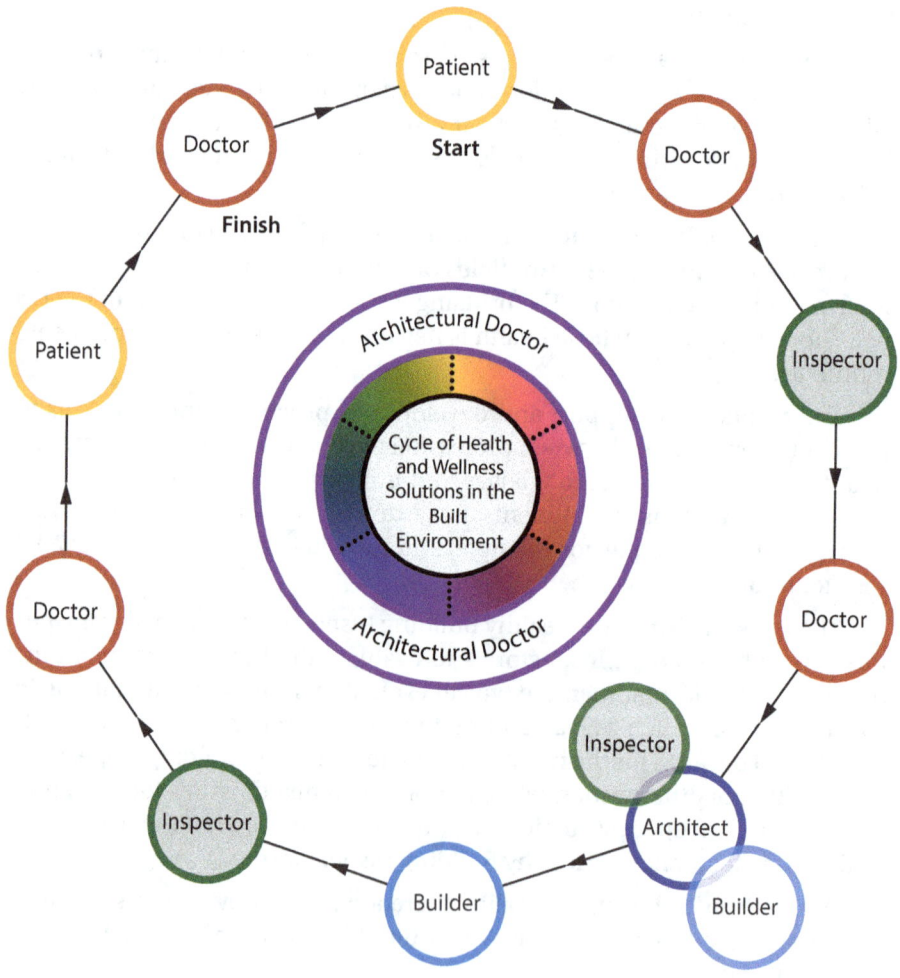

As is noted with these Healthy Building Inspections, the need for an Architectural Doctor to facilitate these processes and help develop these protocols and standards will be an important facet for this field's development.

Combined with the Architectural Medicine System (AMS) in support and development, which is discussed in the next chapter, the Architectural Doctor can provide a bridge between these professions. They will help guide the way to integrate the many facets and people involved in a cohesive system, supporting the goals of health and wellness in the built environment.

An Introduction to the Architectural Doctor

There are many variables and processes required to occur, from the doctor's initial evaluation and ordering of a healthy building inspection to the follow-up summary and meeting of the doctor, inspector, and architect to discuss a solution as an Rx.

With the complexities that these professionals already have in their line of work, this addition of training and systems for solutions might be asking too much to add to their already busy workload.

This is where the introduction of the Architectural Doctor can be of help and support in the process of training, providing integrated solutions, and offering communication to support the entire process. The Architectural Doctor can also be there to support and help the patient in the process. After all, dealing with various professionals, and the fact that this is focusing on their own homes and living places, can often be overwhelming for the patient to navigate.

Doctors working with architects are also not the norm. Having a professional involved that is well versed in both the fields of architecture and medicine can provide a form of translation to bridge these gaps. Supporting this integrated approach and process can help the complete solution process to unfold and proceed successfully.

With the Healthy Building Inspector's involvement, this is another professional not often connected to the medical fields and might not be familiar with many of the health field processes involved.

While the Architectural Doctor does not necessarily have to be either a doctor or an architect in professional accreditation, this new professional is well versed in the nomenclature and processes of each profession. In this manner, the Architectural Doctor can be there for support, can follow up with all of the people involved, and provide integrated solutions that will be required for a successful outcome.

From the initial diagnosis and on-site inspection request from the doctor to the building inspector's steps and the evaluation of the reports and findings of the laboratory results, the Architectural Doctor can help guide each step of the way. And when the process of meeting and working with the architect and builder to provide solutions is included, this too will be another facet of their work.

A critical part of this equation is also the inclusion of the patient in the process. Since it will include both inspections of the home or place of living, and eventual solutions where architects and builders will be involved, there will be many steps in making these positive changes and updates to their buildings.

This is more than the typical Rx that a doctor may prescribe, which can go beyond a pharmaceutical solution or other therapeutic recommendations. It will include inspections at their homes and potentially changing their built environment. One's house is a place of great protection, and when there are changes in one's personal space, it can bring up even more stresses and concerns. If the patient is already dealing with an illness, this can often lead to more stress. And they may already be suffering from an ailment, on top of the tensions of upgrades needed for their home.

This requires the integrated work between professionals and the care and concerns to ensure that the patient, who should be at the core of all of these processes, is adequately cared for and communicated with along the way.

Our homes are known as places of ultimate nurturing and caring for our mental, physical, emotional, and spiritual wellness. It requires a tremendous amount of caring and concern to ensure that this built environment as the patient's support system is not carelessly invaded.

This process will involve the doctor, architect, inspector, and Architectural Doctor to support the methods and support the patient's well being during the process.

The Architectural Doctor can provide this form of integration, especially as these professionals in architecture and medicine become more fluent and familiar in this new system to support the healthy built environment relative to their work.

The good news is that the world of online training, research, and development allows for a digital support system for each of these professionals and the patient. Updates to the process can be evaluated and can inform those involved to access knowledge and information about the results and the solutions.

The Architectural Doctor can provide such training, and the Architectural Medicine Software Solution - ARxMD can also provide the infrastructure to support these processes in a systematic approach.

By providing these digital support systems, the focus can be on the nurturing and caring qualities to support the patient in their health, healing, and wellness. This knowledge and information is not intended to replace the human caring factor. It is instead meant to support this process for better care. It can provide both the science and data of the steps required, along with the artful human caring that can help in the patient's overall healing.

The world of architecture and medicine will also have to recognize the importance of caring and empathy for their patients and clients in these built environment scenarios. In terms of human fear, few factors can have such a significant impact as illness and the topic of changes in one's place of living.

The supportive kindness and caring from these professionals can significantly impact the patient's overall health. In times of duress and stress, this form of empathy can go a long way.

As it's known in the modern world, stress is one of the largest, if not the most significant, sources leading to death.

This focus on compassion during building changes, which are often known as being one of the most stressful events in one's life, can assure that stressors involved can be minimized.

Perhaps one of the most significant additions that can be provided is the support of the patient in each of the many facets of these procedures. The Architectural Doctor can provide both help in training the professionals and support the roundtrip process.

This can appear in many different formats, so while there may not be a perfect equation to define all of these steps, there can be a hub of support for all involved.

The Architectural Doctor – Supporting the Many Facets of Health and Wellness

As discussed in previous chapters, while healthy building is typically geared towards the physical building issues that can cause disease, Architectural Medicine is also based on mental and emotional health and overall well-being — even spiritual wellness.

And as these fields develop more integrations to address health and wellness, several important steps will need to be taken to achieve these goals. Each professional will be required to contemplate these developments, be prepared to comprehend the issues, and take new steps needed to support these objectives. In addressing these facets, the following outlines the topics and questions that each group can begin asking and become more aware of:

- What can the history of these built environment topics define for future trajectories?
- What should the general public know and perhaps demand?
- What should the field of Architecture be aware of?
  - What are some of the main issues?
  - What are some of the solutions to these issues?
  - What might be seen in terms of change for architects and building professionals?
- What should the field of Medicine be aware of?
  - What are some of the main issues?
  - What are some of the solutions to these issues?
  - What might be seen in terms of change for doctors and health professionals?
- What is a Healthy Building Inspector, and what are their roles?
  - What does a Healthy Building Inspector do?
  - Why is it needed and required?
  - Why and how can it help people to live healthier lives?
  - How will they achieve these goals?

The above provides a basic outline of the many topics and questions that will be a part of these integrated solutions. As each profession reviews these questions, the answers need to factor into the equation the involvement of the other professionals. Otherwise, there will be more problems created and a lack of complete solutions achieved.

By going through each of these items, we can address each topic with the appropriate context related to the integrations between professionals. Let's start at the top:

What can the history of these built environment topics define for future trajectories?

In previous chapters, the details of each of the topics of green, sustainable, and healthy building, were discussed along with physical, emotional, and psychological wellness. When you plot the trajectories of each of these topics, what can be found is how our built environment's materials and methods either support better health and wellness or detract from this safety and security.

As more fields begin to recognize the impacts that the built environment has on human and biological health, the process of utilizing this knowledge in practical systems for each professional is going to be critical to achieving positive results for individual and societal health.

What should the general public know and perhaps demand?

As Dr. Weil stated in his book and video *8 Weeks to Optimal Health*, Integrative Medicine's development was moved forward by the general public's requests and demands, not of the medical profession's internal progress. Understandably, the complex discipline of medicine has reservations in making changes. Yet, recognizing what the public wants for their own better health and quality of life is also essential. When people feel empowered in their health and wellness, it signifies a positive trend in knowing thyself, and this is a step towards more wisdom for society at large.

What should the field of Architecture be aware of?

What are some of the main issues?

The evolving process of architecture and the built environment is complex and continues to advance. From newer synthetic materials and chemicals to complex systems that a building depends upon for maintaining mechanical processes, the building is becoming more advanced every year. This means that architectural designs and solutions must consider the impacts these materials and methods have on human health and well being.

What are some of the solutions to these issues?

In recognizing that indoor environments impact physical, emotional, and mental health, the architect and designer of the future will need to have more understanding of the physiological responses to the built environment. This includes a better understanding of human and biological health and how to design and create better solutions for the inhabitants.

What might be seen in terms of change for architects and building professionals?

Perhaps the most significant changes will be the study of human health and how designs can either hinder or support human flourishing. This combination of education and working directly with the medical and health professions to provide better solutions for human wellness, can be major changes for architects and building professionals.

What should the field of Medicine be aware of?
What are some of the main issues?

The topics of the built environment and how these environments impact human health, will be one of the biggest issues for the health and medical fields to recognize. The inclusion of adding built environment factors into their analysis and evaluations for their patient's health can be major changes for doctors and health professionals moving forward.

What are some of the solutions to these issues?

A key solution will be to include social determinants of health and include the patient's building scenarios in their evaluations, which will likely provide better health solutions in providing more whole picture solutions.

What might be seen in terms of change for doctors and health professionals?

Doctors working with factors in the built environment, including working with the Healthy Building Inspector and architects and designers to provide solutions, will likely be a source of major changes. Working with new systems to support these integrations will also be a significant change for health professionals.

What is a Healthy Building Inspector, and what are their roles?
What does a Healthy Building Inspector do?

A Healthy Building Inspector is a professional that addresses building issues in their inspection process. These inspections are focused on the health of the building's occupants. They will provide testing focused on health-related topics and work with doctors and architects in achieving these goals.

Why is it needed?

The complexities of the modern-day building can be a source of many contaminants and pollutants. As these buildings become more complex, there is a need to have professionals provide proper testing that health professionals can utilize to evaluate their patient's health. There will also be a need to have testing and reporting done for both the doctor and the building professionals to test, evaluate, and determine health issues. This includes follow-up inspections after building solutions have been implemented.

Why and how can it help people to live healthier lives?

As buildings become more complex and potentially harmful by increasing diseases and illness, there is a need for these professionals to test and report on topics specific to human health in the built environment. Their work can help to bridge the gaps between the medical and architecture professions.

What do they do, and how will they achieve this?

These inspectors will provide an extended testing process, which can provide a more extensive scope of topics for the health professional to ascertain a patient's health status. The inspectors provide advanced building inspections focused on health issues, and then work with the health and architecture professionals to evaluate the processes and solutions required.

What Does the Architectural Doctor Do, and How Is This Related to Architectural Medicine?

The Architectural Doctor works with the defining principles of Architectural Medicine in providing information and training while supporting the systems and protocols that can help define and create healthier solutions in the built environment.

This process includes the support of standards and protocols that can connect the built environment issues with medical fields. One of the interesting developments in the built environment is based on the latest findings and research from epidemiologists and toxicologists. They are finding that the increasingly complex world of new materials and chemicals has been found to cause health issues.

And a challenge of these findings is how this information finds its way into the professional fields of architecture and medicine. The next stage of challenges is based on translating these issues into practical processes as remedies and solutions in the real world. As more research is provided, there is a need for this information to be introduced and implemented into the real world. This is also where systems are critical for the various professionals involved to have methods in working together. These topics are often complicated, requiring complex involvement to put the many different pieces together in practical formats.

So now that we've discussed these many facets on these topics, the next question might be, "What do we do about improving these issues for human health?"

And that brings us to the topic of the Architectural Doctor, and the systems required to help support and facilitate this process.

The Architectural Doctor – a HyBridge Profession

The ideal of the Architectural Doctor is a professional that is well versed in both the architecture and medicine fields, which can help be a liaison to bridge these two fields.

I call this a HyBridge, as it's combining a *hybrid* model and a *bridge* to connect these two fields. Essentially, the Architectural Doctor is there to help support the integrations between the architecture and medical professionals, with the overall goal to support the health of the general public.

And as all professions require systems, the Architectural Doctor needs this to best support these integrations.

What Systems Would Be Required for These Integrations?

The first and foremost is that doctors and health professionals do not typically consider the built environment in patient health.

And the fact that many people are spending up to 90 percent of their lives indoors, it's a topic that must be addressed if core issues of health and wellness are to be found and corrected. It then leads to the questions of solutions for health created in the built environment.

It requires systems to be created and the recognition of building issues that are related to health evaluations.

To make this complex discussion easier to represent, the following is a flowchart that provides more insights into this process. It includes the steps taken and the involvement of each professional, including the Architectural Doctor.

The first flowchart is the entire diagram as an overview of the complete Architectural Medicine System (AMS) process. The text of the entire chart is extremely small on this version, yet the following graphics provide larger views of the flowchart. After the graphics, there is a link to the Architectural Medicine website to view the entire flowchart online.

Chapter: 15 The Architectural Doctor

The Architectural Medicine System (AMS) Flowchart

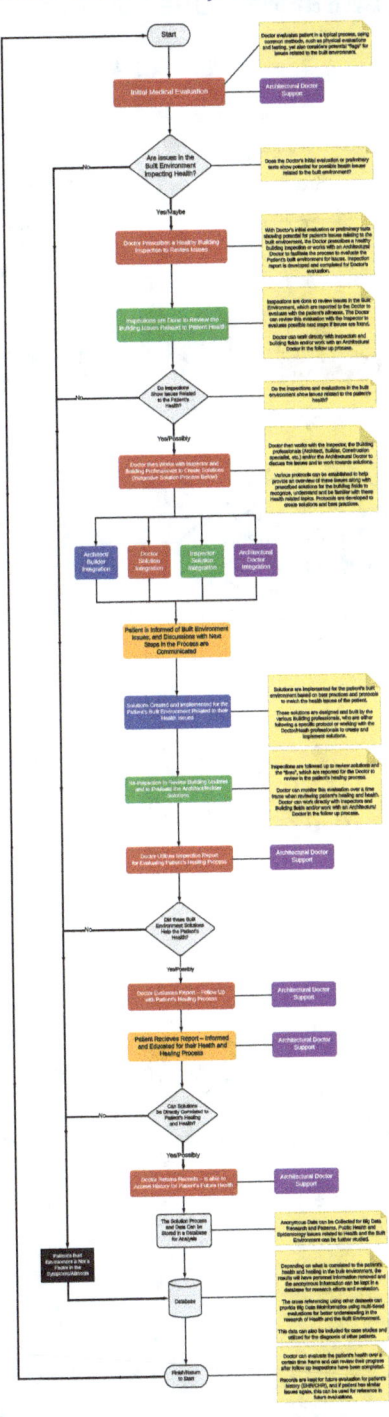

191

Architectural Medicine – Building the Bridge to Wellness

The Architectural Medicine System (AMS) Flowchart
Part 1 of 4

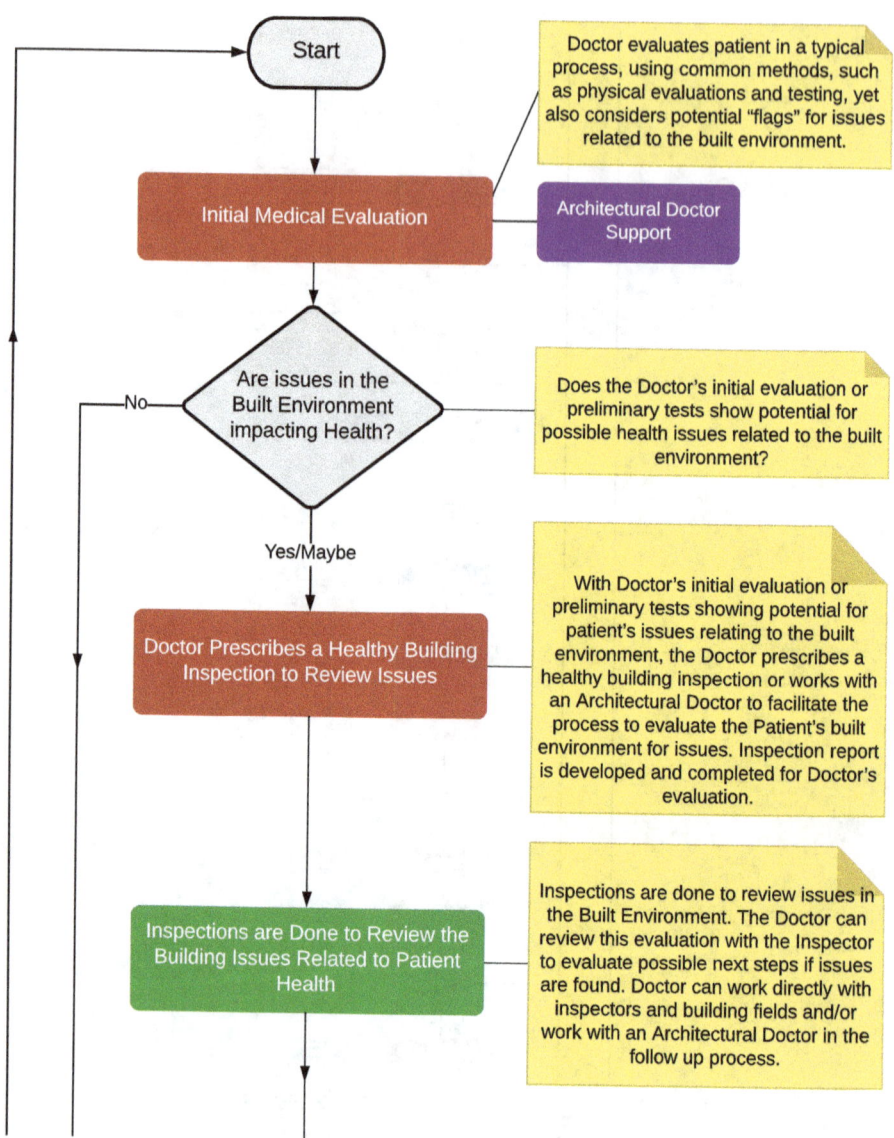

Chapter: 15 — The Architectural Doctor

The Architectural Medicine System (AMS) Flowchart
Part 2 of 4

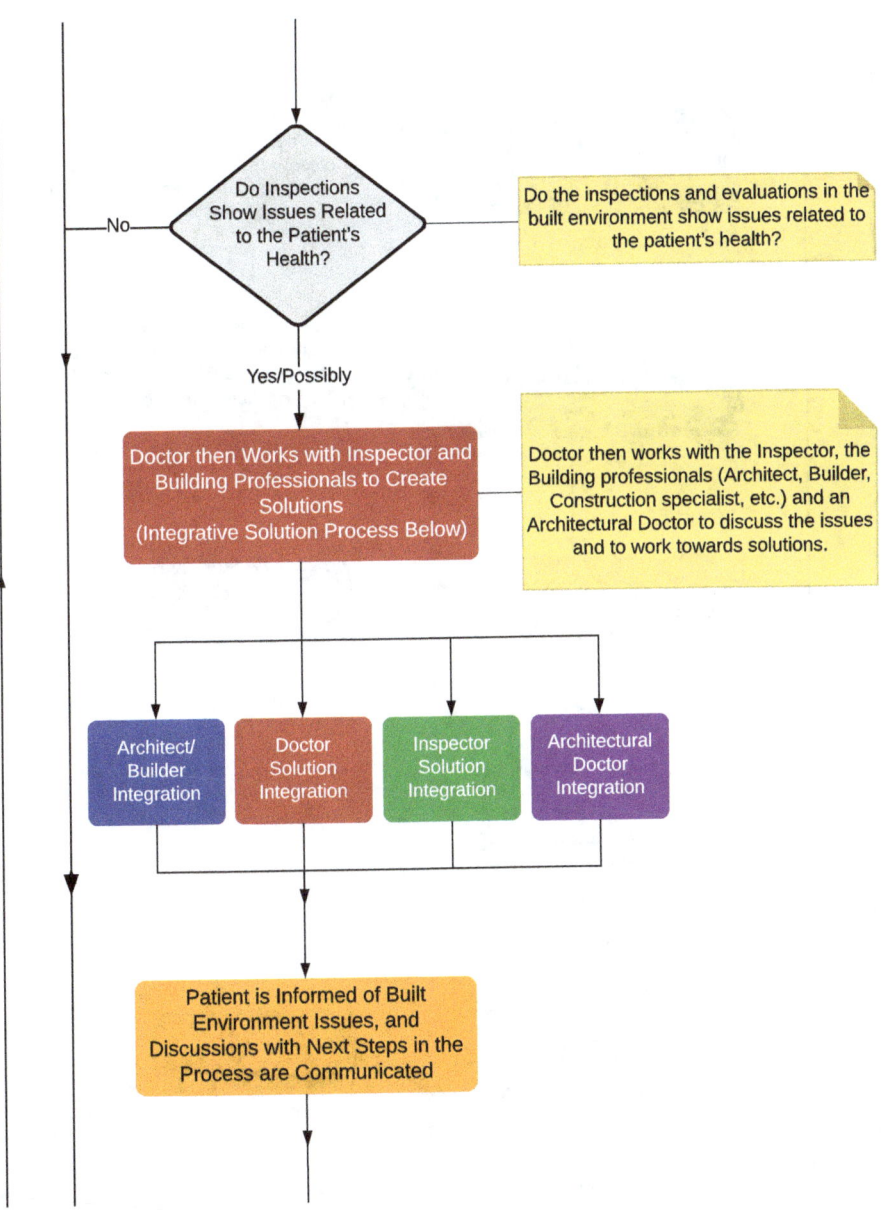

Architectural Medicine – Building the Bridge to Wellness

The Architectural Medicine System (AMS) Flowchart
Part 3 of 4

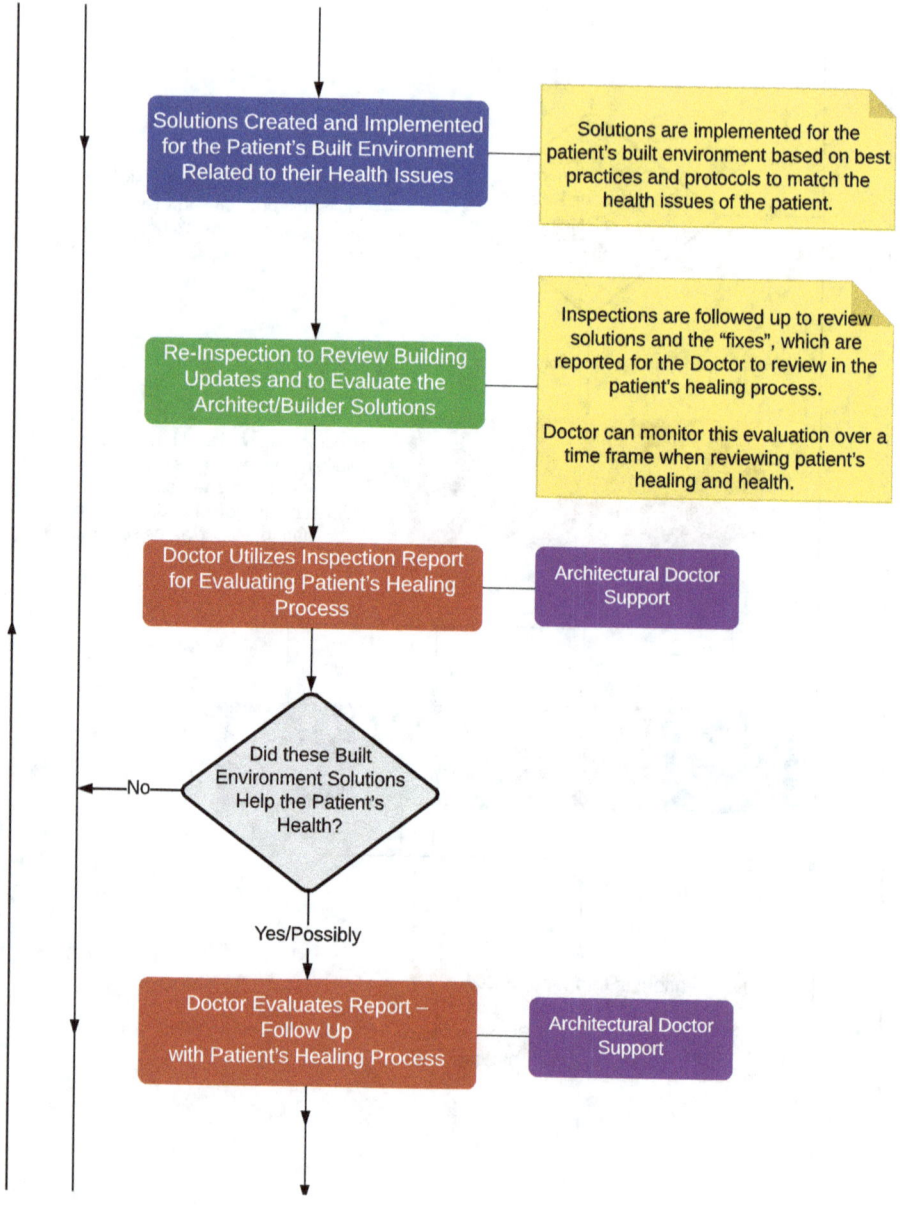

The Architectural Medicine System (AMS) Flowchart

Part 4 of 4

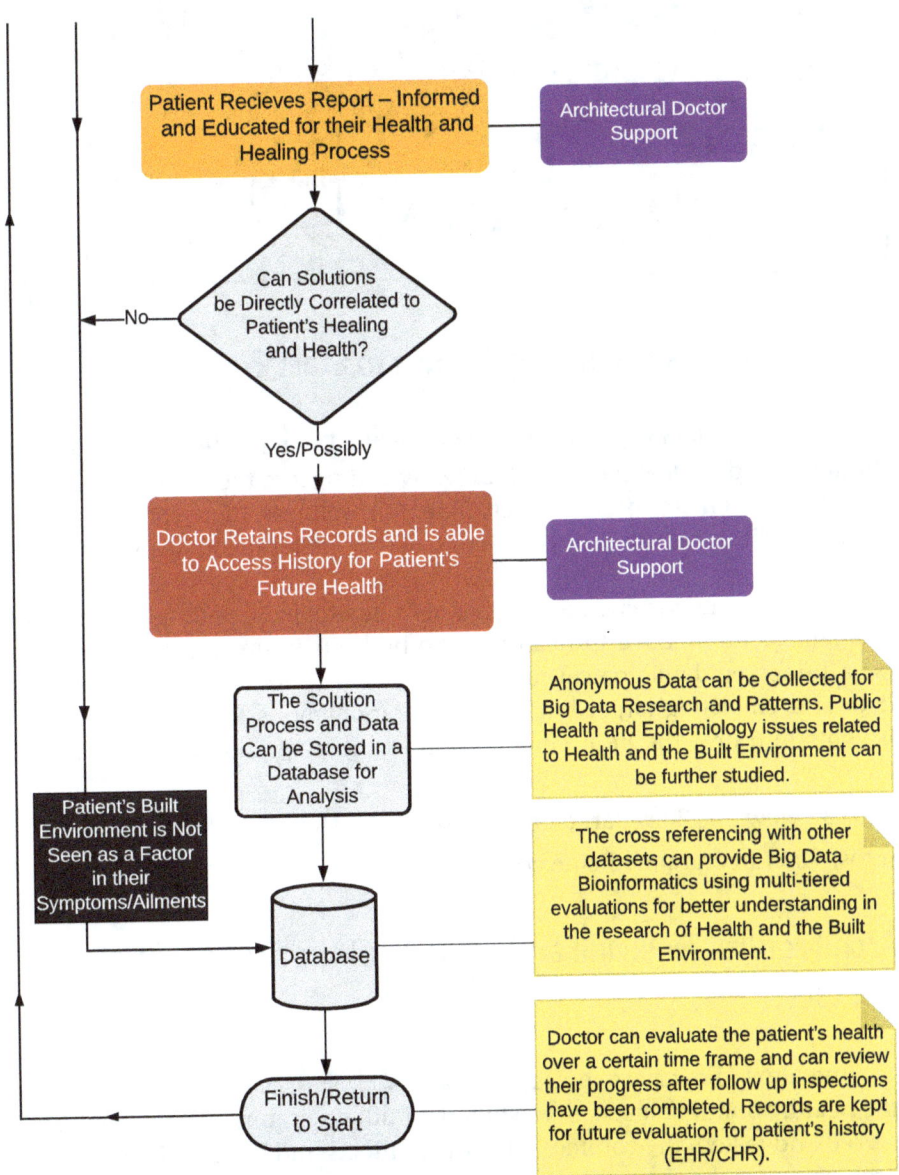

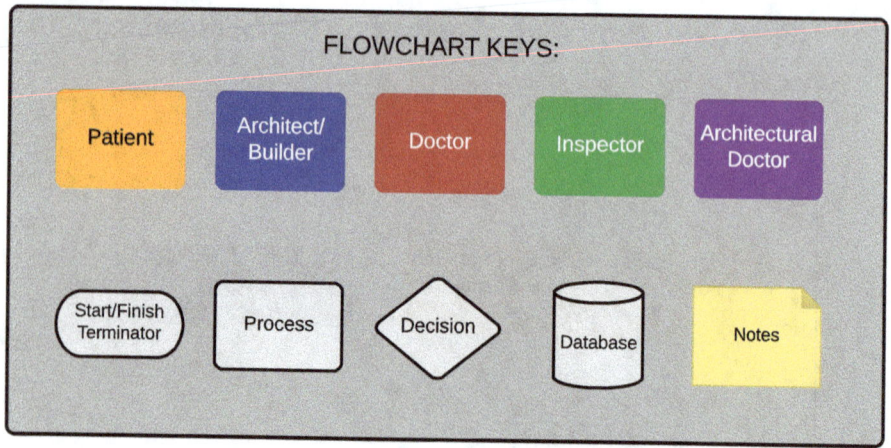

Why Is the Finish Listed as "Return to Start"?

Health is a lifelong process, and as such, the Doctor-Patient connection is about evaluating Health over a lifetime. By adding into the "health equation" how the built environment impacts illness or wellness, there can be a better understanding and, subsequently, control over better health over a lifetime.

In addition to the focus on the individual's health, by providing metrics and evaluating data relative to health in the built environment, there can also be a better epidemiological and public health understanding. Using big data and collecting larger datasets in an anonymous format, can provide insights into how the built environment can impact and influence Health.

You can view this flowchart on our website at the following link: https://architecturalmedicine.com/book/

Architectural Medicine and the Role of the Architectural Doctor

The above flowchart shows the doctors' processes evaluating ailments, the healthy building inspection when the built environment needs to be assessed and tested, the connection with architects and builders in evaluating problems, and the prescriptions or an Rx as recipes for healthier architecture for solutions. The overall structure of this process recognizes the importance of whole systems solutions.

During this entire process, the Architectural Doctor can help support the system itself and can also be there to support each professional. By having these integrated steps, the doctor can include building issues in their patient's evaluations and work with the inspector and building professionals to provide solutions.

As these are complex processes, there are two additional facets to support this workflow. The Architectural Medicine System (AMS) and the Architectural Medicine Software Solution – ARxMD, offer two options to help facilitate these goals. In the following chapters, I will reference each of these subjects, and I will go into more detail on each of these topics in chapters 16 and 18.

The Architectural Doctor can also help define ailments connected to the built environment and the doctor's evaluations in their analysis. This process will also be new for each professional and profession. As the standard systems are often a form of a hierarchical structure, another change will include new methods requiring nodal systems for best solutions.

This new system of integrating architects and doctors with inspectors and building professionals to create healthier built environments can help ensure that each facet of these developments is interconnected for positive results.

Both architects and doctors have a substantial role in working independently to support the best health and wellness through buildings and medical support, respectively. Yet is there anything else that these two professions and groups can create for healthier built environments?

This question brings up the topic mentioned previously, which are the hierarchical and nodal systems. In a later section in this chapter, I will discuss this nodal system in more detail. It is an important topic to define, as the Architectural Doctor's role and this new Architectural Medicine System (AMS) requires new methods and new mindsets in these professions collaborating together.

The Architectural Medicine Flowchart – Steps Involved in Bringing It All Together

Supporting the Connections Between the Doctors, Inspectors, Architects, and Builders:

The above flowchart provides new systems and new workflows involving multiple groups. While flowcharts are often an if-then procedure of decisions that lead to a linear path, the successful iteration of these steps will need to be more cyclical, as mentioned earlier in the book. I define this as a spiracycle, leading towards successful iterations that can continue to develop and improve over time in an upward, positive movement. The steps below outline the basic workflow of this flow chart process:

- Doctor evaluation
- Inspection prescribed
- Inspection reported to Doctor
- Discussions of building issues with Architecture/Building professionals
- Building issues and solutions discussed with the Patient
- Building solutions created
- Building solutions implemented
- Re-Inspection performed and reported to Doctor
- Re-evaluation of health issues for Patient included over time

This cycle is shown in the diagram below:

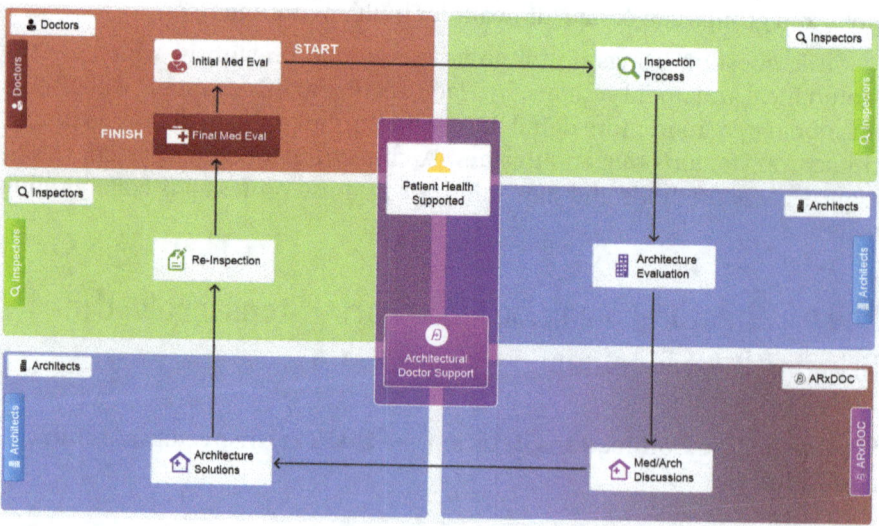

It's important to note that the Architectural Doctor can be involved to support each of these steps appropriately, as can be seen in the graphic. And in the next section, I'll discuss more details on these roles of the Architectural Doctor.

The Architectural Doctor – Health, Healing, and Medicine

In Chapter 4, the definition of medicine and healing was outlined, which I'd like to revisit:

medicine (n.)

c. 1200, "medical treatment, cure, remedy," also used figuratively, of spiritual remedies, from Old French medecine (Modern French médicine) "medicine, art of healing, cure, treatment, potion," from Latin medicina "the healing art, medicine; a remedy," also used figuratively, perhaps originally ars medicina "the medical art," from fem. of medicinus (adj.) "of a doctor," from medicus "a physician" (from PIE root *med- "take appropriate measures.[133]

healing (n.)

"restoration to health," Old English hæling, verbal noun from heal (v.). Figurative sense of "restoration of wholeness" is from early 13c.; meaning "touch that cures" is from 1670s.[134]

heal (v.)

Old English hælan "cure; save; make whole, sound and well," from Proto-Germanic *hailjan (source also of Old Saxon helian, Old Norse heila, Old Frisian hela, Dutch helen, German heilen, Gothic ga-hailjan "to heal, cure"), literally "to make whole," from PIE *kailo- "whole" (see health). Intransitive sense from late 14c. Related: Healed; healing.[135]

health (n.)

Old English hælþ "wholeness, a being whole, sound or well," from Proto-Germanic *hailitho, from PIE *kailo- "whole, uninjured, of good omen" (source also of Old English hal "hale, whole;" Old Norse heill "healthy;" Old English halig, Old Norse helge "holy, sacred;" Old English hælan "to heal"). With Proto-Germanic abstract noun suffix *-itho (see -th (2)). Of physical health in Middle English, but also "prosperity, happiness, welfare; preservation, safety."[136]

As *medicine* is defined in the Oxford dictionary as "the science or practice of the diagnosis, treatment, and prevention of disease," it also focuses on "a substance or preparation used in the treatment of illness."[137]

While many associate a drug as a treatment, if you view how the exterior environment impacts your interior environment or your internal health, you might begin to see how important the state of the external environment affects your health.

And this is not only a factor for maintaining good health, but for healing and wellness. The Architectural Doctor can utilize this process to focus on health and healing in an extended level, which includes the built environment in this complex equation.

By analyzing the built environment, such as physical components that may be causing health issues, and form factors that could also impact emotional and mental wellness, there can be many other variables added into the analysis that can improve health.

When these facets are revealed and addressed, the "medicine" component of architecture can be seen as an essential component for the patient's health and healing and the health of the general public.

This adds an entirely new set of factors into the medical evaluation that has either not existed previously or has only been a small portion of the doctor's analysis and solution process. Topics such as Social Determinants of Health (SDoH) can also be included as part of the doctor's analysis and included in the overall scope of the patient's health.

The Architectural Doctor can support these steps to add social determinants of health into actionable items to be included in both the patient's analysis and for potential solutions.

A New Systems Approach – Connecting Architecture and Medicine

A big part of this book that makes it a bit different from other writing about the healthy built environment is what I've learned in terms of why these concepts and processes don't already exist in the world of building and health.

A big part of this, in my opinion, is that there are very few systems that are in place to achieve these goals. If you follow the latest research on health in the built environment, you will find there is an increasing depth of information defining issues that can provide positive benefits for health professionals in supporting the best health for their patients.

Why haven't these topics become more common, and why haven't the professions integrated this knowledge into their work sooner?

My opinion and experience in these fields are that the current knowledge is scattered, and there are very few systems in place to complete the cycle and processes required to support the end goals. How this research can be applied in a practical format for the medical and architecture fields has been unclear.

The idea of a healthy oriented building inspection and a healthy building or environmental consultant is not new. As discussed in other sections of this book, there are now four to five decades that these have been in existence in some form or another.

What's meant by this is that in terms of doctors and architects having a system in place, akin to say, the process of ordering a blood test or MRI, is practically non-existent. Even if a doctor were to evaluate a patient's condition and see possible connections to the built environment, what would a doctor do about this?

Or suppose you view an architect working with an engineer to review design specifications. In this case, a process and system is in place that allows the architect to proceed with proper analysis and receive the requested results from the engineers. In this manner, the architect is familiar with the systems to work with the engineer and vice versa.

There are systems in place for both professions that allow them to know what the procedures are and proceed with evaluations, from lab testing to engineering evaluations for the doctor and architect.

These procedures, along with the learning processes in school and continuing professional education, have allowed developments to evolve in architecture and medicine.

However, when it comes to health topics related to the built environment, most doctors are not trained nor educated on what to look for. This includes potential red flags and even what to do if the built environment might be the cause of symptoms or conditions.

As well, the architecture field is not trained nor educated about health topics, and even less aware of building processes and materials that may cause health issues and how to resolve such problems.

While there may be a focus on physical building materials and topics such as mold and indoor air quality, other issues are related to health, such as noise and a lack of natural lighting. In the discussions mentioned previously about environmental psychology and neuroscience in architecture, these topics should also include the shapes, forms, and colors in a structure. All of these topics have impacts on physical, mental, and emotional health and well being.

An architect must be aware of these topics and include them in the overall design process, just as ergonomics and anthropometrics are factored into the design equation.

Many gaps exist for each profession, and the most significant gap is probably the lack of systems in place where a doctor can work with an architect and those in the building professions, and vice versa. This lack of systems, lack of education, and training have led to these topics being more conceptual than actionable.

An essential part of Architectural Medicine and the Architectural Doctor is to support these systems, both in terms of education, teaching, and knowledge, in providing these systems. This can support the doctor and architect to work together and utilize this knowledge in their professions. These integrated systems can provide bridges that allow for collaboration.

It is also critical that the many other professionals involved become part of the system, such as a healthy building inspector, where an inspector is trained to look for structural issues in the building and issues related to health. These inspectors are critical in working with the doctors and architects to evaluate and resolve building issues associated with occupant health.

The Healthy Building Inspector as a Key Integrator in This Process

The Healthy Building Inspector is a key integrator in this process and would act as an important piece of the puzzle. Providing the doctor with laboratory results of their evaluations and providing reports for the architect and building professionals support the necessary components for a successful solution process. I go into more details about this role in chapter 17.

Yet, there are still many other professionals, from epidemiologists, toxicologists, and those involved in public health to those in the design and manufacturing of materials. This includes emerging fields such as green chemistry. Each of these professionals can participate in providing a collaborative process for cohesive solutions. They would add their knowledge and research to the list of best practices, yet only if there are sound systems in place to provide this information and expertise in multi-disciplinary formats.

Recipes for Better Health – The New Rx

If you are a medical professional, you're aware that the pharmacist's abbreviation of Rx is the shortened term for the word Recipe.[138] This becomes interesting when this symbol is used to define a recipe as a prescription or Rx for a healthier built environment.

The combination of professionals working together with increasing public awareness to support their health and wellness can produce a demand for professionals to provide solutions.

And these results require an integrated approach and process, from the example in the flow chart of the procedures to the information, education, and training necessary to fulfill these round trip, whole system solutions.

If these systems as prescriptions or an Rx can be put into place and utilized, then the collective collaboration could have a substantial positive impact on well being for public health in the built environment. The synergistic effect this could have on the built environment, focusing on health and wellness, could support a better life for growing populations in current and future contexts.

In Terms of Integrations – What Is Missing?

At this point, there may be questions as to these integrations – questions as to exactly how there can be connections between these two professionals.

At this time, what is missing is a system and an approach that allows the many different professionals to work together in a collaborative format. The Architectural Doctor can help bridge these connections as a liaison to support integrative solutions.

For example, while current building inspectors are trained to evaluate the building's structural integrity, there are currently little to no evaluations completed relative to health.

But why not?

If a doctor were to learn or suspect that a patient's health condition might be caused or conflated by a built environment issue, how would they even know this? And what would a doctor even do if this was suspected?

In our modern-day medicine era, the doctor will commonly have testing requested, from blood work and X-rays to MRIs and other lab tests for analysis. Yet currently, the doctor has no way to order a lab test of their patient's built environment for analysis to review for their patient's health — yet why not?

After all, the average person in the modern world can spend up to 90 percent of their time inside. If there are health issues caused or made worse by some form of contaminant or health issue, how would the doctor even know this? In particular, chronic conditions might benefit from such evaluations, as this could provide greater insight into why these conditions are perpetuating in the patient's health. And topics in the built environment causing stress could be the root of many underlying physiological conditions.

However, currently, there are no building inspection tests that a doctor can request at this time. And even if they did, what would be their ordering process, and who would they be requesting to provide these inspections and reporting?

And this is one of the largest gaps in today's modern world of building, which both Architectural Medicine and the Architectural Doctor strive to bridge.

This bridging requires that the current building inspector either includes in their evaluations or have new professionals for the process of evaluating buildings relative to human health topics. This education process, training, and working with doctors and health professionals would be brand new to the building inspector professionals, yet would be a requirement for such analysis.

While this bridges one-half of the connection between doctors and the built environment, there is also the other half – the architects, builders, and the fields related to architecture.

Currently, few architects would even know the requirements in providing solutions to issues found in these healthy building inspections. And if the doctor considers the reports from the healthy building inspector showing building issues, the current doctor will not just call up an architect to help them and their patient resolve such matters.

These procedures also require the education and training of the architecture professionals, who would be adequately equipped to understand such issues and prepared to design solutions for these building problems.

And this again is where the Architectural Doctor can help connect the doctor, the architect, and the healthy building inspectors in these evaluations and solutions.

The Architectural Doctor is versed in both the architecture and medical fields, enough to understand the concepts and nomenclature, yet would not necessarily be a doctor or architect. These two professions are amongst the most demanding of jobs, and to master both would likely be outside the scope of one person to master.

Yet, the Architectural Doctor would learn enough of these two professions to converse and understand the overall concepts to help integrate the crucial facets of the healthy building inspection.

This process has unveiled many gaps that currently exist and provides some big picture concepts that would ideally be developed moving forward with these connections.

In review, there would be a requirement for a new group of professionals as Healthy Building Inspectors. Along with this new group, the need for education and training for the doctors, architects, and these new Healthy Building Inspectors would be required. This would provide specific instructions for each professional to understand the whole picture while being well versed in their particular portion of this puzzle.

ARxMD Procedures – New Standards and Protocols

The next steps in this process would require some basic standards and protocols. In the same manner that a doctor requests a lab test for blood work or an MRI, there are processes and procedures that are known and followed. These procedures would also have to be created for the doctor to recognize issues based on the patient's condition. Then the doctor would have to request an inspection to be undertaken by the Healthy Building Inspectors.

And then, once there are issues found, the next step would be for the doctor to contact the architects and building professionals to request a process of evaluation, with solutions provided to fix any building issues.

This means that the architects and builders would also have to be educated and trained on such issues to understand how to resolve them.

While there is a recognition between the health and building professionals on topics such as dangerous mold and overlap with respiratory problems relative to asbestos, the interconnections between doctors and architects are limited.

The only other place where these two professionals may have experience working together is in hospital design. In the past 10 to 15 years, designing and developing healthy hospitals has been on the rise.

Yet while these two professions may have experience in hospital design, the issue of requesting a healthy building inspection and providing evaluations and solutions is new for most. Requests to architects and builders for resolving such health issues are not very common or known by most clinical doctors or health professionals.

This is already a lot to digest, yet there is one final topic to include in this development for best practices in achieving these integrated goals. And that is to have best practices and systems that are defined and implemented between these fields. This would allow the doctor to request an inspection, an inspector can provide testing and reporting, and then this information can be appropriately communicated to the architects and building professionals to provide solutions.

These new methods can be supported using ARxMD procedures, using either new standards and protocols or utilizing existing standards as appropriate. ARxMD (pronounced arcs-med) is the Architectural Medicine Software Solution's name and the procedures used by this solution to achieve these goals. These standards can define new protocols or can use current standards that fit these solutions. From SNOMED, ICD, and DSM to the ISO, OSHA, and IFC standards, a number of organizations already have defined standards for the fields of architecture and medicine. The essential part of this process is to help ascertain standards to fit as appropriate, and when there are new standards needed, the ARxMD methods and protocols can be included.

Integrating the Fields of Architecture and Medicine

One crucial question might present itself when contemplating the procedures of integrating the fields of architecture and medicine. And that question is based on how the Architectural Doctor can help to support these connections.

When you view the flowchart listed earlier in this chapter, essential connections need to be created and developed to achieve these steps.

The role of the Architectural Doctor is not merely an additional professional involved in these procedures. They help to interconnect independent professions into interdependent partners to provide these solutions within very complex systems.

And to achieve these integrations, some critical structural methods need to be reviewed to have successful systems moving forward. This includes the adoption of new methods that are more nodal in origin and less hierarchical. To prevent confusion on this topic, let's discuss exactly what is meant by this comment of "nodal" systems.

The Tree Analogy – From Silos to Nodal Integrators

To discuss the topic of the Architectural Doctor and how Architectural Medicine can be a bridge between these two fields for wellness, the nodal integration method can help provide more context. Some of the challenges that prevent existing integrations are professionals that function in a silo. And as this analogy of the metaphorical silo is discussed, it requires a bit of an adaptation.

The silo concept, if one is not familiar with this terminology, is often used to describe professionals that are so focused on one facet of work or a particular granular topic, that it is akin to them being in a large farm silo. A farm silo is a tall vertical structure with no windows, typically used to store grains and harvested crops. It is designed specifically to keep all of the grains or crops in the enclosure with no exposure to the exterior.

Therefore, one who is described as living in a silo is seeing only what they are working on and nothing else, or one who does not integrate with the outside world.

This type of silo view or lack of integration with anything outside of their scope can be why those whose research reaches deep into the topics related to health in the built environment can lack the light of day to provide such information available to the building and health professionals.

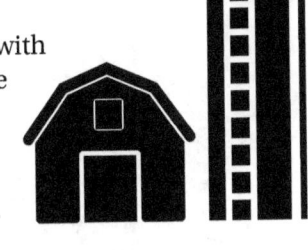

Farmhouse with Silo

However, in moving forward on this topic, I'd like to propose these silos be replaced with another analogy: a *tree* and *nodal* or *neural networks*. This might sound strange to combine a tree analogy with a neural network, yet let me explain this in more detail.

If you look at the components of a tree, consisting of the roots, the tree trunk or stem, and then the branches as the graphic demonstrates, you can recognize these three main parts.

Now, if you take the concept of the silo and exchange this analogy for the roots of a tree, you might see that they have similar characteristics. The silo is an enclosed, separated space where there is no exterior input or exchanges. The person existing in this proverbial silo focuses in-depth on one facet of the whole picture. The roots of a tree can also utilize this same analogy, where they are literally in the ground and cannot see anywhere outside of the single root that they exist within. The root is also digging deeper in-depth and providing more resources to the subject or topic of their focus, so again the analogy fits.

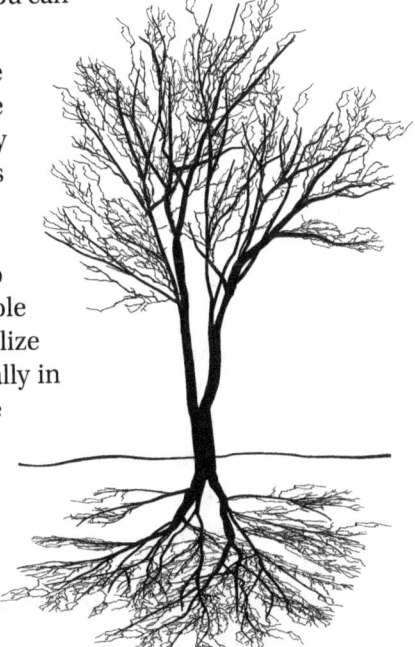

Continue the analogy and view the branches as those professionals that are either actively involved in utilizing these research concepts or developing the end products of this research. You can see the value that the examination of the roots can provide. The branches can often be those generalists taking the research and development and putting this into practice. They are out in the world for all to see and put this research into practical application.

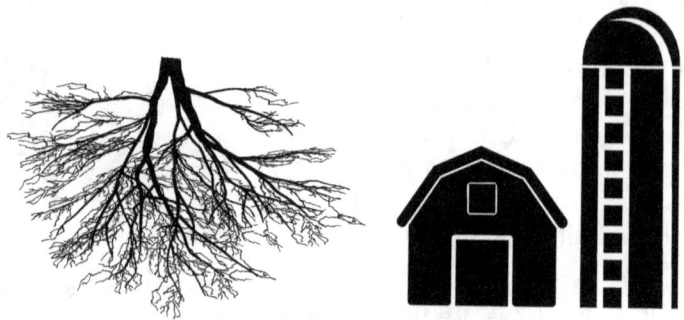

When viewed in this format, you can see that the remainder of the tree is the trunk.

For a tree, the trunk's purpose is to be the conduit and provide integration between the roots and branches. They support the branches and act as a liaison between the roots and the branches. The trunk or stems of trees and plants are there to bring the required nutrients to the branches. Both the roots and the trunk support the branches, which bear fruit and propagate their unique qualities of the tree. Trees and plants also provide photosynthesis through their leaves as energy creation for the entire tree, so the branches send their benefits to the rest of the tree by means of the trunk. The analogy is a symbiotic nature that provides mutual benefit for the entire organism.

While the roots support the branches and the branches also support the roots, many ignore the trunk's essential roles in connecting these two components. In this manner, this tree analogy can also be used in the professional world as well.

As the researchers, the roots can be seen as these proverbial silos, where they dig deep into their own specific field of study and do not see anything else outside of their scope. The tree analogy can provide a better image of this, as anyone knows that the roots cannot view outside of their realm due to the surrounding ground.

As well, the analogy of the branches can often be seen as those who utilize the benefits of this research, such as those in practice as architects and doctors, yet perhaps are not as connected to these deep roots of research.

However, how do these various professionals and this valuable information become connected? How does the roots' research become integrated into the branches' analogy as practicing professionals?

And this is where the analogy comes into full scope. The trunk integrates the many specialists or the roots, with multi-disciplinary knowledge that can parse this information and provide this to the practicing professionals. The integration provided by the trunk or stem is often left out of the equation, resulting in gaps and missing connections.

The Architectural Doctor can provide these liaisons between the architecture and medical fields and the many other facets in these processes, akin to connecting the roots and the branches.

However, in today's modern-day world, these integrators rarely exist to provide such multi-disciplinary knowledge to provide integration as a whole between these two fields. Architectural Medicine recognizes many gaps between architecture and medicine and strives to help bridge these gaps that this tree analogy describes. The results are better systems provided between each field, and this is where the Architectural Doctor becomes paramount.

Silos, Branches, and the Neural Network Model

These branches in both architecture and medicine include the many fields and subfields related to these topics. When you take this separate model of the silo, and reimagine this as a root system of a tree, the visualization can morph into another model defining interconnection as that of nodal neural networks.

If you start with each profession's single topic as a line that branches out into a broader expansion of topics, this image can be seen as the many different facets and professionals involved in these expansive topics of both architecture and medicine.

The key and challenge is to bring these branches back inward and merge these branches back into focus. This can then return to a single branch or a

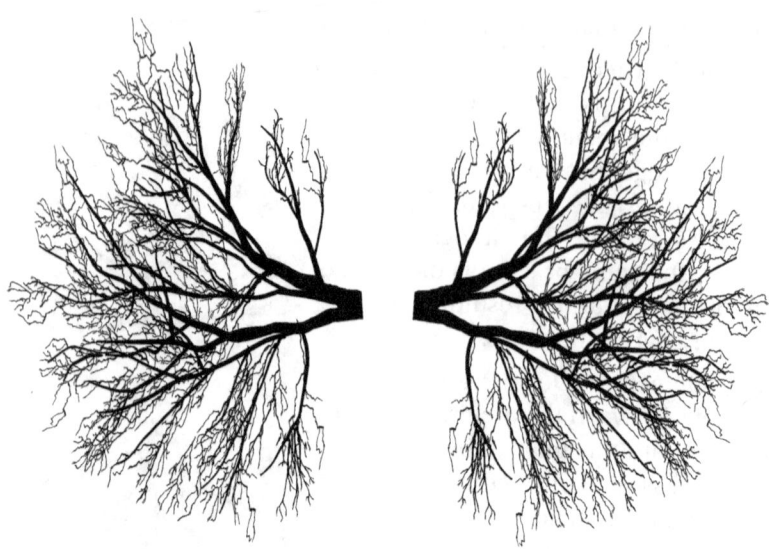

focus that can be discussed without feeling there is a chaotic, disconnected processing that leads to no direction.

If left in this manner, the branching continues to infinity and then leaves a fizzling out effect that just slowly fades away and ends. This leads to information overload or a lack of any valuable knowledge to be implemented.

But if the branching can come back together, to weave and merge these concepts back into a more cohesive understanding, the results can be connectivity and the sharing of complex information.

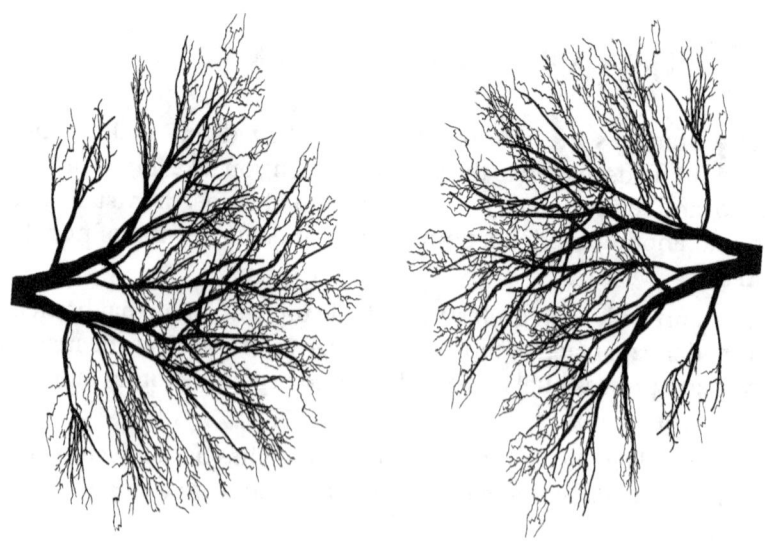

Utilizing the contents from all of these various relevant branches can bring something of substance into an actionable construct. This connection can bring these branches back into a whole. There can then be a better understanding that takes the branching chaos into meaningful information that is manageable, understandable, and usable.

If this were to be seen visually, it might look something like this, which can be viewed as a tree branch merging into the roots or integrating two complex nodes:

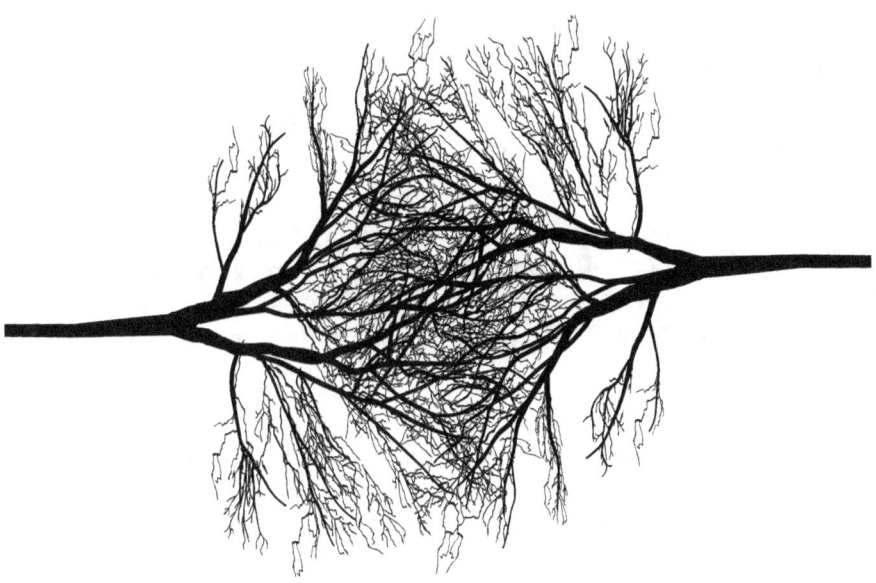

You can then have these concepts and topics branch out and then merge back to a solid idea, much like this integration of the branches merging into the root systems. So, the process begins on one side and then branches out into more facets, yet merges with another complex group.

The other facet is that when these two groups or concepts come together, it also looks like neurons and nerves of the nervous system and many other systems of the body that connect from the macro scale to the micro level.

Perhaps this same process as a visual can be an example of a complex thought process branching out and then entering into a more integrated concept. This visual can define each of these fields' complex developments, and the Architectural Doctor and Architectural Medicine can support these complex subjects to be formulated into manageable and usable processes.

Anastomosis

An example of this interconnectivity can be found in nature called anastomosis.

Anastomosis is the union of branches to intercommunicate or interconnect. The diagram of the tree as an integrator between the root systems and the branches can be utilized to define and describe this interconnectivity between architecture and medicine professionals in a bridging format.

anastomosis (n.)

1: the union of parts or branches (as of streams, blood vessels, or leaf veins) so as to intercommunicate or interconnect

2: a product of anastomosis : Network[139]

in anatomy, "union or intercommunication of the vessels of one system with those of another," 1610s, medical Latin, from Greek anastomosis "outlet, opening," from anastomoein "to open, discharge" (as one sea into another), "to furnish with a mouth," from ana "again, anew" (see ana-) + stoma "mouth" (see stoma).[140]

This connecting between "two vessels, channels, or distinct branches of any kind, by a connecting cross branch" can be used as an example of how these professions can connect and provide literal bridges to gaps and divides between these fields.

The Architectural Doctor is a multi-disciplinary integrator that can help bridge these complex topics between the architecture and medical professionals and help support a process to review, evaluate, and find solutions to many built environment issues impacting health.

They can do so by providing deep-rooted research on these health topics in the built environment and providing practical use of this knowledge for all groups to utilize.

In reviewing the original definition of anastomosis, there are essential functions that these natural processes have that can define these integrations. It was initially defined as "the cross communications between the arteries and veins, or other canals in the animal body; whence to similar cross connections in the sap-vessels of plants, and between rivers or their branches; and now to cross connexions between the separate lines of any branching system, as the branches of trees, the veins of leaves, or the wings of insects."[141]

The Architectural Doctor – Providing Integrative Solutions

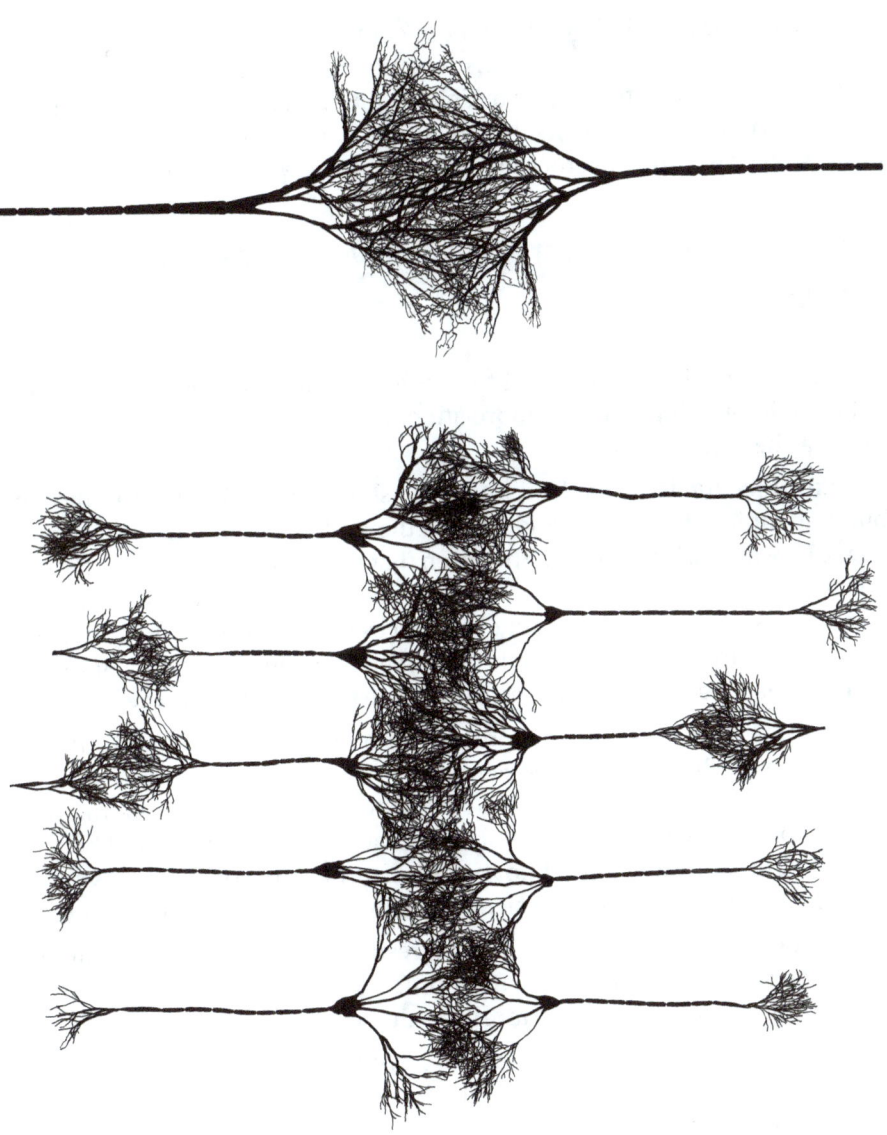

Connecting the Fields of Architecture and Medicine as Nodes in a Neural Network

The Architectural Doctor's purpose is to help support the integration between the doctors and the architects and to increase interconnections between these fields.

This analogy can help provide more context to this new nodal format of working between these professions and providing supportive functionality for both fields. The integrative workings of the Architectural Doctor can be a healthy format for future work, both with this profession and the many other professionals working together to create collaborative solutions.

The Architectural Doctor and the Novel Coronavirus Pandemic

During this time of 2020 and the novel coronavirus pandemic, the topic of health in buildings has had more attention focused on health in buildings than has been in decades.

Not since the issues of lead in paint, asbestos in buildings, and the sick building topics of the 1970s and 80s has the built environment been in such focus. However, a big difference between that time and now is that, back then, mostly, it was a focus on specific building topics. In contrast to today, the subject is focused on people's direct experiences with building issues. And this, combined with the fact that people have been following the Stay at Home initiatives, has made people focus on their living places more than ever.

In some ways, this is a good process for people to contemplate. After all, changes in the building processes require a demand from the general public. And yet, this pandemic has also been extremely challenging for many, as depression and lack of social contact have caused added stress. And being in built environments that might not be as nurturing and comforting as people need, has caused an even more significant increase in stress and anxiety.

As society looks to re-open schools, restaurants, and business buildings of all types, perhaps this connection to health and the built environment's evaluation can become more critically evaluated.

We should have greater abilities to have these buildings inspected and tested, and provide communications between the health and building professionals to achieve these goals.

Can the current coronavirus and the lack of testing be akin to the doctor evaluating health issues without proper tests in the built environment? If the doctor cannot review contaminants that might exist in the built environment negatively impacting human health, how can they provide the best analysis for patient health?

Can this be connected to the importance of systems in providing testing and focusing on the healthy building inspection?

If this pandemic can teach humans anything about the built environment, it should be the increasing impact that buildings have on health and wellness. And not just physical wellness, but mental and emotional well being. It is my hope that the great suffering during his pandemic can provide more significant insights into the human experience and promote better architectural solutions moving forward.

Introduction to the Architectural Medicine Software Solution – ARxMD

As the Architectural Medicine System (AMS) has highlighted the importance of systems, there is another facet of this development to help in this progression.

These new systems would ideally require a type of software system to help the doctor request inspections, inspectors to record testing, the doctor to review and analyze the results, and then subsequent information sent to the architect and building professional to provide solutions.

This software is something that I have been thinking about since 1999. After spending many years contemplating such a solution, the development began and now exists as the Architectural Medicine Software Solution – ARxMD.

This software allows each professional to log in to their dashboard, provide a process to evaluate with guides and protocols, and then assess their piece of the puzzle for best results.

An essential key to this whole process has not yet been adequately discussed, at least in the importance that it merits, and that is the "Patient."

Most of the time, the patient has been ignored by many professionals, with a focus on their work and important processes even if they are related to the patient. Yet, in my opinion, there is no greater focus and attention than to make sure the patient is supported and adequately informed throughout the entire process. Each professional should be helping them to better understand the steps that are taken for solutions.

After all, the whole purpose of this is to create healthier built environments for the occupants, not just to have a process of evaluation to do so without an end goal. The goal is to provide a solution for the patient and provide a healthier built environment to prevent disease and illness and offer solutions for wellness.

Architectural Medicine's whole purpose is to provide a bridge between these professionals to benefit the occupants and society at large. Otherwise, these are just systems in place for the professionals.

Another purpose of the Architectural Doctor is to help the patient navigate these steps and keep them informed and educated for their benefit. They can also help guide them through the process of inspections, evaluations, and potential building changes for solutions.

And because the Architectural Doctor is well versed in each profession, they have the knowledge required to help guide the patient through the process to become educated and informed on these issues and the solution process.

This is one of the critical differences between Architectural Medicine and the Architectural Doctor in reference to other fields discussing the topics of healthy building. As mentioned in other sections of this book, the goal is not to replace these various fields, yet to help integrate the knowledge and processes that are either available or potentially linked to creating a better understanding of health issues in a building.

This is why Architectural Medicine strives to connect the many fields, from biophilia and epidemiology to environmental psychology and neuroscience in architecture.

These fields have valuable information that can help provide a better understanding of the built environment and provide integrations with the many pieces involved in the puzzle. Architectural Medicine strives to put these pieces together to complete the cohesive whole and bridge the gaps to provide solutions where required. The idea of integrating doctors with healthy building inspectors and then working with architects and builders to create solutions is where Architectural Medicine sees opportunities to provide solutions.

The graphics of the nodal and neural networks shown above can provide visual examples of these facets and combine all of this information in a contextually relevant reference, which can be a powerful and supportive system for health and wellness.

The Architectural Doctor and Next Steps

These systems support the more common philosophy in today's day and age, where professionals are more open to collaboration. Professionals are becoming more familiar with multi-disciplinary processes.

The Architectural Doctor's role is one such multi-disciplinary process and has at its core an integrated approach to be knowledgeable about the architecture and medical professions. These new professionals will have an inherent interest in working together to support each of these professions and create positive results for the patient and the population.

This supportive approach can also be essential to help connect the various professions involved in each project. And their help can support the process by allowing each professional to achieve their work while ensuring the other professionals are aware of this work and how these processes may have overlap.

It is critical to have this understanding and knowledge as an Architectural Doctor, especially as these methods are new to other professions involved, helping to provide guidance and support.

The result is professionals that can work together focusing on their specific role while providing an overview for the patient with knowledge of all events. This collaboration can achieve the goals of better health and wellness for the patient and society at large.

By including public health professionals such as epidemiologists and toxicologists into the equation and adding the building professions, trades, and product developers, there can be a cohesive process to find, evaluate, and resolve these building health issues. This integrative approach can create better products, systems, and solutions for the current and future built environment.

An investment in research, development, and collaborative solutions can be utilized to create healthier built environments for future generations to come.

This cohesive process can be defined as the *Architectural Medicine System (AMS)*, and this is discussed in the next chapter...

"It always seems impossible until it's done."

– Nelson Mandela

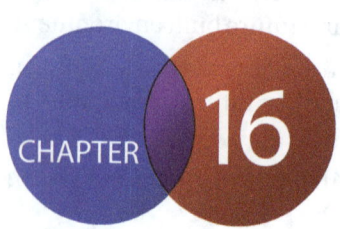

THE ARCHITECTURAL MEDICINE SYSTEM (AMS)

The Pulse of the Healthy Built Environment

Up until this part of the book, there have been discussions on how these processes might function, yet in this chapter, we're going to get into the details of these specifics.

To start, the trajectory of this path has taken time to develop, and while there is much written about the topic of health in the built environment, there have been large gaps in providing solutions.

This is where a system can support the integration of many professions, which can utilize new knowledge and apply research in practical and usable formats.

The key is to have systems in place where each professional can implement this knowledge into their workflows and have solutions that can coordinate with other professionals as a cohesive whole. To achieve this, several important components have to be in place.

The first is each professional's ability to understand these facets and be trained and familiar with processes in achieving these goals. The second is to have standards in place and to be aware of potential issues that each professional might navigate. And the third is to have a system in place for each professional with a functioning system that can provide integrations between different professions.

With these in place, a system can be utilized for providing better solutions for health in the built environment. With this foundation, developing standards, processes, and procedures to achieve the goal of healthier built environments can be built upon.

Social Determinants of Health (SDoH)

Many people involved in public health are aware of a topic called Social Determinants of Health (SDoH). A good definition of this can be found from the World Health Organization (WHO), where they state the following:

"Social Determinants of Health (SDoH) are the conditions in which people are born, grow, work, live, and age, and the wider set of forces and systems shaping the conditions of daily life."[142]

These social determinants of health can be defined as "the economic and social conditions that influence individual and group differences in health status."[143]

The comment above includes the "wider set of forces and systems shaping the conditions of daily life," which can point to the impacts that the built environment can have on health.

The following graphic is by the group goinvo[144], shows the importance of both the built environment and medicine, which together form 18 percent of these determinants of health. In fact, when you view this chart in closer detail, you will see that many of the emotional and psychological factors listed in the other segments can also be included in the topics of Architectural Medicine.

Architectural Medicine – Building the Bridge to Wellness

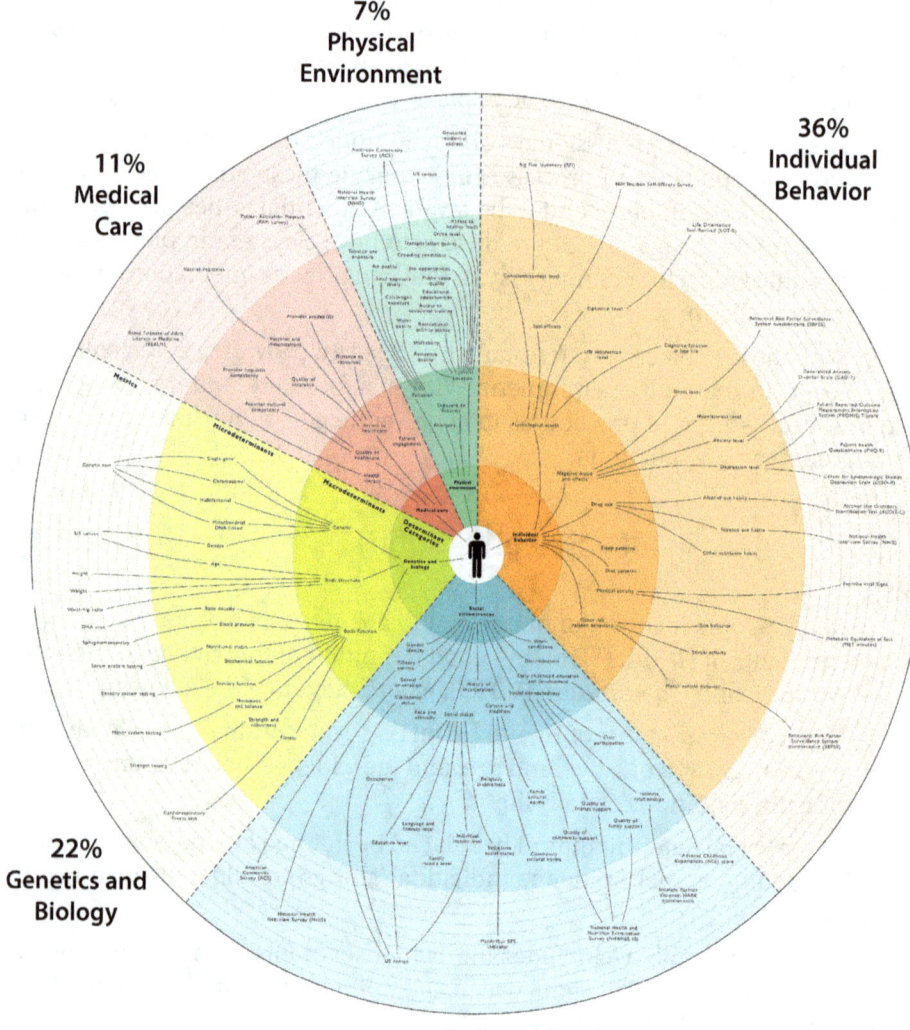

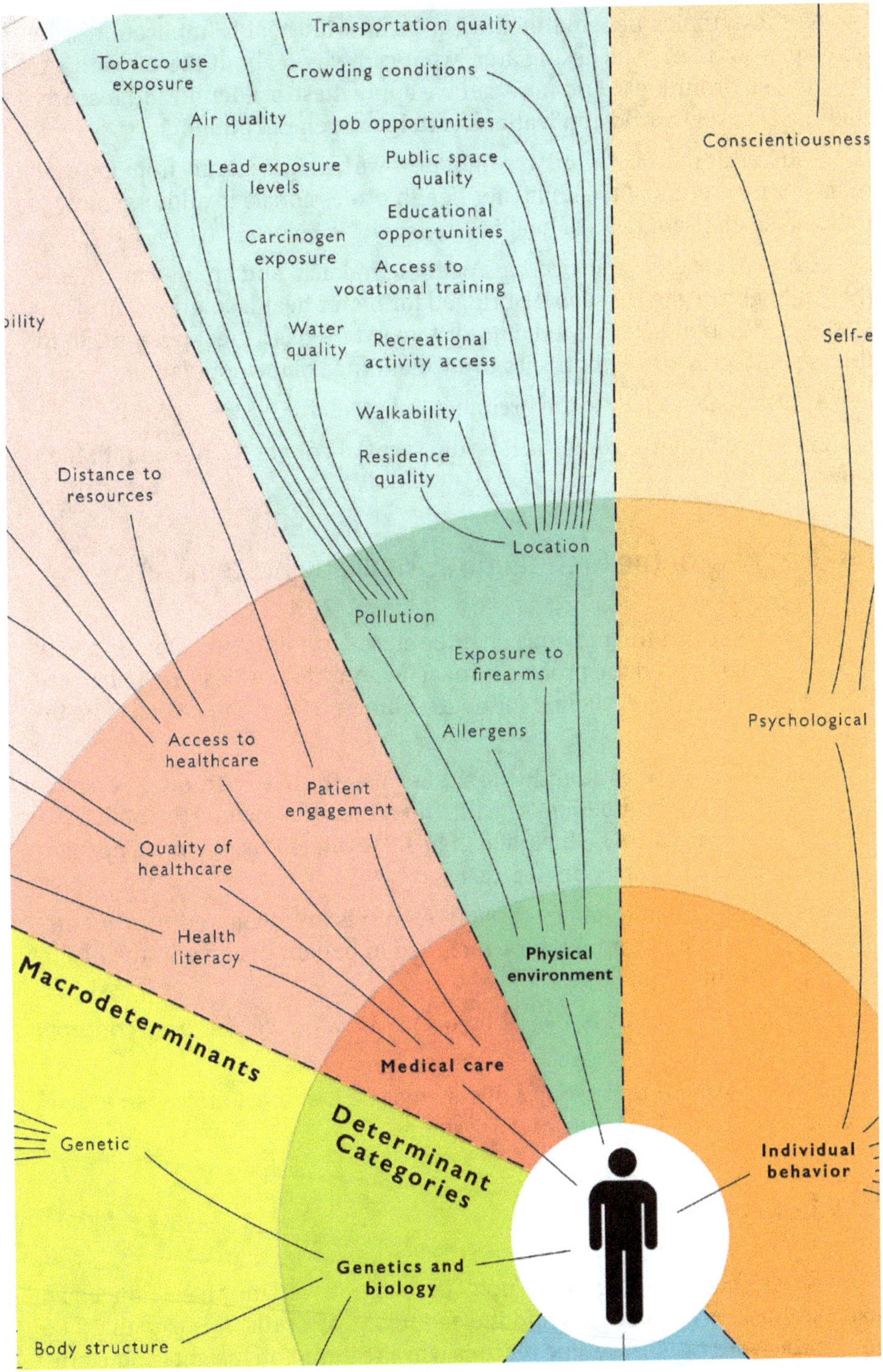

Chapter: 16 — The Architectural Medicine System (AMS)

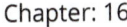

221

As these topics become more of a focus with health implications, the questions some may be asking are, "what can we do about these relative to the built environment? And how can we apply these academic and research findings into real-world applications to help the general public?"

And in this realm, the answer right now varies significantly from location to location in terms of the ability for health professionals to address many of these social determinants of health.

However, as this topic overlaps with the medical and architecture fields, this highlights a gap that can be bridged for better health solutions. And this is where the Architectural Medicine System (AMS) has a great potential to fill this gap and provide better health to a wider range of the population.

And so, what exactly is the Architectural Medicine System (AMS)?

Let's dive into this topic, as it is an essential core of Architectural Medicine.

An Overview of the Architectural Medicine System (AMS)

As discussed in the previous chapter on the Architectural Doctor, a vital flow chart highlighted the processes that currently do not exist. Yet if the built environment is to be evaluated for better human health, this needs to be included.

The flowchart brings attention to the fact that the current models of a physician's analysis of their patient's health often does not include the built environment. And for this to be included in health evaluations, there is a need for integrations that currently do not exist.

The Architectural Medicine System (AMS) is an integrated process that allows the built environment to be included in patient health and the health of the general public at large.

And so, how does this integration occur? How do we put these concepts into reality and practice?

As we delve into these topics of systems, we first must first grasp exactly what a system is and the purpose of systems.

What Are Systems?

If you've been reading to this point in the book, you may have noticed an extensive use of word origins and the etymology of words. It is true that I do love these word origins, yet the reasons why are based on insights and clarity of these meanings. And this includes the origins of the word "system" to provide deeper insights into why such systems are critical in bridging these fields:

system (n.)

1610s, "the whole creation, the universe," from Late Latin systema "an arrangement, system," from Greek systema "organized whole, a whole compounded of parts," from stem of synistanai "to place together, organize, form in order," from syn- "together" (see syn-) + root of histanai "cause to stand," from PIE root *sta- "to stand, make or be firm."[145]

The Oxford Dictionary defines a system as:

I. An organized or connected group of things.

3. a. A group or set of related or associated things perceived or thought of as a unity or complex whole.

d. A collection of natural objects, features, or phenomena considered as or forming a connected or complex whole.[146]

The idea of a large group of professions working together to evaluate, analyze, define, discuss, and then provide solutions for the patient's health is a perfect example of a complex, functional system. This concept of a system as an integrated whole of parts that are placed together for organization, fits into the overall goals of Architectural Medicine.

It also requires many facets to fit together with precision, along with the sharing of data and training that crosses disciplines for quality results.

If you view this as a whole, this process is very complicated. Yet if you take each part and evaluate this for each group involved, it can allow for manageable segments for synergistic benefits.

The key is to provide each group with their segment appropriate for their profession. This part of the puzzle is then connected to the other segments in a meaningful and useful format. And this is where the system itself can provide steps for each profession, yet connect these steps in sharing data and reporting, for a cohesive evaluation.

Systems and Ecosystems

The term ecosystem in the early 21st century has been used as a buzzword to discuss and define many types of "whole systems." What's fascinating about this, at least in my worldview, is the actual definition of an ecosystem:

eco-

word-forming element referring to the environment and man's relation to it, abstracted from ecology, ecological; attested from 1969.[147]

ecology (n.)

1873, oecology, "branch of science dealing with the relationship of living things to their environments," coined in German by German zoologist Ernst Haeckel as Ökologie, from Greek oikos "house, dwelling place, habitation" (from PIE root *weik- (1) "clan") + -logia "study of" (see -logy).[148]

The origins of the word eco are based on the Greek word oikos, which is defined as "house, dwelling place, habitation."[149]

What can be gleaned from this is the use of words with the eco preface as that which refers to our places of habitation – our homes and places of dwelling.

Ponder that for a moment and recognize the power of how a word prefix – often used by many as an off the cuff generalization for whole systems – is defined as a study of our place of habitation, our homes, and places of dwelling.

And this word "system," based on the word origin "syn," which means together, can provide more insights into the Architectural Medicine System itself.

If systems are a combination of many parts and putting them together, then what is the Architectural Medicine System (AMS) putting together?

By providing context for each facet relative to the whole, the many parts can function together correctly. In the flowchart listed in Chapter 15, the first step involves the doctor's evaluation of their patient's condition. In this process, it is recognized that a potential cause of the patient's health issue is related to their built environment.

For there to be a proper evaluation, the next step is for a healthy building inspection to be requested and completed by the healthy building inspector. This requires sharing processes and sharing the patient's necessary information for an inspection to take place. And with these results, along with any laboratory tests, a better picture of the building's health issues can be ascertained. This also includes the inspector's procedures and protocols, which are also new to both the doctor and the typical building inspector.

With all of these new steps needed to achieve these evaluations, a proper functioning system is crucial for its success.

This is just a small component of the bigger picture of the entire Architectural Medicine System (AMS), yet each step along the way is critical for positive results.

Uncharted and New Territory for Architecture and Medicine

In this chapter, I will have to admit that we are going into details where there are some basic protocols that are utilized in the real world and some that are in their infancy. This will be a chapter that is interwoven with experimental and practical processes with much room for development.

And this is also a main goal of Architectural Medicine – to support the development and procedures for health in the built environment moving forward.

In earlier chapters, we discussed some of the histories of these developments. While we have much to learn from this history, we also have more nuances and developments to address in the current day. This chapter will discuss an outline that can be used right away with new steps and goals to achieve in the future.

The Architectural Doctor and the Architectural Medicine System (AMS) – New Systems for Integrative Solutions

In chapter 15, we discussed the Architectural Doctor and the Architectural Medicine flowchart. This flowchart maps the processes from the initial doctor evaluations and the Healthy Building Inspections to the diagnosis of issues found.

This is followed by the subsequent solutions by the architect and building professionals.

To implement these processes in a round trip, start to finish method, we can put these steps into this Architectural Medicine System.

The Architectural Medicine System Diagram and Overview

The graphic below shows the initial flowchart process in chapter 15 that has been reconfigured as a circular diagram:

Architectural Medicine – Building the Bridge to Wellness

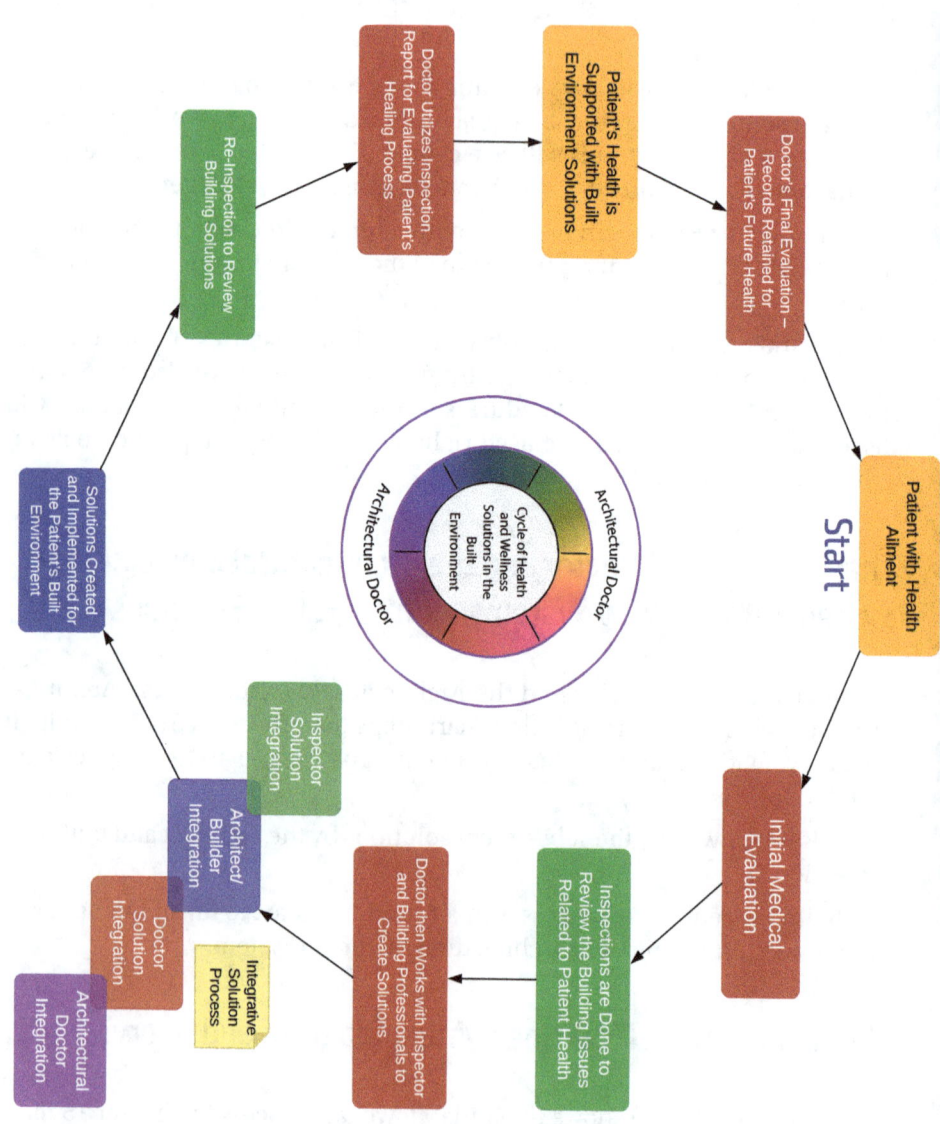

Chapter: 16 — The Architectural Medicine System (AMS)

These steps can then be shown in a more simplified process, as shown in the diagram below:

The Architectural Medicine System (AMS) Process

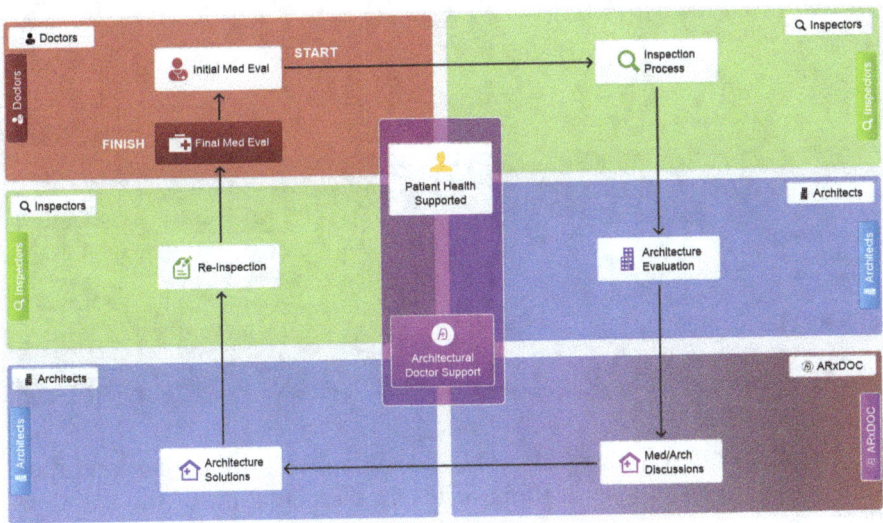

The Architectural Medicine System Steps Taken From Initial Doctor Visit to Final Building Solutions

This graphic shows the system's simple process from start to finish, beginning with the doctor's initial evaluations.

This system provides the synthesis or the system's creation towards connecting the two primary professions of architecture and medicine focused on health.

These steps lead to the Healthy Building Inspection process. When issues are found in the built environment, these reports are then sent from the inspector to the doctor and the Architectural Doctor for evaluation. This leads to the next steps of discussions with an architect, the building professionals, and the Architectural Doctor for cohesive support with plans for solutions.

These steps can be shown below in the swimlane diagram. Each professional is shown in horizontal lines, yet with the interconnections and processes between each professional:

The Architectural Medicine System (AMS) Swimlane Diagram

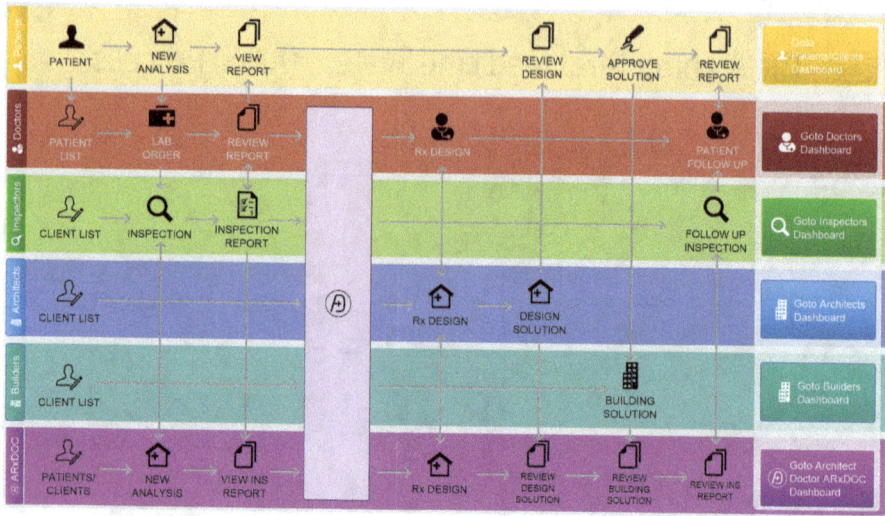

The subsequent phases include discussions with the patient and these built environment issues, leading to the implementation of the solutions. These problems will then be resolved by designs from the architect and builders and implemented by building professionals.

A follow up inspection will then ensure that the issues were resolved, and if any re-testing is required it is completed at this time. These follow up reports are then provided to the doctor and Architectural Doctor for final evaluation. These issues and fixes can be discussed with the patient in their current and long-term health evaluations.

Where Do We Start in Implementing These Evaluations of the Built Environment?

Now that an introduction to the system has been provided, the next step is to discuss the details of what exactly is evaluated in the built environment relative to the patient's health.

As discussed earlier, we reviewed human health and wellness in three main facets:

- Physical Evaluations and Diagnosis
- Emotional Evaluations and Diagnosis
- Mental/Psychological Evaluations and Diagnosis

Chapter: 16   The Architectural Medicine System (AMS)

The following is an initial list of built environment topics that can cause health issues:

- Indoor Air Quality-Lack of Fresh Air
- CO/CO2-High levels of Carbon Monoxide, Carbon Dioxide
- Radon
- Toxicity of Materials such as:
    - Lead and other Heavy Metals
    - Asbestos
    - Pesticides
    - Volatile Organic Compounds (VOCs)
    - Toxic Chemicals
- Mold/Moisture Issues
- Temperature/Humidity
    - Uncomfortably Hot/Cold
    - Uncomfortably Dry/Humid
- Water Quality
- Noises/Loud Sounds
- Lighting Issues/Lack of Natural Lighting
- Indoor Air Particulates
    - Material Particulates
    - Cigarette Smoke
    - Pollution
- Material Colors – Colors causing negative psychological and emotional responses
- Shapes and forms of structures – Physiologically induced issues/Neuroscience – increased stress
- Reduced exposure to Nature – Lack of trees, water, natural sounds, greenery

The above list can have many different impacts on physical, emotional, and mental or psychological health and wellness, resulting in some of the conditions listed below:

Physical Ailments:
- Respiratory/Asthma (Respiratory ailments)
- Endocrine related issues
- Toxicity issues
- Neurology issues
- Skin disorders

Emotional Ailments:
- Mental disturbances based on certain shapes and forms (see Neuroscience of Architecture, Environmental Psychology, and Architectural Phenomenology)
- Depression
- Neurology issues
- Toxicity issues

Mental/Psychological Ailments:
- Mental disturbances based on certain shapes and forms (see Neuroscience of Architecture, Environmental Psychology, and Architectural Phenomenology)
- Depression
- Neurology issues
- Toxicity issues

At first, there may seem like a similar list of topics for each group of ailments. The case may often be that a doctor, psychologist or therapist, and neuroscientist may see all of the same conditions and have differing opinions and vantage points regarding the physiological results.

This is not to say that there won't be various causes of these ailments, yet how many will be diagnosed because of issues in the built environment?

And when you view all of these different facets that may be connected to patient health, how can these be determined by the physician or the mental or emotional health experts?

And this is a core reason why this system requires many professionals to work together to provide cohesive solutions in evaluations to support solutions for the patient.

In many ways, these are the many pieces of the jigsaw puzzle that can help the professionals provide a whole solution for their patient's wellness.

Dividing the Puzzle Pieces for Evaluation – Putting Them Back Together for Wellness

While the reality is that you cannot separate the physical, emotional, and mental facets in evaluations of the whole person, some steps can be broken down into different pieces of a puzzle to help in the evaluation and diagnosis process. Once these pieces are reviewed independently, they can be put back together for the healing process for optimal human health.

To begin this process, we will start with some of the physical ailments that a doctor and health professional may include in their analysis when working with their patients.

Healthy Building Inspections and Integrative Systems Solutions

The physical components of the built environment that can be evaluated range in scope from some common issues of asbestos and lead in paints and products to the more complex topics such as VOCs and pesticides.

And this is where we get into new territory for many health professionals. While there are many ways to review and order lab testing, such as blood tests, X-rays, and MRIs, how many medical and health professionals will order or request a building inspection focused on health-related topics?

And how many health professionals would be comfortable providing an Rx for a patient's building?

What's needed in this scenario is the addition of the Healthy Building Inspection, and an evaluation process for the doctor and physician to include these potential issues for their patient's health analysis.

To achieve the goal of helping and supporting the patient's health, it will require new training for the doctor and the architect with these new approaches, including the implementation of the new role of the Healthy Building Inspector. This will require new processes and systems in place for the Doctor to request these inspections and request reporting that can provide lab test results from the built environment. It also means that there needs to be room for improvement for these new processes and systems to be implemented.

A key part of these new processes is to have systems in place for these professionals to work together and include this new professional, the Healthy Building Inspector.

I will continue to discuss the Architectural Medicine System (AMS) steps in chapter 18, along with the Architectural Medicine Software Solution – ARx-MD.

Before we get into the role of this new Healthy Building Inspector professional and the details of what they provide to this puzzle, let's continue the overview of the Architectural Medicine System (AMS) in terms of the emotional and mental or psychological facets of the built environment.

Environmental Psychology & Neuroscience in Architecture

In addition to the physical issues that a doctor can include in their patient's analysis, there are also the emotional and psychological impacts that the built environment can have on occupants.

In this next segment, I will comment about these facets of health and include how they can be integrated into the Architectural Medicine System (AMS) for wellness.

There have been many developments focusing on both emotional and mental impacts of the built environment, with Environmental Psychology and Neuroscience of Architecture being two leaders in these developments.

The concerns and thoughts of how a building impacts emotional and mental wellness is not new. After all, architects and medical professionals from as far back as Hippocrates and Vitruvius, along with the famous Florence Nightingale developments and research, have included concerns as to how buildings impact health.

The excellent book by Juhani Pallassma, *The Eyes of the Skin*, discusses the topic of "Architecture and the Senses." The book focuses on the subject of Architectural Phenomenology, which has an emphasis on the human experience.

There are volumes of writings on Architectural Phenomenology. Yet, an overview of this subject can be defined as "both a current aspect of philosophy influencing contemporary architecture and a field of academic research into the experience of built space and of building materials in their sensory aspects."[150]

And the sensory aspects are where the emotions and the mental and psychological facets become very interesting in the current day, where neuroscience can view the brain's physiological responses to spaces, shapes, and environments.

There has been less scientific feedback with these evaluations in the past, and previously this has been more based on how a designer or architect felt that these spaces would make people feel.

However, in the past several decades, neuroscience research has continued to provide insights into how design elements have a physiological impact.

The research by Moshe Bar and Maital Neta published in Neuropsychologia titled "Visual elements of subjective preference modulate amygdala activation" is particularly interesting.

A quote from their paper states, "Using human neuroimaging...we report that the amygdala, a brain structure that is involved in fear processing and has been shown to exhibit activation level that is proportional to arousal in general, is significantly more active for everyday sharp objects (e.g., a sofa with sharp corners) compared with their curved contour counterparts."[151]

Their research on the fMRI amygdala activity showed "behavioral results that provide initial support for the link between the sharpness of the contour and threat perception."[152] And their findings stated that "our brains might be organized to extract these basic contour elements rapidly for deriving an early warning signal in the presence of potential danger."[153]

In essence, if the environment and surrounding objects and shapes are sharp in form and of harder materials, then there is a probability that the body's physiology would respond to this as a threat in the brain center. Perhaps this is not a conscious recognition, yet either way, it can produce an increased stress level in the body.

If people live in this type of constant stress, as either high level or low-level stress, the body makes little difference between them. The body views this as stress, and being that the number one factor of death in the US – and other locations around the world – is related to stress, this adds a component of health that many often ignore or are unaware of.

This means that there are many health-related issues in many people's everyday lives impacted by the built environment that are not only ignored but also unreported to the medical professions.

For this reason, this topic can make a profound difference in such a large amount of the population for better health and wellness.

A big question might be how these factors in the built environment can be analyzed, evaluated, and communicated to the medical professions and patients.

Now that we've discussed the Architectural Medicine System (AMS), let's talk more about the *Healthy Building Inspector* and how this system functions in the next chapter...

"Quality is the best business plan"

– John Lasseter

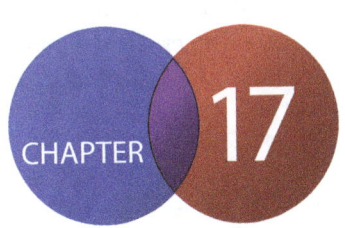

THE HEALTHY BUILDING INSPECTOR

As I've mentioned throughout this book, an essential part of creating healthier built environments is to have systems. And along with systems is the need for those to support the procedures of the systems.

In this chapter, we're going to talk about the topic of the Healthy Building Inspection and those who can properly achieve these goals.

In this case, it's important to note that the average building inspection in the US and other sections of the world is done to ensure the building's structural integrity. These inspections, in most cases, do not specifically evaluate the building in terms of issues related to occupant health.

I state "specifically," as there are inspections implemented where if issues are found, they can also be helpful to flag potential health issues. These include lead paint, asbestos identified, and other problems such as faulty HVAC systems that can also impact health via air quality.

Yet these are only a few topics that are evaluated, and there are many other issues that could be negatively impacting human health that are not tested and, too often, go unrecognized. They are certainly not part of the standard inspection, which means the building's inhabitants are also unaware of possible issues.

This, of course, is not to fault of the current inspectors and inspections. After all, this is what the standards have been, and they are doing their work to that standard.

Yet can these inspections be taken to another level to specifically look for built environment issues related to health issues? And if yes, how would this be done, and what would they evaluate?

The awareness of Sick Building Syndrome (SBS) and Building Related Illness (BRI) that began in the 1980s and 1990s formed a basic understanding of how health issues could impact occupants.

However, it has not been embraced across the board of the professional world as being relevant in making many changes. Therefore, creating an approach such as the Healthy Building Inspection to address such issues has not seemed to be an essential priority in the building world.

The Healthy Building Inspector & the Healthy Building Inspection

As I've mentioned throughout this book, the key to many these issues is the creation of systems to provide cohesive processes and solutions to evaluate the issues and resolve the problems. Until this time, there have not been systems in place between the architecture and medical professions to provide these solutions.

On the one hand, there are some professions that utilize commercial building standards, such as in the US, there is OSHA – the Occupational Safety and Health Administration. This group was created to "ensure safe and healthful working conditions for working men and women by setting and enforcing standards and by providing training, outreach, education and assistance."[154] This organization is mainly focused on industry and the workplace.

On the other hand, some offer inspections that look at the potential health issues in homes and built environments that are not necessarily industrial or commercial spaces. They have often been working on their own, striving to provide information and solutions for clients as independent environmental consultants. And this is extremely difficult to do for individuals, as it requires a large amount of knowledge and an even more considerable amount of education to provide to the client.

This work also requires the training of various professionals to provide solutions. For many decades now, this group of individuals would often help clients with building issues such as mold and volatile organic compounds (VOCs) before there was professional consensus that these were health issues.

The coronavirus pandemic of 2020 has brought the topic of health and wellness in the built environment into clarity that has not ever happened before in our modern time. While the pandemic of 1918 was undoubtedly close in timing relative to today, based on the rearview mirror of historical pandemics, this topic has been out of sight and out of mind for most.

Yet, as the current scenario has made this concept of a pandemic a harsh reality, this is when the potential for change in people's lives is often most relative and possible.

As people strive to get back to normalcy and spend time outside of their homes, the recognition of ensuring a building is safe from contaminants has never been higher on the list of priorities in the modern day time as it is now.

The question is, how can we know if these built environments, such as buildings for work, retail, shopping, and in other homes, are safe from the coronavirus? And how can this be measured and resolved?

The Healthy Building Inspection can help provide such solutions, and in the following steps, we will go into more details as to how this will work. This includes issues from the coronavirus to the many other topics that impact physical, mental, and emotional health in the built environment.

Industrial Hygiene Professionals, Environmental Inspections, and the Healthy Building Inspector

Before I go any further into these specific processes and protocols on the healthy building inspection, I think it's important to note two other professionals that focus on building issues related to health. The topics of inspecting buildings for pollutants, hazards, and other factors that cause health issues overlap with two other groups mentioned in chapter 11. And these are the Industrial Hygiene professionals and the Environmental Inspectors.

The first group is mainly focused on industry, as the name references, and the latter is often focused on residences. These fields are important facets in the topics of health in buildings, and have a history of importance in terms of the Healthy Building Inspection.

The industrial hygienist is a professional field with certifications on a national level in the US and worldwide. On the other hand, environmental inspectors are often professionals that have gathered knowledge from many sources and work to fill gaps in the building inspection fields to include human and biological health. As I mentioned previously, the professional building inspection is focused on the building's structural integrity and the mechanical aspects of the building. These inspections are often not focused on diagnosing issues related to potential health issues.

The American Industrial Hygiene Association (AIHA) defines Industrial hygienists as "scientists and engineers committed to protecting the health and safety of people in the workplace and the community. The industrial hygienist is part of a broader family of professionals often referred to collectively as the practice of occupational and environmental health and safety."[155]

The International Occupational Hygiene Association (IOHA) defines its mission as "enhancing the international network of occupational hygiene organisations that promote, develop and improve occupational hygiene worldwide, providing a safe and healthy working environment for all."[156]

As can be recognized in the above statements, there is undoubtedly a focus on building health and safety. Yet, in my experience, this is often specialized for commercial and industrial buildings.

On the contrary, the environmental inspector is often an individual that offers an extension to the typical building inspection, with the added focus on health issues in residential construction. Over the years, this has included topics such as mold and moisture issues, pesticides in structures, and issues related to chemical exposures such as Radon, VOCs, and the many synthetic materials and products that can pollute indoor air quality. These issues can cause a wide range of health problems, from asthma and respiratory problems to endocrine and nervous system issues.

In my own experiences, many of these environmental inspectors provide services to people who have not been able to find solutions from the medical community in typical formats. And as such, the lack of medical professionals having the knowledge of building issues related to health problems is part of the origins of the Healthy Building Inspector.

In my opinion, it would be great to have these Industrial Hygienists work directly with the medical and architectural community to support the health evaluations for residential and commercial industries. Yet, for now, the focus of these organizations seems to be directed towards industry. Obviously, their work is extremely valuable and important. It is my hope that more bridges between these professionals can support better health for all occupants of buildings – both commercial and residential structures.

The Exposome and Exposomics

These building evaluations can also support the development of the exposome, where the data retrieved in evaluations can be included in big data analytics to combine external exposure analysis with "internal assessment methods" in supporting exposomics.[157]

As stated by the US National Institute for Occupational Safety and Health (NIOSH), "a key factor in describing the exposome is the ability to accurately measure exposures and effect of exposures."[158]

The research of environmental exposures for long-term health is certainly a valuable health assessment in the built environment. And while biomarkers to categorize these exposures are still being evaluated, the fact that individuals and groups are focused on this as long term health issues is a step in the right direction.

The European Union's project HEALS – Health and Environment-wide Associations based on Large Population Surveys, aims to "elucidate the human exposome."[159] By utilizing human biomonitoring (HBM) it can provide a "valuable tool for understanding the magnitude of human exposure from all pathways and sources."

In 2018, HEALS published "Biomarkers of exposure in environment" which strived to summarize the availability of biomarkers of exposure (BoE) for a "broad range of environmental stressors and exposure determinants."[160]

This research on environmental stressors and exposure determinants can help support the science of the Healthy Building Inspection and the evaluation processes required to achieve these goals.

The Healthy Building Inspector, the industrial hygienist, and the environmental inspector can gather data on environmental exposures, which can be powerful bioinformatics for health professionals in supporting health evaluations.

These healthy building inspections and appropriate procedures can gather data for more detailed analytics to contribute to the exposome research. And part of this process is to utilize the big data of available data collection using software to support these inspections. I will get to the ARxMD software solution in the next chapter, yet for now, this topic flows into the inspection process itself.

The Healthy Building Inspection

A key element to this system is to have "Healthy Building Inspectors" trained to provide inspections focused on health. These new inspectors also need to be aware of the systems that doctors and health professionals expect in following the proper procedures and reporting in these health professions.

The first step is to require these three facets:

1. Healthy Building Inspectors
2. Training of these new inspectors
3. Protocols, processes, and reporting that will fit into the systems of the health professions

The next step in this process of the doctor recognizing an ailment as possibly related to a built environment issue is to have a need for systems in place to work with healthy building inspectors trained, and hopefully in the future, certified.

In this way, the medical professional can order a building inspection with health specifications in testing and then receive a report and summary from the inspector about the issues found. This would be done in the same manner that a doctor orders a blood test or an X-ray. They can request the testing reports, which can be sent from the inspectors to the laboratory professionals and then reported to the doctor. In this manner, the doctor has more information from their patient's built environment offering better insights in evaluating their health.

Yet right now, the profession of medicine is not typically connected to the field of architecture and building in this manner. So at this time, there is a need for both a field of building inspectors that can evaluate structures based on health, and there is also a need for protocols to be put into place to support this integration between doctors and inspectors for round trip solutions.

As discussed in Chapter 15 with the Architectural Medicine flowchart, the evaluation process of the doctor and medical professional is required for the next steps to take place. With these steps, the doctor also needs to have the ability to order such building inspections.

What's required next to have a group of professionals as building inspectors who understand the necessary inspections required to evaluate health-related issues. While some inspectors and consultants do this type of work in the US for residential buildings, only a few do this with a high level of integrated training focused on health. In places such as Europe, as in Germany, Switzerland, and a few other locations worldwide, they do offer such professional inspections in the field of Bau Biologie, where there are some options in place for health-related building inspections.

Many of these healthy building inspections are done in collaboration with the support of doctors who are more open to integrative approaches within these modalities. The training of health issues in buildings in certain places in Europe is not only more commonplace, yet more accepted and understood by certain doctors.

However, even with this greater awareness, there is still a need for doctors to have connections with each professional. And this includes the processes and knowledge of working with them to achieve the proper diagnosis to benefit their patients.

In this realm, providing these inspections for building health issues, the following is a list of requirements to achieve these collective goals:

The second step is to provide these three facets for the Healthy Building Inspection:

1. The processes, protocols, and technology to achieve these inspections – testing, equipment, laboratory results, standards, reporting, etc.
2. The connection between professions – to work together for cohesive analysis
3. The interest in creating healthier built environments – supply-demand

As I finish up the writing of this book, it is the year 2020, and the world is experiencing the global pandemic of the novel coronavirus. This has led to the Stay At Home initiatives, and people are staying in one place in one building for several months at a time – and often all of the time.

This situation brings awareness to the impacts that the built environment has on one's health – physically, emotionally, and mentally. Spending so much time inside for prolonged periods can often force people to recognize the impact of their built spaces. It can increase awareness of how their built environment impacts their lives and possibly increase demand for better health designs moving forward.

In order to bring things back to "normal," there must be health procedures and processes in the built environments of workplaces, retail stores, and the many public and private buildings to ensure the health of the masses. As people return to spending more time in large groups inside buildings, there must be processes required and implemented to ensure the populations' health.

And this leads to the topics of how to achieve these goals, both as processes and protocols.

As mentioned previously, what is currently missing from this important equation are those who can evaluate health in the built environment, and this is where the concept of the Healthy Building Inspector becomes important.

This new profession, combined with the Healthy Building Inspection, can provide better metrics through testing, evaluations, and relevant protocols to ensure that these buildings are safe. And while you may have thought the building inspector's profession was already set to do this work, the reality is that the average building inspection ensures the building's structural integrity, not the health impacts of the building on its occupants.

The healthy building inspection can include many physical and material issues in the structure that can cause health issues and problems, including impacts on the occupant's emotional and psychological well being.

Below is a list of inspection topics that are focused on the health and safety of the occupants:

- Air Quality
- Volatile Organic Compounds – VOCs
- Mold
- Lighting – Natural/Artificial
- Sound – Noise
- Material Toxicity
- Thermal imaging/Temperature analysis
- Pressure testing – positive/negative pressure
- HVAC systems for health
- Water quality for health

Along with the physical issues, there may also be issues impacting the inhabitants' emotional and psychological wellness.

For the emotional and psychological impacts of the built environment, the healthy building inspector can work with psychologists and environmental psychologists, as well as neuroscientists and neuropsychologists.

Processes and Procedures for the Healthy Building Inspector

The healthy building inspector will have many variables to navigate, yet all of their procedures will follow a general pattern:

- Inspection setup process
- Systems and processes of working with the medical fields and medical professionals
- Inspection using standards and protocols
- Systems and processes of working with the architecture/building fields and architecture/building professionals

The associations and organizations for international standards and protocols can work with the medical, architecture, and other health and construction professionals with their subsequent professional organizations. This includes organizations such as the American Institute of Architects (AIA), the American Medical Association (AMA), the American Psychological Association (APA), and the many other groups and organizations involved in this large scope of topics.

These groups can span an extensive range from psychologists, environmental psychologists, and neuroscientists to public health professionals, toxicologists, epidemiologists, and other professionals. These professional organizations can collaborate for integrative solutions for better health in the built environment.

Healthy Building Inspectors Working With the AIA and AMA

A large bonus would be if these groups would also work with the architecture groups, such as the AIA, and the medical groups, such as the AMA, to work on standards and protocols that cross-reference all organizations and yet are defined for their specific profession. Please note that these are the US organizations representing these topics. Yet, it would be even better if groups in all parts of the world specific to their regions would also work together for global standards.

In terms of working together, the following is a brief overview that these organizations could help to define, working with the Healthy Building Inspectors:

- Set standards and protocols for the medical professionals (AMA, etc.) relative to health in the built environment
- Define procedures for the medical professionals to recognize ailments related to the built environment
- Define processes to work with the inspectors and building professionals
- Set standards and protocols for the architecture professionals (AIA, etc.) relative to health in the built environment
- Define procedures for the architecture professionals to recognize health issues and solutions related to the built environment
- Define processes to work with the inspectors and medical professionals

We have discussed the medical component in how the healthy building inspectors would work with the medical professionals, yet what happens after this step?

And this question segues into the subsequent discussion, bringing the architecture professionals into the equation.

The Architectural Solution Component

While the healthy building inspection is certainly a requirement to gain insights and a better understanding of these evaluations, another facet of the puzzle is still needed.

And that process is the architectural solution component. It's an excellent start to have an inspector evaluate a structure and provide reports on issues found, yet there is still the need to solve these built environment issues.

Currently, few architects are well-versed in the component of health in the built environment. And even less who are truly focused on health for their occupants. This is not because architects don't care. It's mainly due to the lack of training they have had as architects. You can't expect a doctor to know about the specifics of building processes, and at the same time, you can't expect architects to know about health and medicine specifics.

Yet, there are essential interconnections that must be developed to create healthier built environments and fix architecture that requires healthier building solutions.

So again, there are two components to this process that need some attention. The first is that architects and builders need to have better training on topics related to health in buildings, and then there is a need for the architecture professionals to work together with the medical professionals.

The first part of this equation, of architects being better versed on healthier building solutions, already has some great information outlets. Groups such as the Healthy Building Network and architects who are already working with medical professionals in healthy hospital development already have insights into this process.

Organizations such as the Center for Health Design, which offers an Evidence-Based Design Accreditation and Certification (EDAC)[161], provide more information for building and health professionals to bridge this gap for better health solutions in architecture.

And as of now, while there is an increasing collective base of information from research in the past ten years than perhaps in the past thirty-plus years, there are still connections between the fields of architecture and medicine that will need more comprehensive support systems.

For instance, when the doctor can order a healthy building inspection and receive a report with a summary of recommendations, what is the doctor and patient to do with that information?

Ideally, when the doctor receives this information about the negative built environment issues, they would likely want to write a prescription of some form similar to other ailments for which they prescribe.

However, at this time, there really isn't a prescription or an Rx for a health-related solution in the built environment.

That said, an Rx or prescription is actually a good place for us to discuss this topic of building solutions for health. An Rx is actually shorthand for a recipe, or at least this is a common recognition for the Rx symbol's origins that can be reviewed below:

Rx

1580s, "medical prescription," from Middle French récipé (15c.), from Latin recipe "take!," second person imperative singular of recipere "to take" (see receive); word written by physicians at the head of prescriptions. Figurative use from 1640s. The original sense survives only in the pharmacist's abbreviation Rx.[162]

As you can see, this shorthand for recipe as Rx is based on the concept of the prescription being something that you take or is given to help with the ailment.

This Rx or Recipe for a healthy building solution would address a health-related issue causing or impacting a patient's ailment.

It would be more apropos as some form of building solution for health. This Rx as a recipe, where an architect and designer would be versed on health-related topics, is trained on issues of health to ensure that their building designs and solutions are literally built into these solutions.

These Rx designs can provide blueprints as solutions for the issues found, and act similarly to a doctor providing an Rx as a supplement or prescription.

These solutions could include topics such as materials and functionality, such as ensuring that fresh air is introduced appropriately into HVAC systems. It can consist of the inclusion of air filters that are not just there to protect the HVAC equipment but also focus on supporting and protecting human health.

Many people don't realize that in Heating, Ventilation, and Air Conditioning (HVAC) systems with filters, filtration is not specifically for Indoor Air Quality (IAQ) issues for human health. The filters are there mainly to protect the HVAC systems' equipment and machinery from particulates large enough to cause problems in the fans and other operating parts of the machinery.

This is a far cry from the necessary air filters that would be ideal for filtering contaminants for human health. Yet particulates are just one factor for indoor air quality (IAQ), where there are also issues that should include concerns about toxins and pathogens, along with pesticides and other chemicals.

Materials in the building can break down over time and can then be recirculated as smaller particulates through the HVAC systems in homes and business buildings. These particulates can be organic or non-organic, each creating different forms of health issues that can negatively impact the respiratory, immune, and endocrine systems.

Many other factors may be causing health issues, from mold and moisture-related matters in the physical form to topics that impact emotional and psychological problems such as shapes, forms, and colors. This includes the topics of noise and a lack of natural lighting. These can all cause health-related issues in terms of physical as well as psychological, and emotional wellness.

The benefit of architects, designers, and builders having training in these topics and issues, brings both awareness in the design-build process and provides a basis for solutions. These solutions as recipes can then be supplied as blueprint prescriptions. As such, it can mimic the Rx from a doctor and medical professional translated as a built environment solution.

There are many variables in this process, and they include the architecture and medicine professionals working together on these health-related issues in buildings. This, of course, consists of the building inspectors as an integral part of the equation.

In the previous two chapters, we discussed the Architectural Doctor and the Architectural Medicine System (AMS). All of these professionals working together towards a common goal of better health in buildings can provide powerful solutions for the future of wellness.

Integrated Standards, Systems, and Solutions for Healthier Built Environments

Creating integrated standards and systems for professionals to work together allows for the process to function interdependently with each professional. It also allows each field to analyze and develop solutions for better health in buildings.

This includes the setting of standards for the healthy building inspector and the Architectural Doctor, and this is where the ARxMD standards, protocols, and processes enter into the process.

ARxMD Standards, Protocols, and Processes

As we will discuss in the next chapter, ARxMD is the name of the Architectural Medicine Software Solution, yet it also outlines the standards, protocols, and processes for these solutions.

Pronounced "arcs-med," this term can help define and support standards that bridge the fields of architecture and medicine. Having these standards can provide guidance in evaluating patients, buildings, and the many processes that link these topics together for more clarity in the process, from evaluation to solutions.

While there are standards and protocols for certain facets of health in buildings, they are often specific to a profession and sometimes siloed for each group. This can make it challenging to have any standard metrics, especially when it comes to the cross-over between architecture and medicine disciplines.

In the next chapter, these topics of standards and processes will be discussed in more detail.

Earlier in the book, I mentioned that one of the critical insights as I became more involved in creating healthier built environments was the lack of systems.

And what this means to me, specifically, is a lack of a doctor's capability to include issues in the patient's built environment that might be impacting their health in a negative format. During my process in striving to create healthier built environments and being involved with inspections and construction of such buildings, there was a huge gap that seemed as wide as the Grand Canyon.

But all the while, the key takeaway was the simple idea that without systems, the process itself would be extremely challenging to achieve, especially on a large scale. The challenges of not having an inspector to evaluate health issues in the built environment, and doctors who could not specify a building inspection for health, would lead to more challenges for the occupants of buildings as patients. Adding architects not being involved in providing solutions is often too big of a gap to achieve without any systems in place.

In this scenario, what would have to happen without such a system is that a doctor or medical professional would have to find an environmental building inspector or environmental consultant. In the US, some strive to find issues in the built environment related to health problems that are often off the radar based on the typical building inspection. They aim to find health issues in the built environment, often referred to as environmental building consultants or environmental inspectors.

While many of these environmental building consultants have worked to bridge these gaps and provide healthier building evaluations, it has often been a challenging process.

Even the procedure of supplying education and information has been challenging due to the many different professionals involved and the enormous scope of the content.

However, as can be imagined, the processes and systems of achieving these goals are incredibly complex. Many began to provide these services in the 1990s and early 2000s. Even the capabilities of technology using computer systems, databases, applications, and online video were tremendously expensive to create in the late 90s and 2000s. It was very expensive to author this content and provide it to the various professionals and professional channels involved.

My work over the years has seen many of these gaps in systems, and I've taken that time to learn about these topics over several decades. And in 2011, when I came up with the term Architectural Medicine and the Architectural Doctor, I had already had foundations of processes in my mind to put into a system.

The idea of this began for me in the late 90s, as I was doing some of this work hands-on. I knew that a digital clipboard or tablet of some sort as a mobile computer could help guide me through these processes and be utilized for "how-to" guides. This, along with the actual documenting of the inspections to input the results, would provide a better reporting system.

At the time, I called this the Electronic Clip Board or the Datalog software approach. Not exactly the "roll off your tongue" in naming, but the core purpose was to provide a way to capture data of inspections and evaluations. In this manner, you would then have the ability to connect this to other computers and view it in digital format for assessments. You could then create reports for medical professionals and the client, and this device could be utilized as a way for these inspections focused on health to have guidelines and structure for the process itself.

However, I would have to work on these processes in a bit of a vacuum first, and I also had a lot to learn about how the various professionals functioned. I knew about the architecture, building, and construction fields and learned a lot about the inspection processes, yet the medical field took more time to comprehend its methods.

Luckily, many of these topics of digital integration in the medical systems were just beginning. It's only been in the last ten to fifteen years that the EHR's have become standards for both hospitals and doctors. The common Electronic Health Record (EHR) has become more common, yet even this process is not something that the average person as a patient is truly familiar with.

Along with the slow process of architecture fields going digital, it has provided some time for these systems to develop, which will be a requirement for these multi-disciplinary interconnections.

This process provided some time for the slow-moving systems to be better understood and evaluate how the Architectural Medicine process would be integrated into these systems.

And how will Architectural Medicine integrate into medical, architecture, and inspection systems and processes?

The *Architectural Medicine Software Solution – ARxMD* provides an application and training process to bridge these divides to support and provide information for round trip solutions.

How can this be provided for all professionals involved?

That's a good question, and in the next chapter, I discuss this topic...

"A spirit with a vision, is a dream with a mission."

– Neil Peart

THE ARCHITECTURAL MEDICINE SOFTWARE SOLUTION – ARxMD

In previous chapters, we discussed the many facets involved in creating the healthy built environment and the new professionals – the Architectural Doctor and the Healthy Building Inspector.

This, along with the Architectural Medicine System (AMS), begins to form a foundation for providing the people and the systems to create these solutions for the healthier built environment.

The next step in this process is providing the necessary structures to allow all of these activities to function together.

The Doctor, Architect, Healthy Building Inspector, and the Architectural Doctor – New Systems and Solutions

The past twenty years have shown many changes and updates in the format of digital and electronic record keeping. The Electronic Health Record (EHR) and the CHR (Comprehensive Health Record) have brought the world of medical paperwork into the digital age.

In the US, the Centers for Disease Control and Prevention (CDC) enacted the Meaningful Use standards in 2009 defined by the "Health Information Technology for Economic and Clinical Health (HITECH) Act."[163]

The CDC defines *meaningful use* as "the use of certified EHR technology in a meaningful manner (for example electronic prescribing); ensuring that the certified EHR technology connects in a manner that provides for the electronic exchange of health information to improve the quality of care."[164]

This helped support the transition of a paper-based medical system to an electronic or digital process. In this process, data sharing and data exchange between different medical systems, hospitals, and health professionals was the end goal.

While still a work in progress in the US and worldwide, the electronic sharing of data has brought the possibility of integrated systems to another level. These new systems can allow for software to be developed to support many various healthcare system factions. These systems range in scope from ordering and receiving test results to the sharing of examinations between health professionals without needing to be in the same network or even on the same continent.

And these new processes create opportunities for new systems to be added, integrated, and updated in formats that previously would have been extremely challenging.

An Evolution in the Architecture & Construction Fields

What's particularly interesting about the medical and health fields' history updating to electronic records is that a slow digital evolution in the architecture and construction fields has also been occurring.

The public knowledge and concerns with these Electronic Health Records

(EHR) have allowed these updates to be more transparent and popularized in developments. However, behind the scenes in the worlds of building and construction, another evolution has been happening: the digitization of the architecture fields.

From the developments of Computer-Aided Design (CAD) from the 1980s onward to the early 2000s, a data exchange movement has been slowly developing called Building Information Modeling or BIM as it is known today. The roots of this began in the early 1990s as a group of leaders in the fields of software for building created an organization to outline standards for the interoperability of data files. This group began to develop a standardized, digital description of the built environment called the Industry Foundation Classes or IFC.[165][166]

Today these standards, which the buildingSMART International organization oversees, provide vendor-neutral standards that are usable "across a wide range of hardware devices, software platforms, and interfaces for many different use cases."[167]

This data exchange can allow many building professionals to all work together, from architects, structural engineers, and construction (AEC) professionals to mechanical, electrical, and plumbing (MEP) professionals. They can import the latest designs to add their part of the building development in their software and then export these updates back to the architect and construction management team in real-time – or mostly real-time if the solutions are hosted in a cloud platform.

Essentially, the world of architecture has been slowly creating infrastructures to exchange this data electronically to enable these construction professionals to work together.

In a similar format to the Electronic Health Record exchanges, these digital construction systems have also developed for better interoperability.

And this is where the integration between these new professionals and the Architectural Medicine System (AMS) can enter into the equation with greater possibilities.

With all of these new facets involved, as the Architectural Doctor and the Healthy Building Inspector, the advent of these electronic systems can be supported using new software solutions.

This is where the *Architectural Medicine Software Solution – ARxMD* enters into the picture.

Chapter: 18   The Architectural Medicine Software Solution — ARxMD

What is the Architectural Medicine Software Solution – ARxMD?

Once you outline the lack of systems that have existed between the medical and architecture fields and recognize the importance of such systems, the next step and question might be, "What can be done to help implement these systems?"

If you followed along the trajectory of topics in this book, you might now be asking the question, "how would this Architectural Medicine System (AMS) function?"

And this is where the Architectural Medicine System (AMS) meets the actionable of the Architectural Medicine Software Solution – ARxMD.

ARxMD, pronounced "arcs-med," is a software solution that provides the nuts and bolts of implementing the system. It is how the processes can function between the many professionals involved, including the information to the patient as the general public.

How ARxMD Came to Be and Why Is It Important?

This software concept is a big part of what first began my path towards Architectural Medicine. As I've mentioned earlier in the book, this idea originated in 1999 when I first had the idea of what I called the electronic clipboard. As I've said earlier in this book, it's a good thing the name changed, as the electronic clipboard does not quite have the same word or brand recognition as the ubiquity branding of the portable tablet – the iPad.

Yet essentially, a mobile tablet as a device for professionals to use in the field and on-site is exactly what would have been ideal back then. At the time, I struggled with paper and clipboards to provide inspections, evaluations, reporting and referencing for all of this new information I was learning.

As the goal to create healthy built environments is extremely complex, having a mobile electronic device with the capability to record the testing and evaluations would have been very helpful. And as the modern tablets of today have powerful computing capabilities, there is a lot more that can be done than merely recording data for reporting.

The Architectural Medicine Software Solution ARxMD provides several features that can provide a cohesive solution for each of the professionals involved. And of course, this includes the focus of providing the best health and wellness for the patient.

How Do We Get There? How Do We Create Healthier Built Environments?

While the systems and processes discussed in this book may seem to be either complex or daunting in scope, the alternative is to not work in some form of unison. The past thirty-plus years of this process has shown to me that a lack of integrations as a team can end up being precarious at best. So, if there is to be a different outcome, then there will need to be a different approach. And taking a proactive approach and taking the initiative for planned benefits seems to be a wise choice, at least in my book.

This process of reverse-engineering the desired goal, along with a forward-thinking design mindset, can help define and then create an action plan to achieve those goals. The lack of current systems to have these various professional fields working together is a roadblock to achieving any form of integrative solutions.

As mentioned earlier, with the advent of integrative medicine and a proposed approach of integrative architecture, combining these two developing fields that are open to change and willing to embrace more integrative approaches opens the doors for these professionals to work together in a synergistic format for exponentially beneficial results.

Next Steps and How Systems Can Be More Integrated to Support the Architectural Medicine Process

By defining six main groups, there can be processes put into place to help the evaluations of buildings and the development of procedures with an integrated systems approach:

- Patients
- Architects
- Doctors
- Inspectors
- Builders
- Architectural Doctor

Chapter: 18 — The Architectural Medicine Software Solution — ARxMD

The Architectural Doctor can be included as a unique component, as they can provide support in differing levels of involvement depending on the circumstances.

Some may find the listing of "Patients" in this list to be surprising. After all, they are not professionals, so why would they be listed and involved in the procedure process?

The simple answer is that they are the focal point for all of this work. Not including them or eliminating them from any processes, protocols, and procedures is going against their better health goals.

While they may not be involved in all decisions and may not be in the discussions for many of the protocols, they should be a part of the systems approach and be a critical part of creating healthier built environments.

How Does ARxMD Work and What Is Involved?

First, the software provides several vital functions that allow the Architectural Medicine System (AMS) to be implemented.

From a big picture viewpoint, it allows the many different professionals to work together and provides a platform for each professional to work with independently and interdependently. It can give an overview of the processes and provide details of each step along the way.

The second part provides each professional a platform to utilize and achieve their facet of the work from a very granular perspective.

For the doctor, the software allows them to request a building inspection when they see health issues with their patient – potentially related to their built environment. This can provide the physician with a system and procedures to better evaluate their patient's conditions.

The software can then provide a mechanism to create an inspection and then allow for the Healthy Building Inspector's integration process.

The testing and collecting of data to analyze the patient's built environment can then be recorded and sent back to the doctor. This data can be reviewed by the doctor and the Architectural Doctor, leading to integrative, multi-disciplinary discussions with the architect and builders to evaluate and provide solutions.

The third part is that the software provides an overview, with guidelines for each professional's procedures. This can be extremely helpful when the doctor and architect's complex professions already have many methods and protocols to follow.

Electronic Health Records, SNOMED, ICD, DSM, LOINC, HL7, IFC, BIM, and ARxMD

The fourth part of this software system is the ability to provide proper communication, data, and procedures for each step of the way. It can send and receive this data to other HealthCare systems using standards that are familiar within the medical community.

By using the Electronic Health Record (EHR) and Comprehensive Health Record (CHR) in synchronization with Hospital Information Systems (HIS), the Architectural Medicine Software Solution can integrate with current medical systems.

This process includes the standards of SNOMED, ICD, DSM, and LOINC codes for laboratory testing and expands the scope of these electronic records to incorporate this into more comprehensive information.

For those unfamiliar with these acronyms, here's a quick listing of common healthcare and architecture nomenclature:

Architecture Acronyms:

BIM – Building Information Modeling

CAD – Computer-Aided Design

CAE – Computer-Aided Engineering

CAM – Computer-Aided Manufacturing

IFC – Industry Foundation Classes

COBie – Construction Operations Building information exchange

Medical Acronyms:

CPT – Current Procedural Terminology

SNOMED – Systematized Nomenclature of Medicine

ICD – International Classification of Diseases

DSM – Diagnostic and Statistical Manual of Mental Disorders

LOINC – Logical Observation Identifiers Names and Codes

HIPAA – Health Insurance Portability and Accountability Act

HL7 – Health Level Seven

The relatively new concept of the CHR as a comprehensive record can include the built environment and, for example, the social determinants of health as a tool for doctors to utilize for their patient's optimal health.

While this built environment testing may be recorded directly on location, some tests may be sent to laboratories for analysis. In this manner, the same testing processes will utilize LOINC codes used in current medical lab testing. By using the ARxMD platform, this data can be shared with other systems using the common Health Level Seven (HL7) exchange standards.

It is critically important to ensure that this data and information is transferred in a secured format, and so to achieve this, the software will utilize HL7 processes. ARxMD uses the HL7 FHIR (Fast Healthcare Interoperability Resources), the latest standard provided by the HL7 organization, to exchange data using common RESTful API practices.

And while this topic may be new to many, the key is that it allows an exchange of data with many different platforms, not just the Electronic Medical Record (EMR) system or a Hospital Information System (HIS).

It allows for different systems to share and exchange data in a safe and secured format. The FHIR standard was "designed to enable information exchange to support the provision of healthcare in a wide variety of settings."[168] As of this writing, the most up to date version of HL7 is FHIR version 4.

While it's not currently common to use between the architecture and medical platforms, this wide variety of settings provides EHR data to be exchanged and shared. There are many software processes currently used by architects that can be integrated for this use, such as BIM. With the advent of the advanced HL7 FHIR version, the modern web-based suite of API technology can provide interoperability between modern architecture and construction software systems.

The Architectural Medicine Software Solution ARxMD is implementing these new procedures to provide supportive solutions for the architectural fields to connect with the medical fields.

This ability to share data using HL7 FHIR can be seen as the fifth part of this system to provide round trip processes, and an exchange of data can be utilized for best decision making for all involved.

This system can provide preliminary analysis for the doctor and final evaluations to utilize as a Comprehensive Health Record (CHR) from the pre-inspection to the post-inspection process.

And the sixth and final step in this system is – if consent from the patient is received – the data can be anonymized and sent to a health data repository.

This data can be analyzed and evaluated by public health professionals, epidemiologists, toxicologists, green chemists, building material manufacturers, and many others that can utilize this data to better understand built environments in relation to health.

These results can then provide insights for medical and architecture professionals and offer valuable insights into overall population health.

When analyzed, this data can also help determine standards for materials and methods to support healthier built environments for all.

And while all of this, in theory, might sound logical, let's dive into some of these details to see what this software looks like and how it functions.

The Architectural Medicine Software Solution – ARxMD in Use

First, let me state that this software is still a work in progress, and right now, it is in a testing as a pilot program to a select group. The final writing of this book is in the fall of 2020, and the plan is to have the pilot program implemented during the winter of 2020 into 2021. As the world is in a global pandemic from the novel coronavirus, this is both a tumultuous time to launch a new system yet also a timely opportunity to provide better health systems and metrics in the built environment.

There are six main segments of the software, and the graphic below highlights the workflow process to help show each segment:

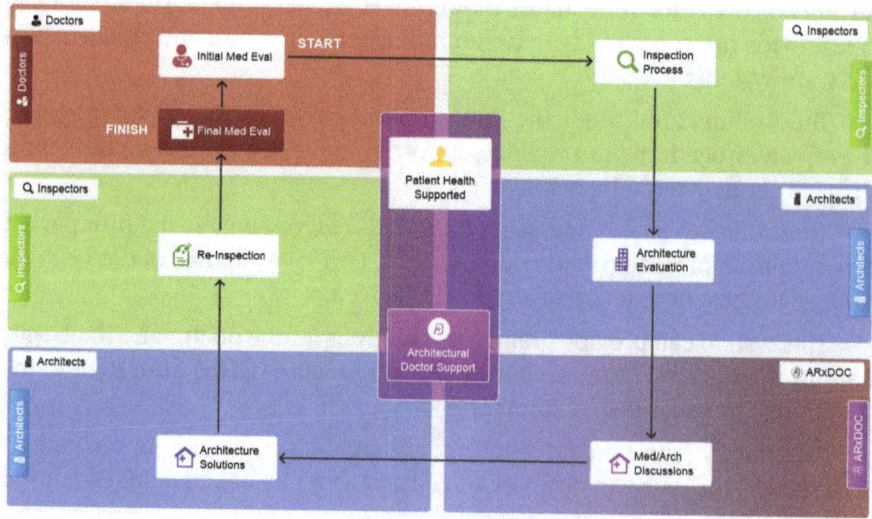

Chapter: 18   The Architectural Medicine Software Solution — ARxMD

As you can see, each profession has its individual procedures, and in this manner, the software follows this structure.

To discuss this in more detail, let's take a look at this swimlane diagram to show how the flowchart shown earlier in chapter 15 can be implemented for each professional involved:

ARxMD – Swimlane Diagram of Processes

While the swimlane shows a dynamic and sometimes non-linear process, it does have a structured format that can be viewed in the following steps:

- During the evaluation of the Patient, the Doctor requests a building inspection based on conditions that are possibly related to the Patient's built environment
- Inspector receives a request(s) to inspect the building and proceeds with the inspection(s)
- Inspection data is recorded directly on-site or sent to the laboratory for test results
- Inspection data is reported and sent to the Electronic Medical Records (EMR) system for the Doctor and Architectural Doctor to review

- Doctor and Architectural Doctor work together and discuss issues related to health found in the built environment
- Patient is informed by Doctor or Architectural Doctor about the built environment issues
- Architects & Builders are included in the discussions when issues are found and need to be resolved
- Architect-Builder provides building solutions for the group to review
- Communication with Patient is provided by Doctor, Architectural Doctor, and Architect about the overall issues and solutions
- Solutions are approved for Builder to complete
- Builders implement solutions and properly fix the built environment issues
- Re-inspection of the built environment is completed and re-testing recorded
- Report on the re-inspection is provided to the Doctor and Architectural Doctor for evaluation
- Patient's health is reviewed after these healthy building re-inspections have been completed, and Patient's health is monitored over time
- * Data is anonymized and sent to a Clinical Data Repository (CDR) or Clinical Data Warehouse (CDW) for data analysis

It is critically important to note that data is only collected as anonymous data and only after there is consent from the patient with full agreement. In the US, full HIPAA compliance is vital.[169]

The software provides a cohesive system for each professional to follow, implement, record, and exchange contextually appropriate data with the other professionals. In this format, each professional can provide their part of the process for completion.

In summary, the end goal is to provide an initial screening of issues that may be seen in the patient's health conditions relative to their built environment. Then inspections are completed to allow the doctor to analyze these issues.

This is where the Architectural Doctor can be supportive in the overall process. And then, a building analysis includes the architect and builders to provide solutions. After solutions are approved and implemented, the eventual re-inspection provides the doctor with updated reports. These updates allow the doctor to evaluate their patient's long-term health.

The Clinical Data Repository (CDR) for data analysis can also provide insights and updates with new findings, which can then be included for each professional's education and training. This provides an iterative process to improve evaluations and leads to better solutions over time. As discussed earlier in the book, this form of a spiracycle process can iterate for beneficial developments over time.

Software Application Views – Inspector, Doctor, Architectural Doctor, and Architect

Now that we've discussed the theoretical aspects of this process, it's time to get into the details of how this functions in real-world scenarios.

The first image of the six main segments of the software shows an overview of the ARxMD software cycle, starting at the top left, where the patient visits the doctor and then continues clockwise to the inspector. It continues to the architect and then the doctor, architect, Architectural Doctor, and the inspector's collaborative process if their feedback can be of value. It continues to the architect and builder providing the solutions for issues found and then a re-inspection to confirm changes have been fixed. These reports then return to the doctor and the Architectural Doctor, if required, to evaluate the patient's health for both short and long-term analysis.

The interface of the doctor's portal of the Architectural Medicine Software Solution - ARxMD consists of the main screen in a common CRM or EMR format when going to their portal page or dashboard.

The ARxMD screen is likely familiar in that it consists of the common Customer Relationship Management (CRM) fields. It is likely what health professionals view when they log into their Electronic Medical Record (EMR) system or their Health Information System (HIS).

It's important to note that the doctors and health professionals may not be accessing the ARxMD software and instead might be utilizing their own EMR or HIS system. As mentioned earlier, due to the advancement of the HL7 FHIR mapping process, the necessary information can be exchanged between systems.

Architectural Medicine – Building the Bridge to Wellness

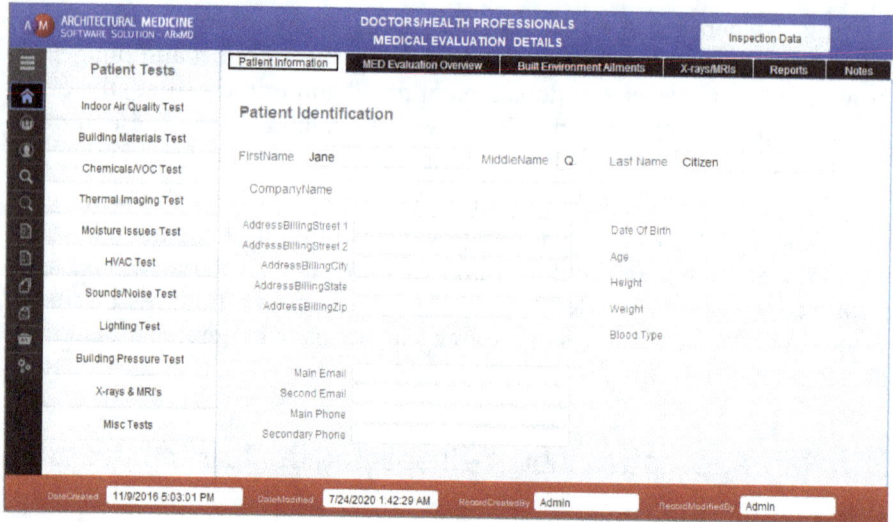

In this doctor's ARxMD portal, the doctor has the ability to record the ailments of their patient, which might be caused by the patient's built environment. They can then request an inspection using the proper coding. This process is similar to a doctor requesting a blood analysis or an MRI or X-ray, yet the request is sent to a different group of professionals.

A building analysis or observation request can use a common medical process, using the SNOMED and ICD codes for appropriate conditions. The relevant LOINC codes would be recorded from the lab testing completed by the inspector.

However, there will also be a need for additional SNOMED, ICD, DSM, and LOINC codes that will be in alignment with these building issues and laboratory results.

At the time of this writing, there are some SNOMED and LOINC codes that describe and define assorted built environment issues based on the social determinants of health topics. So, where there is an overlap between codes, they can be utilized appropriately.

Where there are new codes to be developed, we will discuss the topic of the ARxMD standards and protocols later in this chapter.

When a patient's condition may require further building inspection, the doctor can now request this to be completed by the inspector. Once the request is routed to the inspector, the software sends a message using the secure HL7 protocols, and the inspector receives this request.

The benefit of using HL7 is that only specific information that has been appropriately mapped is sent to the inspector, which can alleviate any HIPAA compliance concerns. In this way, only the Patient Identification (PID) information such as name, address, and the requested inspections are sent to the inspector to do their job.

The advanced mapping features of HL7 FHIR allow the exchange of complex data between systems in a bi-directional format. Therefore, once the inspection is completed, the results can be sent back to the doctor for review.

The Healthy Building Inspection Process Using the ARxMD Software

This exchange of data and request sent to the Healthy Building Inspector results in the next step, which is the actual inspection of the patient's built environment.

To show this in more detail, when you view the swimlane diagram and follow the process of the inspector, the steps involved can vary depending upon the built environment issues. This can range from Indoor Air Quality (IAQ) problems and particulates to problems with materials, VOCs, and other pollutants.

The software shows the inspection details for guidance in gathering this data to support the inspection process. By providing specific instructions focused on building health issues, certain inspections can be performed related to these health ailments.

As mentioned previously in this book, most building inspections around the world focus on the structural integrity of the building and not on human health.

Some structural inspections can overlap with health issues, such as building moisture issues and HVAC system problems. While these can sometimes flag potential health issues, the concern is often not focused on human health. Therefore, many building issues might be negatively impacting human health without the occupants being aware of such factors.

The Healthy Building Inspection focuses on these health problems and starts with a big picture view, literally, of the building plot plan. It then focuses on each facet of the building with a more detailed evaluation.

In the ARxMD software, there is also an interface for the Healthy Building Inspector as they begin their evaluations:

Architectural Medicine Software Solution – ARxMD
Healthy Building Inspector Views

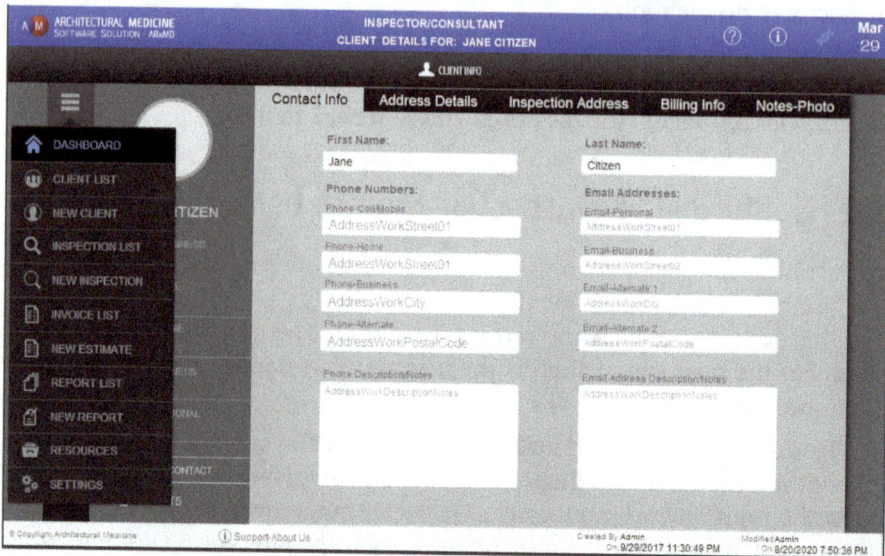

Inspection Process and Steps for Evaluating the Built Environment for Health

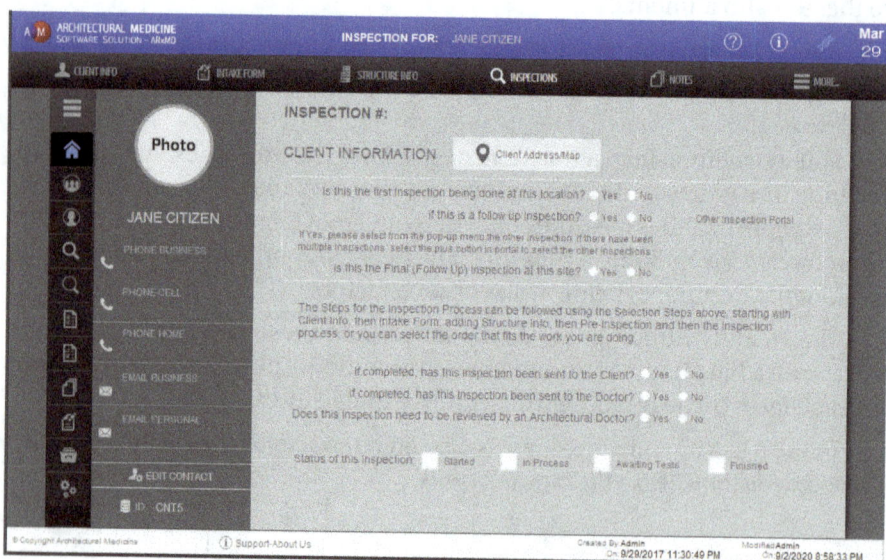

Once the patient's information has been sent to the inspector and an inspection date and time are set, the inspection process begins. Below is the interface for the start of the inspection process:

The software guides the inspector through the processes, from the pre-inspection and inspection to the room analysis and various testing modalities.

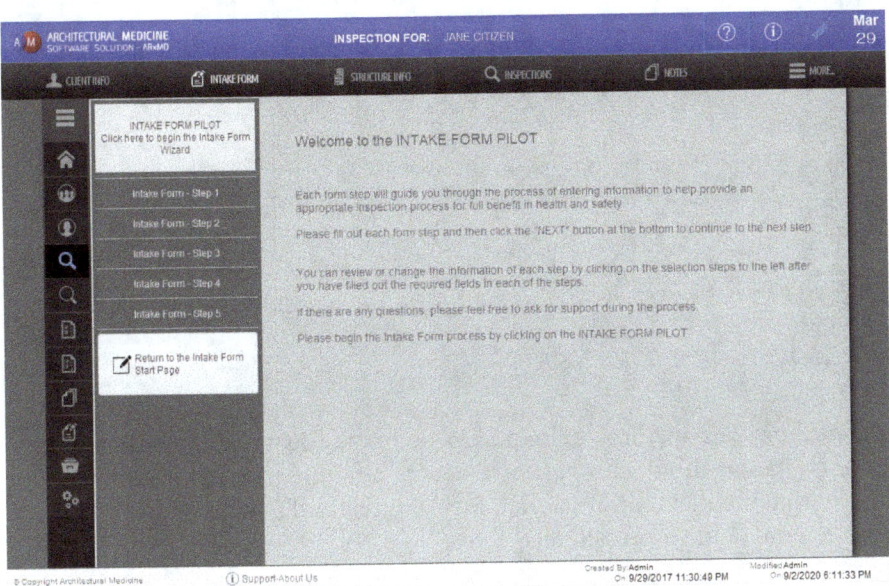

This reporting and raw data are recorded into the ARxMD software, and where appropriate, sent to labs for testing results. When tests are confirmed, they are sent to the ARxMD platform using the relevant LOINC codes using HL7 protocols.

The Evaluation of Inspection Results by the Doctor & Architectural Doctor

Once the inspection results are completed, the data and reports are then sent back to the doctor and Architectural Doctor for review.

In time, with additional education and training for the medical fields, this review can have better support with help from the Architectural Doctor. However, as this field begins to embrace additional data, the Architectural Doctor can support the doctor, especially if the MD is a general practitioner and would benefit from this additional support.

Architectural Medicine – Building the Bridge to Wellness

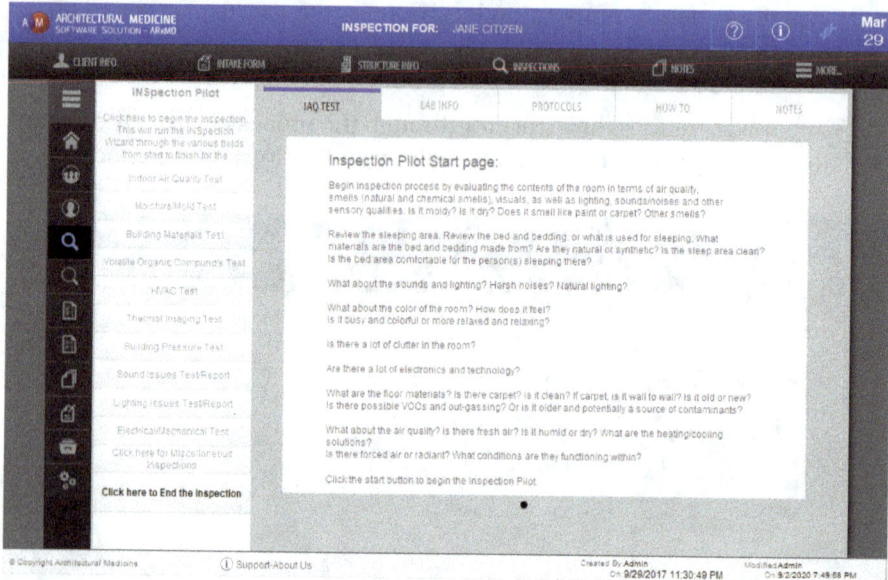

As time goes on, the Architectural Doctor may become a specialized practitioner. Just as the doctor can be listed as a family medical professional or an internal medicine professional, the Architectural Doctor may become the external medicine professional.

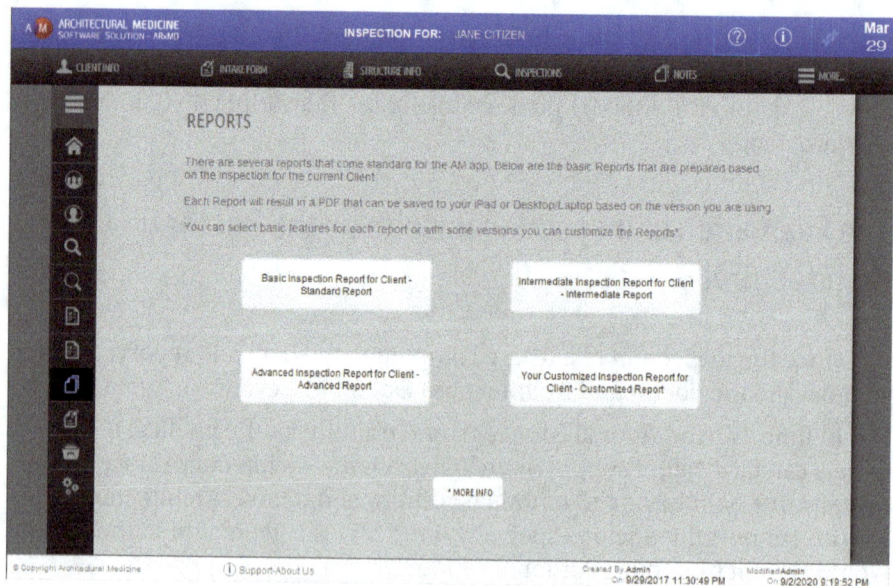

In tandem, these two professionals can support internal and external medicine to achieve the goals of Architectural Medicine to support optimal health and wellness.

Initially, the Architectural Doctor can evaluate the inspection reports and guide medical professionals to achieve their work. The Architectural Doctor can also support the doctor and the patient by assisting in the next steps if and when issues are found.

The Collaboration Process Between Doctor, Architect, Inspector, and Architectural Doctor

When there are issues found that are impacting the patient's health in their building, the next step is to involve the building professionals. Therefore, there is an ARxMD software segment for these architects and building professionals to access these inspection reports.

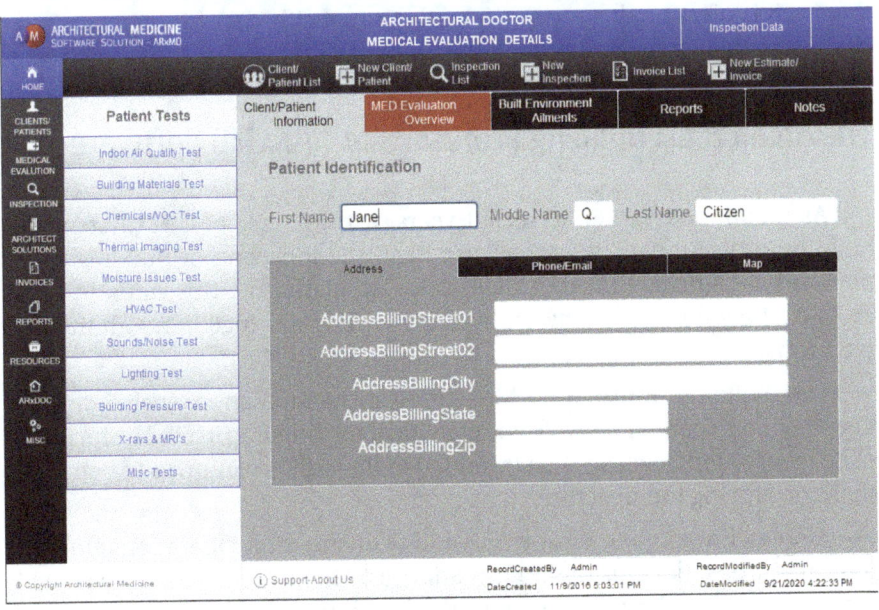

It is crucial to ensure that all of these professionals can work together in a collaborative process during these findings, ensuring that the communication of the issues is clear. This includes the building solution itself, as well as the subsequent steps to implement the process.

These next steps will depend upon the building professionals to review the building issues and provide solutions for these problems.

The interface for the architect and builder's view in their portal provides the appropriate building piece of the puzzle for review and analysis. As stated in previous sections, currently, there are limited connections between architectural and medical software, especially with these topics related to health and medicine workflows. And so, the ARxMD portal that the architects and builders view right now may extend to connect to their software in the near future with the appropriate API and technology integrations. The ARxMD platform can extend its interconnectivity to provide such solutions.

These new HL7 connections can allow for exchanges of data in the future, where the building professionals working on CAD/BIM drawings can provide these building solutions in digital format to be exchanged with the ARxMD software. In the future, these updates can be sent from the ARxMD platform to other professionals for review.

The benefit of the ARxMD software setup is that each portal is customized for each professional. In this manner, the architect and building professionals have customized fields for their work, while the doctor and inspector have fields and layouts appropriate for their work. There are standard fields that each professional can view, yet only the specific data for their use is exchanged between the different platforms.

The Architect & Building Professional – ARxMD Software

As mentioned earlier, in recent years, with the use of CAD systems for building professionals, there has also been the inclusion of Building Information Modeling or BIM with these software platforms. This can also be an excellent way for these software systems to function together with medical platforms.

This Building Information Modeling can include an extensive range of data fields and content as well as metadata of the building itself. The inclusion of health-related data can then be added to these BIM platforms to benefit all those occupying the structure.

Along with another acronym COBie (Construction Operations Building information exchange), this information can help Facility Managers (FM) maintain the building systems and the building's health over time. COBie is an international standard relating to managed asset information, including space and equipment. It provides electronic management to help facility managers maintain the building systems. With the ability for these systems to expand and include additional data, the information of the building's health can also be included.

The building professionals' software interface will provide views they can use to review building issues and record their solutions. These layouts offer details and supportive information to help them understand the health issues and what must be resolved.

By utilizing this information, they can evaluate the building issues and provide their solutions directly in the software. This way, there can be an understanding of precisely what will be required for resolving the problems and the steps needed to achieve this.

When the work is completed, the updated content can be saved to the ARxMD platform. This data can be exchanged and sent to the doctor and the rest of the professionals involved for review and follow up.

The Re-Inspection Process Using the ARxMD Software

After these issues have been resolved, the next step is to update the doctor and the Architectural Doctor to review the solutions. When they receive the updates to this work, they can notify the Healthy Building Inspector to follow up with a re-inspection to ensure that the work has been correctly implemented. The inspectors can provide re-testing of initial issues, using the initial test as a baseline. The updated results are then compared with the initial reporting.

These test results can be provided again through the laboratory systems using LOINC codes or can be entered as direct measurements on-site.

The data is then synced to the other ARxMD segments for other professionals to review. Or the data can be exchanged to an EMR or HIS to ensure that the solutions were successful.

The Informed Patient Is a Patient Educated for Their Own Best Health

Another essential component of the ARxMD software is the patient's ability to receive and review these results. This allows them to be informed by the doctor, Architectural Doctor, and the other health professionals involved in this process. It can also ensure that the patient knows the issues that impact their health and can learn more about these topics.

After all, if the patient is not aware of the issues, they cannot contribute to their good health. And when you scale this individual knowledge to the masses, it is either an empowering process for the public or a large-scale detriment to the overall health infrastructure in built environments.

The ARxMD software can sync this data to the patient's Electronic Health Record (EHR) or Comprehensive Health Record (CHR). This information can be accessible for them to review in different formats. Ensuring that the proper HIPAA compliance is followed using HL7, this information can be exchanged with the appropriate health systems and remain secure for their current and future review.

ARxMD Standards - Naming Conventions and Working With Current Standardized Systems, Nomenclature, and APIs

For those in the medical profession or those familiar with the vocation recognize there are many standards and naming conventions to support the various medical processes.

The CPT (Current Procedural Terminology) is the common terminology system used in the US. As mentioned earlier in the chapter, there is the ICD – International Statistical Classification of Diseases and Related Health Problems, and SNOMED – Systematized Nomenclature of Medicine. These are two of the more commonly known standards in the medical profession that define and classify diseases.

For laboratory testing and terminology, there is LOINC – Logical Observation Identifiers Names and Codes, and then there is also the DSM – Diagnostic and Statistical Manual of Mental Disorders, which is the standard used in the mental health professions.

While there is overlap between all of these medical terms systems, the use of one particular system over another includes several variables. Sometimes the choice is based on the specific profession, and other times it may be based on their geographic location. However, for Architectural Medicine and the ARxMD software, all data mapping between other systems will utilize the industry-standard Health Level 7 (HL7) protocols.

As of this writing, the current state of these standards is the ICD-10, SNOMED CT, and the DSM-5, along with the HL7 FHIR version 4. According to the World Health Organization (WHO), the ICD-11 is in process and will more closely coincide with SNOMED CT when it comes into effect on January 1, 2022.[170]

These protocols and processes allow health professionals to exchange data with one another and enable computer systems to integrate this data within various EMR platforms.

The field of architecture also has specific acronyms, nomenclature, and standards. It would seem like a good idea to have the standards on building health – inspections, analysis, protocols, and processes, along with the architecture solutions – to be in sync with these medical systems.

The Architectural Doctor's process and the Healthy Building Inspector will help develop and standardize these services, tests, evaluations, reporting, and the integrations of these procedures into these medical systems.

My thought is that if these processes and services are not defined and integrated, then the potential of health-related issues in the built environment adequately included and addressed will be precarious.

The Architectural Doctor and the Healthy Building Inspector's goal is to develop such standards and support the process. And the Architectural Medicine Software Solution is set to support this integrative process in a functional format.

These standards, bridging the gaps between the architecture and medical fields, can be defined as the *ARxMD standards, processes, and protocols*. Following the software's naming convention, these standards can be utilized and integrated into the ARxMD software to provide a template for each professional's methods.

It will also include education and provide information to both the architecture and medical communities. With the proper knowledge and processes implemented, this can strengthen the connection for more cohesive solutions.

The following diagram shows the round trip, cyclical or spiracycle as I call it, process of the basic functions of the system.

Essentially, this spiracycle is another format of the more in-depth flow chart of this evaluation process shown in chapter 15. You can view the larger version of this flowchart in chapter 15 or at the following website link:

https://architecturalmedicine.com/book/

As you can see, there is a dependency for each of the different professionals working together. Typically, these two primary professionals, that of the doctor and the architect, may have never worked together at all in the past.

With the inclusion of the two new professionals, the Architectural Doctor and the Healthy Building Inspector, these ARxMD protocols and processes allow for proper integration, which is critical for success.

As each of these topics is addressed for each professional, the requirement of using standards for testing protocols and data analysis in real-world scenarios can provide more integrative solutions.

The doctor will need to have processes that include these facets of the

Architectural Medicine – Building the Bridge to Wellness

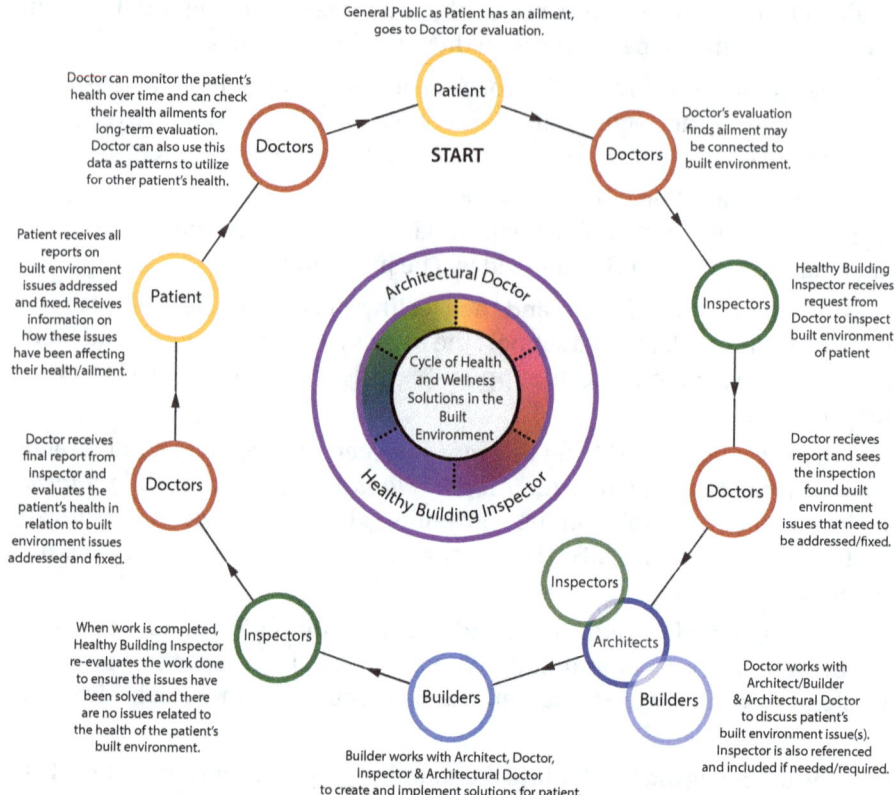

built environment. As well, architects will also need to be more well versed on health issues in the built environment and have proper processes to achieve these goals.

Including Mental and Emotional Health Evaluations in the Built Environment

And as if these steps are not enough complexity, there will also be at least two other professionals that may be involved — the Psychologist and the Neuroscientist.

In today's world, the idea of a psychologist involved in the built environment is sometimes defined as an Environmental Psychologist. While I've written about these topics in earlier chapters, in this book, I will not go into too many details. That said, I will reference two great resources for further reading. That is the work of Dr. Daniel Stokols at the University of California Irvine and Dr. Dak Kopec, who is a professor of architecture at the University of Nevada.

Chapter: 18   The Architectural Medicine Software Solution — ARxMD

Dr. Stokol's environmental psychology online course from a decade ago is still available for free through iTunes, and Dr. Kopec's book *Environmental Psychology for Design* are both great resources for those seeking more information about this field.

Another exciting development is the focus of neuroscience in architecture. This is also referenced as NeuroArchitecture, and a leading institution in this work is the Academy of Neuroscience for Architecture (ANFA). Their website defines the ANFA mission "to promote and advance knowledge that links neuroscience research to a growing understanding of human responses to the built environment."[171]

They have several resources available for more reading and learning about this emerging field on their website: https://www.anfarch.org/

I list both of these professions in this section due to the importance of including them in this equation for healthier built environment solutions. Just as the doctor as an MD can request an inspection as a building Rx for their patient, the psychologist and neuroscientist can also be included in this process to support emotional, mental, and psychological health for patients. Their work can provide an essential part of the ARxMD standards and use the ARxMD software in working with other professionals.

Product Manufacturers, Green Chemists, and Product Designers – Inclusion in the Solutions Process

And perhaps as a final step in the big picture process, and a key component in creating healthier built environments, is the inclusion of a large group of professionals in a wide range of fields across both architecture and medicine.

This includes professionals such as epidemiologists and toxicologists, as well as those in the emerging fields of green chemistry, biomimicry, geoinformatics, and neuroscience of architecture.

While these are not typically common groups working directly with the fields of architecture and medicine, they will play a critical role if health is indeed a focal point for the future of architecture.

The density of populations in smaller regions of cities requires a greater understanding of epidemiology and public health. Health impacts on cities will be exponentially larger in resulting illnesses and the potential for improving health in the future.

Fields such as Bioinformatics and the topic of big data can also play an important role, that is, if there is enough data to be analyzed and reviewed.

Architectural Medicine – Building the Bridge to Wellness

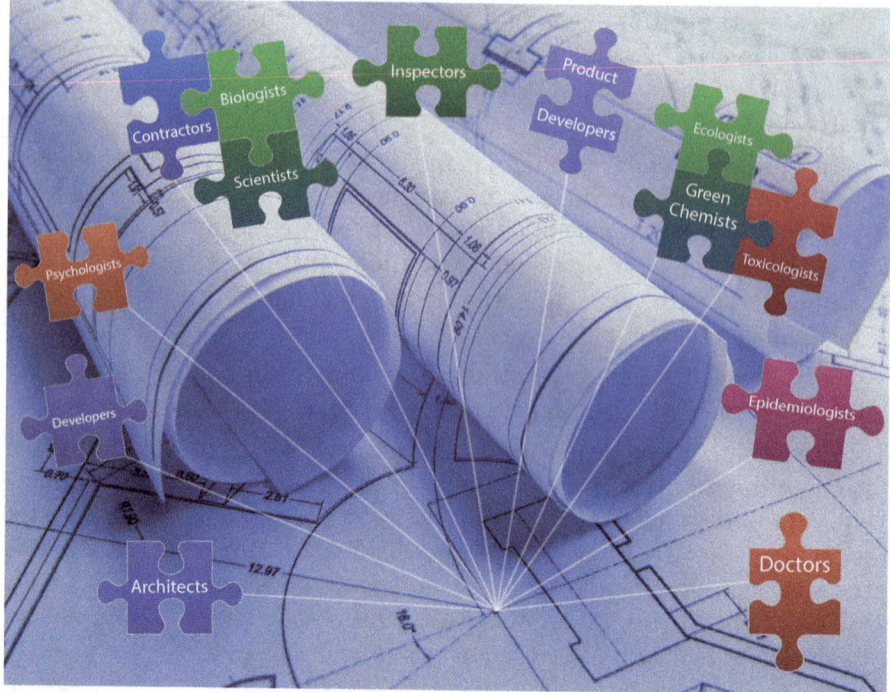

This points the way to the increasing potential of sensory devices in larger areas of the population, such as cities, combined with sensory devices on each person. This data can provide the individual with personal metrics to understand and contribute data for the larger populace when such anonymized data is evaluated.

Just as the first epidemiology strategy of John Snow showed that data metrics could provide clues to sources of illness, the strategy of big data in built environments can support clues and patterns of disease based on pollution and toxicity sources.

The process of setting up more organized sensory devices citywide can be helpful, along with providing individuals with sensors to monitor air quality and other metrics related to health.

And this is where the big data of the Architectural Medicine Software Solution – ARxMD can help support these health criteria in the built environment for professionals to evaluate and study. Having data anonymized and analyzed of these building health metrics, finding issues, and working on better solutions can become a full circle process.

A Clinical Data Repository (CDR) or Clinical Data Warehouse (CDW) can provide the foundation of research to help bridge these gaps and to find better solutions for future wellness and quality of life — from the individual to the larger populations.

A CDR/CDW can provide the raw data for analysis on a large scale to be analyzed and reviewed by professionals in public health, epidemiology, toxicology, and those researching links between the environment and human and biological health.

Some companies have been testing and developing personal health devices and have begun to ship their products in the past several years, such as the company tzoa based initially in Canada. Their personal device to measure air quality, combined with other devices such as the advanced Fitbit version and the Apple watch, can bring together personal data for evaluation.

This personal data, combined with sensory data in cities externally located on buildings, and sensors to measure an extensive range of data from inside buildings, can be put together to show an enormous scope of patterns related to health.

These metrics and patterns can be utilized to monitor potential health issues and provide warnings where applicable. It can be instrumental in monitoring areas of pollution that need attention.

As the EHR, or CHR allows for more comprehensive data, more information can be collected for an individual's health. Some of these metrics can be included, such as environmental data to provide an exposome of health over a lifetime.

The Architectural Medicine Software Solution can keep this information up to date and allow the user to review as to where they live and any sensory devices they have on their person (i.e. Fitbit, tzoa, Apple watch).

By having this data, public health professionals can keep track of large-scale health-related issues, especially if there are geolocated areas that are problematic.

All of this data collection and sharing also requires several issues to be reviewed. One is the fact that the individual will feel supported enough to trust the data shared is anonymized. And the second is to be empowered sufficiently to buy devices that can potentially provide them with the information they can benefit from. The third is to share this data in the greater scope, where they are comfortable that this data will be utilized for their interest and provided for best health processes to be evaluated. These updates can then be shared accordingly across the professions of architecture and medicine.

This trust is also critical moving forward. It is the responsibility of architecture, medicine, and other professions to ensure that this data is protected and utilized to benefit society.

The thoughtfulness and Hippocratic oath of medicine's "first, do no harm" as *primum non nocere* must become a mantra and dedication that is respected and adopted by architecture and other professionals whose involvement requires their integrity to protect society's health. While the original Hippocratic oath does not explicitly state this "do no harm" verbatim,[172][173] medicine's general approach includes this ethics. This is critical in terms of personal data and health related to the built environments. The inclusion of the other professions and the built environment offers a more extensive scope of this topic, yet should be taken as seriously as their patients' and clients' health and well-being. Just as the importance of a building is appropriately engineered to remain standing, and the importance of the doctor to provide healing and health to their patients, it should also be the goal to empower their patients and provide the best health possible for all clients.

Architecture and medicine have vital roles in the health and wellness of society. As professionals practicing on behalf of the public, there must be serious attention paid to these health topics in the built environment for current and future generations.

The decisions made now have an even longer tail of impact than in recorded history, as humanity has greater power to impact the planetary environment and the built environment than ever before. If steps are not seriously taken to properly evaluate all of these many facets, including how they synergistically work together for harm or benefit, merely depending on the outcome to simply work out positively is both irresponsible and misleading.

While ethics prevent us from evaluating the impact of chemicals on humans, the irony is that we are already guinea pigs of testing in many ways on a large scale level. Many may not realize that of the thousands of chemicals used in products, very few have been tested adequately in terms of human health. And even less have been tested when combined in real-world scenarios.

The drawback to this is twofold. The first is that it's harming people's health, which is the most important. And two, there is no evaluation or data collection of these scenarios, so we are not learning anything significant about these issues. Therefore, we cannot appropriately respond to a better understanding of these products and make any beneficial changes.

In the end, if we are not wise to act in proactive formats, humanity at large will be the guinea pigs of testing, and future generations will be at the mercy of the long tail results.

That seems neither intelligent nor wise.

Chapter: 18   The Architectural Medicine Software Solution — ARxMD

While the perfection of a utopia may not be achievable, the result of taking the time, energy, and effort in health-focused decisions can help reach a level of excellence.

And that level of excellence can yield results that provide a technologically better future for generations, as well as a better future in human-based terms – physically, mentally, emotionally, and spiritually.

In my mind's eye, these seem both wise and fitting ideals to strive to achieve. By taking the steps of Architectural Medicine and utilizing an Architectural Doctor's process towards supporting these goals is, to me, an effort worthy and forward-thinking for a better future.

An Aside – a History of ARxMD

The lack of systems between the architecture and medical professionals has meant that the process has often been an uphill battle for those working to help provide healthier built environments.

Over the past several decades in the US and worldwide, environmental consultants and environmental inspectors have strived to provide healthier solutions.

Each time a new project began for this type of consultant, the information and education process started from scratch. And because they were often brought into the building equation well after the design process had been completed, there was often friction between this consultant, inspectors, architects, and the other building professionals.

My experience and that of others in this realm brought my attention to these issues and led to the Architectural Medicine System (AMS) and ARxMD software development.

As I've mentioned throughout this book, the common building inspection and evaluation in the pre-2000s into the first decade of the 21st century were typically done on paper with a clipboard.

And this experience led me to realize the challenges of doing these environmental consultations and inspections. The ability to provide information, data, and reporting to the client and the many other professionals involved was extremely challenging.

While my experiences led to this frustration, a particular moment in 1999 led to the seed of the Architectural Medicine System (AMS) and the Architectural Medicine Software Solution – ARxMD.

The Development and Origins of the ARxMD Software and Standards

This software solution and process is actually near and dear to my heart. It's taken 25 years to develop these concepts into an overall system. While I consider myself an architect by nature, this development process in a systems architect's role is more in line with my latest work.

The Architectural Medicine Software Solution – ARxMD originated through my challenges and frustrations in striving to support healthier built environments, as I sought to be more involved in contributing to these developments.

While my involvement in architecture began as a teenager in the construction field and as an architectural engineering student in college, my search for an architectural world that I felt more in tune with has led me on this path.

In the late '80s and early '90s, architecture was not very interested, at least for the masses, in the concepts of green, healthy, and sustainable building. It wasn't until 1993 that I became aware of the professional activity in these emerging fields while attending an Eco-Design Conference held in New York City.

I was amongst a small group of people who participated in this event and had the great fortune to spend several days with some of the pioneers in these fields. Among those who spoke at this event were William McDonough, James Wines, Paul Bierman Lytle, and some of the people who I ended up working with to co-create Integrated Environmental Solutions and H3Environmental – Mary Cordaro and Kathryn Metz.

The now-famous speech by Steve Jobs at the Stanford commencement, in many ways, sums up many experiences in my life. It can also explain how this Architectural Medicine Software Solution came to be. Even if you're not a fan of the late Mr. Jobs, you might glean some nuggets of wisdom from this speech, especially where he states:

"you can't connect the dots looking forward; you can only connect them looking backward. So, you have to trust that the dots will somehow connect in your future."[174]

For me, this has been my truth. Throughout my life, from my involvement working in construction and working at a health center to the many other jobs involved with architecture focused on healthy, sustainable building, these puzzle pieces have all consolidated into Architectural Medicine. All of these facets of my life, including my work in the worlds of technology, have led me on this path.

One of my mentors, the swiss architect Bosco Büeler, often noted as the godfather of Bau Biologie said something that has stayed with me for the past two decades. About twenty years ago, after I shared with him my frustrations of trying to develop more opportunities in the US for healthier, greener, and more sustainable building – which often fell on deaf ears – he told me the following. He said that often in life, you can't always go directly from point A to point B. Sometimes you have to follow the path and process of sailing, where you have to "tack"[175] back and forth to eventually arrive at your destination.

For me, this tacking back and forth has meant that I've worked in many different fields to experience many facets of life. After many years of experience, the benefit has now come together into the Architectural Medicine System (AMS) and the ARxMD software and solutions.

The Architectural Medicine Software Solution began out of my frustrations. Over the years, I have taken many courses and learned many facets focusing on a career in the healthy, green, and sustainable building fields. Yet I soon learned why many who had previously tried this path had not continued, or at least done so on a less scalable level. I found a lack of interconnections between the fields, whether the architecture and medical fields or the building and public health fields. The lack of connections has led to significant challenges in creating these multi-disciplinary solutions.

Each group seemed unaware of the full attention they should have on the built environment in their unique roles. Therefore, someone such as a healthy building consultant or environmental inspector was an outsider and never really fit into their systems.

This, combined with a lack of supportive training and business systems in an environmental consultant's role, meant everything is done from scratch for every project. And the process of running a business, along with training and educating so many people with such wide-ranging topics, has led this field to consist of only a small handful of people.

All of my experiences have provided insights into the importance of systems and groups working together with similar goals. A systems approach providing standards for working together across professions can help deliver better health and wellness solutions.

During the late 90s, I traveled around the US and studied and worked with different professionals who were developing a mixture of sustainable, green, and healthy building solutions. However, they were often isolated and outside of the mainstream. Luckily, I learned more about these pioneers and visited them due to the internet and online groups.

In the spring of '99, I was en-route to Arizona to learn straw bale construction and natural plasters with the Steens in southern Arizona. The builders and authors, Bill and Athena Steen are among a small group of pioneers who developed many strawbale construction techniques in the '90s to the current day. Their book *The Straw Bale House*, which includes the innovators David Bainbridge and David Eisenberg, provides a vast resource for those venturing to build with this rediscovered building material.

As I was picking up my friend and previous business colleague Mary Cordaro from the Tucson airport, I saw a massive billboard advertisement for home inspections. The sign was an ad for home inspections that included a large clipboard denoting the inspection process.

I had just spent the previous few years working on my education and pathway to this new field of healthy building development and environmental consulting, and an idea emerged. With my recent purchase of a laptop, I immediately found this analog clipboard topic as great potential in a digital solution.

I asked myself, "what if there was a digital tablet that could provide a healthy building consultant with information and training that can be used on-site? What if this could be developed for healthy building reference, and record the intake forms for consulting and inspection results to then provide as reports for clients?"

This began the birth of the software idea, and soon after, I began writing an overview of this process that I titled "The Electronic Clip Board or the Datalog software approach." The idea was to have an electronic clipboard as a tablet and software as a database to reference and create these intakes, testing, and reporting.

This also came from the feedback I had received from a few people who were doing environmental consulting work and healthy building inspections. They often spent a lot of time with paperwork for the intake forms and reporting the inspections. This was in addition to the often lengthy process of educating and informing their clients.

I thought using this kind of electronic tablet could provide digital solutions to these processes and provide some guidance and references – especially for someone learning all of these big topics that needed to be easily referenced.

The initial idea began in a basic format, and I started implementing some of these ideas as I developed the software for both companies that I had co-formed – Integrated Environmental Solutions and H3Environmental. However, the true vision of an application of such complexity of ARxMD at that time of the late 1990s and early 2000s was complicated and expensive to develop. And while I did not expect it to take as long as it has, it's taken a tremendous amount of time to put together these integrated concepts into a functional model.

This also required years of additional learning in the technology and computing worlds to create such software. Fortunately, over time the current hardware and software options are now available to achieve these goals and are also affordable. The advent of modern software integrations and hardware such as the iPad and tablets have allowed the Architectural Medicine Software Solution to become a reality. It's currently in the process of being available for multiple platforms to use for a range of professionals.

And the hopeful result is that this software can support those striving to contribute to these solutions for better health and wellness in the built environment. These systems and the software can offer more structure and procedures to follow and have a smaller learning curve than what I had to navigate twenty-five to thirty years ago.

Creating these systems gives professionals the potential to access information on these topics at their fingertips with processes and protocols to follow for their profession. It can also support connections between medicine, architecture, inspectors, and building professionals working together for a round trip process as a whole system.

The general public's ability to access this information can empower the populations for their better health. The reports created by these professionals can be available for them to review. In this way, they can become more educated about these topics and have access to resources to learn about these issues for better health education.

ARxMD Follow up and Conclusion

One of the most critical facets of my learning was to witness and experience the challenges of having no connections between the worlds of architecture, building, medicine, and inspection professionals. While the patient as the client may be up to date or inquisitive on these health topics in the built environment, there have often been challenges where professionals either aren't aware of these factors or don't know how to resolve them.

The construction field is often challenged with new products. They usually don't have the best support in learning these more recent products and processes. Sometimes professionals have some information about these issues yet have no protocols, systems, or solutions to offer.

Often there is a lot of education and information required from the consultant to provide such information, some of which are rejected and some accepted. Overall, the professionals involved in these newer processes and products are often weary on behalf of their familiarity with new products while maintaining their professionalism.

The case was that too often, the time required to orchestrate these solutions for better health in the built environment either fell on deaf ears or went nowhere due to the complexities involved in these newer processes.

So, the Architectural Medicine System (AMS) goals and the Architectural Medicine Software Solution ARxMD are to help bridge those gaps and help support those involved. It is intended to ensure they have the best solutions, and access to their profession's protocols and procedures. It provides the required integration to work with other professionals along with the patient.

All of this requires each professional to be involved and be responsible for their part. If this can be followed through, then the result is a group of professionals working with the patient to find and resolve issues for the patient's best health.

And as this process scales to larger groups of people, what this translates to is better health of the individual and better health for the community and society.

When this can scale up to city-level benefit, then healthier cities can be created and maintained over time. This leads to a future that supports better health and wellness in the built environment, and in my opinion, that's a future worth planning for.

The updates to these systems can provide a foundation of better building solutions for the DNA of healthier cities. This DNA of buildings and the DNA of cities was referenced earlier in the book. And at this stage of writing, it should be more clear as to the importance of these processes in achieving these goals.

While the current version of the ARxMD software has been developed over time with input from many different sources, it is still in its infancy. In terms of future development to grow into a more robust solution, the addition of new components and integrations will provide better support moving forward.

It is meant to be a collaborative process and will depend upon many different professionals' support along the way. With this mantra, I invite you to contribute, add comments, and recommendations on how it can be made better. And, if you are a professional, it can allow you to be more productive and supportive in creating healthier built environments.

Chapter: 18   The Architectural Medicine Software Solution — ARxMD

More information on the Architectural Medicine Software Solution is available on our website, with more details about ARxMD and options for use. You can find a link on our home page or use this link:

https://architecturalmedicine.com/arxmd

Since these whole systems of cycles or spiracycles can lead to an iterative process, the next question may be, "where do we go from here, and what is the future of health and wellness in architecture?" And this is a perfect segue into the next chapter...

> "Do not go where the path may lead,
> go instead where there is no path and leave a trail."
>
> – Ralph Waldo Emerson

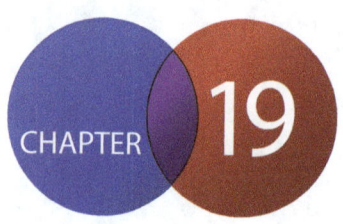

THE DNA OF CITIES & PARAMETRIC ARCHITECTURE

Over the many years of my life, from childhood to adulthood, there has been something consistent in the building fields that I've experienced my entire life. Whenever I have discussed architecture with architects, builders, or contractors, I don't recall ever having a single conversation about the critical role architecture plays in nurturing human beings.

In my college years, I began to think about this topic with more clarity, especially as I learned more about the architecture profession and the building methods of other species and creatures on this planet. Time and time again, in the natural world, I've learned about nature's process of building shelter for nurturing, specially created for their offspring. The many creatures on this planet intend to build a shelter for safety with the intent of developing nurturing environments.

Designing Nurturing Places and Spaces – The DNA of Cities and Parametric or Curvilinear Architecture

The history of human shelter and architecture has changed quite a bit over time. With the history of hunter-gatherer societies, some of these groups consisted of the women building shelter, which changed in dynamic when agrarian life became more common.

From women creating shelter to men being those who often are the builders, the agrarian lifestyle brought changes to the human building processes. This change in dynamic shows a possible timeline when architecture became more about a statement of place instead of a place focused on nurturing.

Now, to be clear, I'm not critical of this for the sake of criticism, yet in the context of shelter as buildings for wellness, this is quite important. This is also not to say that men cannot create nurturing architecture. But it can point to the reality that if you look around at the world of architecture, more so than not, the buildings' discussions are less about their ability to provide nurturing environments and more about other topics – often based on the intellectualism of function and form.

Again, not a negative by itself, yet when you consider the scale that the built environment has grown to be, the lack of something as important as nurturing also scales exponentially – either for the better or for worse.

My point is the lack of attention to this important topic has defined many centuries of architecture that has not focused on nurturing nor thriving for populations in society. And this, in many ways, is likely the reason why the topic of health and wellness in the built environment is not common in today's age of architecture.

The truth of this statement, and perhaps irony, is that instead of today's architecture being a strong point of security focused on health, it is common for people to be proud of these structures more so as objects. And this lack of attention to health has led many buildings to become toxic.

I began to learn this mantra at an early age, where men were supposed to be proud of showing no emotions or striving to have no feelings. By the time male children have had years of practice on this topic, it's no wonder that when they grow up to become architects and builders, this mantra is maintained to become a badge of courage. And since the fields of building and construction have a large percentage of male workers, this equates to a culture founded on this mindset.

Yet when you think about it, removing one's emotions can also impact what's required to evaluate a space and place as to whether or not it is safe on these sensory levels. Obviously, it's crucial that the structural integrity of a building provides shelter and is not going to fall down. This, of course, is essential, yet to be tuned out of your feelings means that you also cannot evaluate issues in these same spaces with one's senses.

And this has led to many buildings as places that can stand up to weather and the natural elements, but in doing so, without empathy and emotional intelligence, have created toxic environments.

The goal would be to achieve this shelter and security in ways that do not create toxic environments. If you cannot sense these health issues, then striving to achieve this very goal of providing shelter and security can be at odds with these goals.

And to make sure that the sensitivity to gender roles is clear, this is more so a description of masculine and feminine rather than gender. I've worked with many sensitive males and also worked with females in the building fields, so it would be wrong to state that nurturing is inherently gender-based.

Yet if you, like me, have spent time around construction projects, you know that they are rarely nurturing environments – to put it mildly.

There can be a balance between these two topics of shelter and security while also providing healthy, nurturing qualities. There are ways to ensure that the building provides the necessary structural integrity and protection, yet can be nurturing and caring for those living within these structures.

It does, however, take the recognition of these issues, which requires awareness of these topics to begin with. And then, it requires the openness to find solutions to both current and future designs that embrace both security, safety, and nurturing as a whole.

After all, if you cannot create safe and nurturing structures, you cannot expect to have built environments that support optimal health and wellness.

For me, I was very fortunate to grow up in an environment that was both tough and filled with sports, yet I also spent a significant amount of time in nature and the natural world as a nurturing element. It has been no picnic to strive to bridge these divides, yet as I've gotten older, I've begun to see these different worlds in both an intellectual and sensing format. I've had a foot in each world recognizing these topics, and have worked towards solutions that, in my mind, are both logical and sensible.

A lifetime of navigating these worlds of opposites has supported the ideals of Architectural Medicine. If I can help contribute to these solutions for current and future generations, then I see it as hardships alchemized into a worthwhile pursuit.

The idea that our homes and living places greatly impact our well being is often overlooked until people do not have a home or place for shelter. The notion that architecture can nurture may be strange to people, yet this might reflect how little people are aware of their built environment and their bodies.

When people become more aware of their places and spaces, and how they feel and think in these spaces, a glimpse of this power can be revealed.

Yet much of modern-day design is focused more on the latest fads and design motifs than they are on creating nurturing designs.

The study in the 1980s by Dr. Urlich, which had a positive impact on healing for those patients with a window allowing views of nature — such as trees and large open natural spaces — showed how this supported healing in hospitals.[176] This has forever changed the mindset and approach to hospital design.

This nurturing and healing topic is not often discussed, yet is perhaps one of the essential facets to review in future designs. The concept of architecture or buildings being nurturing can often seem strange.

Yet, the reality is that when we have shelter as homes and places of work where we feel comfortable, it can allow for nurturing that reduces stress and improves the quality of life. This, in turn, can lead to better overall well being.

Chronic stress is often quoted as a proxy as the number one source of death in the modern world.[177] [178] The idea that you can design spaces and places to reduce stress might be more important than people are recognizing.

What is the DNA of Healthy, Green, and Sustainable Cities for Well Being?

As today's populations continue to gather in urban areas, some critical facets of architecture should be viewed in a closer context. While urban locations are of great focus today, there are some vital issues to evaluate based on rural buildings.

What do rural buildings have to do with urban skyscrapers?

This may sound strange, but the reality is that the urban landscape often takes its DNA from rural buildings. Let's review an example to show how this is possible.

If you look at the origins of most cities, you can rewind back to a time when there was no city there at all, even to the point when no houses and not even a single structure existed. The natural existence of all cities is…nature.

If you go into the rural environments of yesteryear or even today, you will typically find a familiar design landscape. Everywhere around the world, the rural landscape is similar. It begins with a structure built for either home or work, or in many cases, as a farmhouse, so it often includes both. It starts with one structure, and then soon after this, another building is added, perhaps as storage or a farmhouse or even a garage or shed.

Yet if you look at how this rural landscape morphs into a suburban area and then an urban landscape, it all starts with that single structure. Then a second and a third building is added. Initially, these buildings may be several acres away from each other, yet the type of these buildings as homes, farmhouses, and sheds typically have a similar design. And this design in both aesthetics and functioning is the eventual DNA of a city.

If you take that single building and look closer, what do you see? What are the aesthetics of the structure? Does the design strive to fit in with the natural environment, or does it look like a box that has just been plopped down onto the land?

What about the way it functions? As an example, how does it receive its water? What does it do with its waste and sewage? What do the people living there do with the products that they use in daily life? Does it become recycled or repurposed, or does it become garbage? What about energy? Where is that coming from? Is it from a local power grid, or is it from a renewable energy source such as solar power? What materials are used to build the structure? Are they local materials? How were these materials produced? And how did they get to the location?

These are some common questions that can lead to more specific details, such as, what is the impact that the structure has on the environment? How does it handle the local weather and storms? Is it designed to be energy efficient, or are these afterthoughts? Does the structure require more energy to provide artificial lighting and heating and other "air conditioning" solutions?

These are important questions to evaluate because this single house often becomes the template of other structures and eventually the DNA of the city. Because as most rural developments progress, it begins with one building, and then another building that is relatively similar if not the same. These buildings multiply over time as somewhat identical copies of each other. Once there are enough of these buildings, then it's defined as a sub-urban environment. From this development, the buildings become larger, closer together, and the population becomes more dense until it is an urban city.

The landscape that started with a single building can eventually become a city. Yet by the time it is a city, the evaluation of these issues and topics is much more difficult to either manage or change to become more environmentally interdependent. And if you look at most cities around the world, they are essentially similar in how they function. The aesthetics may be slightly different in terms of the type of high rise or skyscraper. Yet, many of the functionalities from the power sources to water and waste and other municipalities follow the path of the original structures of these rural areas.

We are now at a point in time where human impact on the environment, ecology, and "places" has a global level of impact, not just local. So if we are to make changes to how these cities can coexist with the natural environment of both the local areas and the global planet, then reviewing the DNA of this first building is critical.

The question may begin with, "what does a healthy, green, and sustainable city look like?". And as the question becomes asked, the result of this can be an analysis of a single building. The next question might be, "can this design scale up to a city in a healthy, green, and sustainable format?"

This is how the rural building landscape, which mostly appears to be open land with a small building on a vast area of land, can become the DNA of the densest cities in the world.

The design aesthetics, along with the functionality of this architecture, is critical. Can this single building support good health — physically, mentally, and emotionally? What about the systems of the building, can they be mutually interconnected with the environment in which they exist? How does the building utilize water, power, and waste? How do the daily functions of the building and its occupants impact the local environment? Are they mutually in accordance with each other, or is the structure eroding the natural landscape and degrading the location's ecological balance?

Does the building fit into the natural environment, or does it overcome the location or, worse, completely ignore its impact on the surroundings?

Does the architecture support the psychological and emotional wellness of the occupants? How about the physical characteristics of the structure? Are they helping or harming the health of the inhabitants?

These are all critical questions in today's day and age of architecture. And with the advent of today's emerging fields of environmental psychology and neuroscience of architecture, these design questions also include the occupants' health in terms of physical, mental, and emotional well being.

The scalability of this rural structure as the modern-day city's DNA is a fractal pattern of the future. Just as Christopher Alexander's *Pattern Language* examines, these patterns in architecture will define the future of cities.

What kind of future will we choose to design and build?

The DNA of Healthy, Green, and Sustainable Cities Begins with the Single Structure

There have been many positive movements and changes to the architecture and building fields to make the built environment more energy-efficient and sustainable. And the developments in healthy hospital designs have provided healthier built environments for the patients and health professionals alike.

With these topics becoming more common and more important for the future of humanity and the planet, these developments need to be more pro-active and implemented more quickly.

The other factor in this equation is the growth of populations and the fact that larger numbers of people are now moving to and living in urban environments. So the process of making large-scale changes is critical.

Yet, how do these changes happen? And what small steps can be taken to achieve these goals?

The reality of this process is that if we are to make significant changes, there must be cohesive changes. Making a little change here and there is always positive, yet to have the large-scale updates that are needed requires a considerable transformation.

Many say that humans don't like change, but I think that's a misnomer. While it's true that many don't like change at all, if the average person were given 100 million dollars, their lives would change, and I don't think most people would be upset with these changes. No, the changes we don't like are those that we don't embrace and cause a negative response.

So, there are two things to note about this. One is to find a way to reframe these changes that people would embrace as positive, and the second is to outline what some of these changes are – at least enough to provide a framework of understanding. An approach to this is to see the single structure as part of the DNA of global architecture. To add to this equation, it shouldn't just be the architects, designers, and builders championing these changes. If the general public doesn't demand that these upgrades are made, then the supply of the building professionals will fall flat.

So this process requires at least the following three topics:

- The general public demanding healthy, green, and sustainable buildings
- The building and construction professionals become well versed in solutions to create these healthy, green, and sustainable buildings
- The concept of each structure as the DNA of the city must be recognized

Just as our DNA defines the structure of our entire bodies, the DNA of each structure defines the resulting DNA of the city. A city is a composition of many structures, so while these designs and aesthetics may be different, the function of these structures and the approach of these designs must embrace health, energy efficiency, and sustainability.

The good news about these developments is that the effects of these changes are both synergistic and wide-spreading. Just as the synergy of pollution of the Cuyahoga river resulted in the river spontaneously combusting, the opposite is true as well, and the positive synergy of these new design approaches can yield excellent benefits. These benefits are broad in scope, from the local health of each structure's occupants to the entire eco-system of the planet. When one change is made with benefit in synergy with many other beneficial changes, the cohesive and collaborative results are enormous.

These changes help benefit not just the local ecology, but the health of the global planet and its many creatures and organisms. This includes the health of the oceans and water sources, which has become an increasing concern over the past several decades. The health of the forests, oceans, and plant and animal life is not just good stewardship as humans, it is critical to conserve, preserve and take care of for our own good health.

The reality is that humans depend on a healthy environment, and we should strive to protect and take care of planetary health. Since buildings and cities have such a big impact on the natural environment and ecology, we need to pay attention to this. And as we focus more on planetary health, we must have critical thinking approaches to understanding the negative impacts the building process has on ecological, biological, and human health.

Another facet of good news is that when we begin to do this, we start to see how human built environments impact natural habitats. And this understanding can help us design and build solutions that do not harm or destroy these environments for humans and the entire biology of the planet.

However, it does require us to recognize these impacts and be honest with the destruction that we can create in building structures. There needs to be an honest look at what negatives the current building practices and approaches have on the environment and human health.

Once we can understand these issues, we can then begin to design and engineer appropriate solutions.

If we can see these issues, problems, and solutions from a coherent and intelligent viewpoint, we can begin applying wisdom to solutions.

These solutions can become the DNA of a new building approach and process, from materials and methods to design and engineering.

When the function and forms of the built environment consider the occupant's health – physically, mentally, and emotionally, and applies this knowledge in ways that are energy efficient and sustainable for future generations, then we can apply the DNA of wisdom to the built environment for all living beings.

This is the DNA of new houses, new developments, and new cities. It is the same DNA, yet with the creativity of our own DNA as humans, where only four different DNA options can create billions of different possibilities.

So while some may be concerned about the lack of options, it instead can provide greater opportunities. To know that when the resulting variations are created, they will still have the same genetics to ensure that the topics of healthy, green, and sustainable building methods are all embedded into the coding of the architecture of the future.

And that's a change that most people can be happy and hopeful about...

The Future of Health and Wellness in Architecture

In the book *De Architectura*, Vitruvius wrote, "for if a man be placed flat on his back, with his hands and feet extended, and a pair of compasses centered at his navel, the fingers and toes of his two hands and feet will touch the circumference of a circle described therefrom. And just as the human body yields a circular outline, so too a square figure may be found from it."[179]

The Vitruvian Man illustration that Leonardo da Vinci drew is arguably one of the most famous descriptions of Vitruvius' writing, yet how many times have you viewed this diagram and asked, "who is Vitruvius and why did he outline this description to begin with?"

| Chapter: 19 | The DNA of Cities & Parametric Architecture |

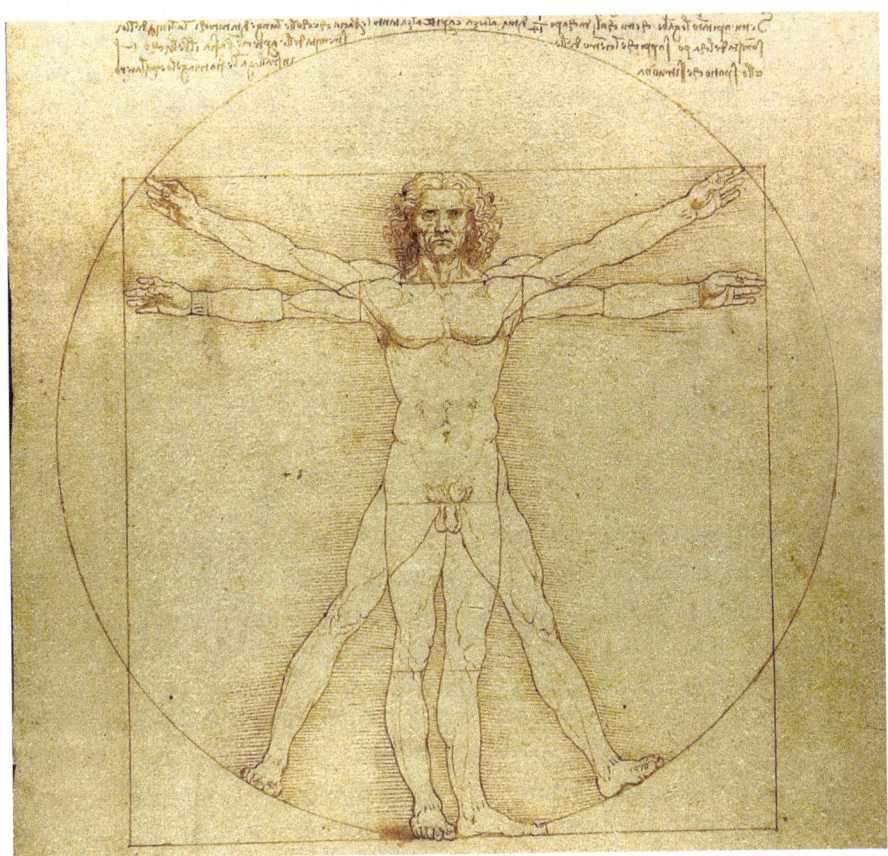

Artist: Leonardo da Vinci – c. 1490 – Photo: Luc Viatour – https://Lucnix.be

The Vitruvian Man – Vitruvius and da Vinci

Vitruvius, the architect from the 1st century BC, and his writings on architecture are amongst the earliest in recorded history. An interesting note to Vitruvius as an architect is his comments as to medicine and health.

Vitruvius's interest in the proportions of the human body, complete with precise measurements and elaborate geometrical relationships, was his approach to understanding human proportions. In his viewpoint, architecture is essentially an imitation of nature. He believed that understanding the body's proportions leads to a better grasp of desirable proportions in buildings.

He stated, "The architect should be equipped with knowledge of many branches of study and varied kinds of learning, for it is by his judgment that all work done by the other arts is put to test."[180]

"The architect should also have a knowledge of the study of medicine on account of the questions of climates, air, the healthiness and unhealthiness of sites...for without these considerations the healthiness of a dwelling cannot be assured."[181]

While many have noted that the process has been to square the circle, I'd like to focus more on the circle itself. I do so because of the natural proportions that are both described by Vitruvius and outlined by da Vinci – literally.

And this leads to the conversations of circular and curving designs compared to the square and rectangular designs in architecture.

What Is Parametric or Curvilinear Architecture and How Is It Connected to Health?

While much of this book has not focused on specific architectural designs or styles, one design style can be discussed relative to health.

In this chapter, I will discuss Parametric Architecture, Parametric Design or Parametricism, and the many definitions relative to the proliferation of curvilinear designs in the 21st century. I'm specifically going to discuss the possible connections between these designs and health and explore these connections relative to Architectural Medicine.

This topic focuses on architecture with curving shapes and forms, which can also be defined as "Curvilinear Architecture," as opposed to the common building forms in a more rectangular or rectilinear building form. The topic of parametric design can be categorized as computational design and has an overlap with algorithmic design. I will discuss more of these details later in the chapter.

Parametric Architecture or Parametric Design is not new, yet there has been a tremendous increase in architectural designs worldwide of this style in the past twenty years. There are many discussions and differing viewpoints on the definition of Parametric Architecture. By providing some history of this topic with past and current developments, I will delve into this subject and explore this important topic for the built environment in the 21st century.

Parametric Architecture or Curving Architecture

To start with, there are a few different labels discussing this topic, from parametric architecture and parametric design to parametricism. The first two have practically the same overlap in definition, with parametric architecture often listed as a segment of parametric design. The term parametricism has its own distinct yet similar definition that I will also explore later in this chapter.

The simple definition of parametric design is shapes and forms that have a curving nature, often similar to a parabola or other flowing forms in the shape of arcs.

These forms can include the arcs of entryways or the structure's entire profile in the form of flowing curves.

Good examples of these designs are the TWA Building at New York's JFK airport and the Ingalls Rink at Yale, both by Eero Saarinen.[182] The works of Antoni Gaudi, Frank Gehry's Guggenheim in Bilbao Spain, and the designs of Zaha Hadid are other good examples of these forms.

Antoni Gaudi's work can be viewed as an early example of designs based on these curving forms, which can be graphed based on a set of "parameters" much like a parabola or other conical cross-sections would create. And while Gaudi may not have used mathematical formulas to achieve these shapes, he did create the forms of Sagrada Familia based on the catenary curve by hanging chains from the ceiling of his design studio to determine these shapes.

By using these hanging chains, he then inverted these arcs to define his design forms. Essentially, he based these shapes as a physical connotation to the mathematical equivalent of such parameters.

In the mid 20th century, designers and engineers, such as Frei Otto, would create these curving designs by utilizing mathematical equations as "parameters" to engineer these curves and forms.

Parametric Design – First Look — Just the Math

The term "parameter" is a key term to this design approach. The use of the word in this sense can be based on the mathematical "parameter." This can be defined as the following:

"in mathematics, a variable for which the range of possible values identifies a collection of distinct cases in a problem. Any equation expressed in terms of parameters is a parametric equation."[183]

If you're a math professional or advocate, this definition may make perfect sense, yet for others, this can be fuzzy as to what exactly this means.

What this is essentially defining is a curving line or form.

It is essentially an arc defined by a set of parameters or numbers whose shapes can be defined in an equation.

The Oxford dictionary defines a parameter as "a constant occurring in the equation of a curve or surface, by the variation of which the equation is made to represent a family of such curves or surfaces."[184]

This definition is significant if you are to use a computer to define and engineer these shapes. In modern-day computing and current Computer-Aided Drawing (CAD) programs, these curves and forms can now be graphed in three dimensions as architectural forms.

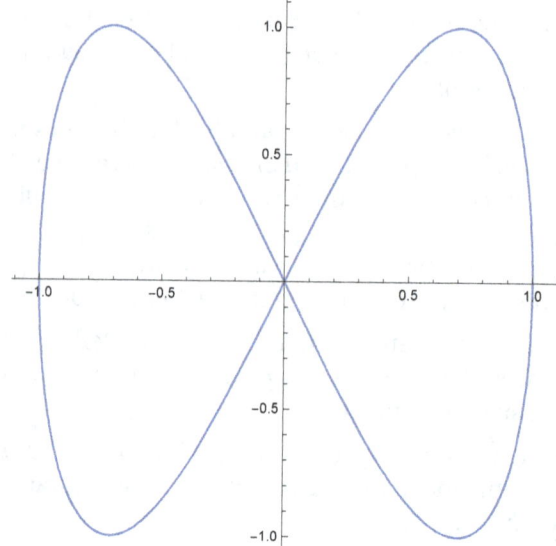

The ability to utilize software applications also allows the engineering of these forms to be evaluated. These CAD drawings can then be fabricated using CAE and CAM – Computer-Aided Engineering and Manufacturing.

The ability to design, engineer, and fabricate these forms using the computer, is likely a significant reason why there are so many architectural designs utilizing these curving forms today. In the past, the amount of manual labor that would be required to both engineer and manufacture these shapes from stone, steel, aluminum, and other materials would be cost-prohibitive.

The computing factor is an important topic related to parametric design. These forms are now created on computers instead of the hand drawings and physical experiments done by Gaudi and other designers in pre-computer times.

And this is why parametric design has often become synonymous with mathematics as algorithms, as opposed to many historical designs that were hand-drawn.

This viewpoint that computational designs are a fad as a style is, in my opinion, a short-sided view on parametric design, and I discuss these thoughts later in this writing.

A Deeper Dive Into the Math – Computational and Algorithmic Designs

Before I get into the math details, let me take a moment to discuss the topics of computational and algorithmic designs relative to parametric design. What are the differences?

There are many terms used to define designs created using computers, and these are typically categorized as computational design. From Computer-Aided Drawing (CAD) to Parametric Design, each of these utilizes computers to achieve results using hardware and software platforms. There are many similarities between parametric and algorithmic design processes.

An algorithm is defined as "a procedure for solving a mathematical problem (as of finding the greatest common divisor) in a finite number of steps that frequently involves repetition of an operation."[185]

However, the algorithm does not explicitly state that math procedures will be parametric in form and shape. Therefore, you can say that parametric design is a type of algorithmic design, which can be defined as computational design. In this next section, we will explore more details of the math involved in these computational designs.

If you don't have an interest in a deeper dive into the math, you can skip to the next section.

To help bring more clarity and depth to this topic, let's explore two other definitions related to parametric design based on analytic geometry and mathematical analysis on parameters.

In analytic geometry, curves are often given as the image of some function. The argument of the function is invariably called "the parameter."[186]

A circle of radius 1 centered at the origin can be specified in more than one form:

- *implicit* form, the curve is all points (x,y) that satisfy the relation $x^{2}+y^{2} = 1$
- *parametric* form, the curve is all points (cos(t), sin(t)), when t varies over some set of values, like [0, 2π), or (-∞, ∞):

(x, y) = (cos *t*, sin *t*)
where *t* is the parameter.

Hence these equations, which might be called functions elsewhere, are in analytic geometry characterized as parametric equations, and the independent variables are considered parameters.

In mathematical analysis, integrals dependent on a parameter are often considered. These are of the form:

$$F(t) = \int_{x_0(t)}^{x_1(t)} f(x;t)\, dx$$ [187]

"In this formula, *t* is the argument of the function F, and on the right-hand side, the parameter on which the integral depends. When evaluating the integral, *t* is held constant, and so it is considered to be a parameter. If we are interested in the value of F for different values of *t*, we then consider *t* to be a variable."[188]

The advanced mathematics platform Wolfram defines parameter as such:

"the term *parameter* is used in a number of ways in mathematics. In general, mathematical functions may have a number of arguments. Arguments that are typically varied when plotting, performing mathematical operations, etc., are termed "variables," while those that are not explicitly varied in situations of interest are termed *parameters*."[189]

For example, in the standard equation of an ellipse:

$$(x^2/a^2)+(y^2/b^2)=1$$

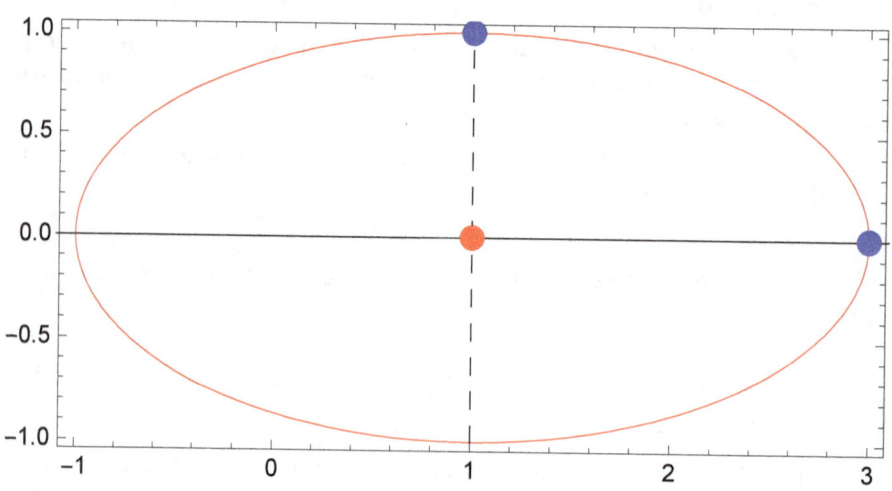

Assuming a >= b, the foci are (+-c, 0) for c = $\sqrt{a^2 - b^2}$, the standard parametric equation is:

(x, y) = (a cos(*t*), b sin(*t*)) for 0 <= *t* <= 2π

"**x** and **y** are generally considered variables and **a** and **b** are considered parameters. The decision on which arguments to consider variables and which to consider parameters may be historical or may be based on the application under consideration."

However, the nature of a mathematical function may change depending on which choice is made.

And so the term Parametric Design is based on the various parameters that define the curving nature of these designs as lines or forms.

Parametricism and Parametric Architecture – What's the Difference?

As with many other fields, there are often differing definitions of a similar topic, and so is the case for this topic as well. Parametric Architecture also has another title, which is called *Parametricism*.

In a segment on the history of Parametricism, it's stated that it, "emerged as a theory-driven avant-garde design movement in the early 1990s, with its earliest practitioners - Greg Lynn, Jesse Reiser, Lars Spuybroek, Kas Oosterhuis among many others – harnessing and adapting the then new digital animation software and other advanced computational processes that had been introduced within architecture much earlier by pioneers like John Frazer and Paul Coates, but that only spread to make an impact within avant-garde architecture in the last 10-15 years."[190]

Patrik Schumacher of the Zaha Hadid design group has said he "believes the work of Frei Otto is a precursor of Parametricism." He comments that Frei "used physical processes as simulations and design engines to 'find' form rather than to draw conventional or invented forms."[191]

I was incredibly fortunate to learn of Frei Otto's work in the late 80s and early 90s when I found the book *The work of Frei Otto*, by Ludwig Glaeser in my local book store. I was amazed and inspired by the flowing forms of these designs. In the years since that time, I've both cherished and referenced the book, especially as current CAD systems have advanced to enable these parametric forms to be actualized.

The term *Parametricism* was coined in 2008 by Patrik Schumacher, an architectural partner of Zaha Hadid. In reference to parameterization, his definition of parametricism is "a style within contemporary avant-garde architecture, promoted as a successor to post-modern architecture and modern architecture. Parametricism has its origin in parametric design, which is based on the constraints in a parametric equation. Parametricism relies on programs, algorithms, and computers to manipulate equations for design purposes."[192]

This definition coincides with the "Parametric equation" topic, which is defined in the Wolfram library as:

"a parametric equation defines a group of quantities as functions of one or more independent variables called parameters. Parametric equations are commonly used to express the coordinates of the points that make up a geometric object such as a curve or surface, in which case the equations are collectively called a parametric representation or parameterization (alternatively spelled as parametrisation) of the object."[193]

If you're familiar with calculus, you may recognize that many of these equations are based on the process of determining the curving form of lines and the areas underneath these curves. Using these mathematic equations, curves can be created in 3D software systems such as CATIA, Rhino/Grasshopper, Nemetschek, and some of the newer versions of AutoDesk's offerings such as Revit.

According to Schumacher, "parametricism is an autopoiesis, or a self-referential system, in which all the elements are interlinked and an outside influence that changes in one alters all the others."[194]

These interconnections of objects, shapes, and forms in a parametric format can create structures and architecture with curving forms as nodal connections. As mentioned in chapter 15, nodal connectivity can support a non-hierarchical system of processes, including the functionality of parametric design.

In many ways, these parametric designs can be defined as "curving architecture" or "curvilinear architecture." This juxtaposes the typical architecture from the 20th century and earlier, from the rectangular shapes of the Parthenon to the rectilinear designs of most homes and skyscrapers in today's designs.

What Do Curving Shapes and Mathematical Forms Have to Do With Health and Wellness?

If you asked a child to draw a house in the modern world, they would likely draw a square or rectangular box with a triangle roof as a half square. This typically includes a rectangle as a door and a square window or two. Along with a rectangular-shaped chimney and perhaps a long linear fence in the basic shape of a rectangle, this is probably similar to how they view the symbol of a house.

And this viewpoint as a "symbol" of a house can be quite profound in terms of how a building is viewed in a child's or adult's psyche. If these architectural objects are seen as symbols based on squares and rectangles, how does that impact the view of nature and the world they live in?

This may not seem like a big deal until you take the time to realize that very little in nature is shaped this way. Your body mostly curves and is not square or rectangular in any form. Most of the natural world is curvilinear, whether it be human and animal, or the shapes and designs of landscapes.

Most of the world is curving. Even your internal structure as a skeleton has a natural curving format. Your skull, spine, and rib cage are based on curves, and while many of your bones are linear, the bones do have a slightly curving shape. They also have a curving design as individual bones, with a larger portion of the bone at the ends with thinner interiors, which creates a curving shape and not just a straight line. And your spine is a combination of many individual vertebrae that allow the body to twist, turn, and flex in curving formations.

This is particularly important in terms of the human connection to the natural world. Without a sense of connection to the natural world and oneself, how can humans feel connected to nature? And if you can't feel connected to the natural world, can't it be challenging to see the importance of conserving and taking care of, and living with, nature?

This topic is one of the main focal points of *Biophilia*, which is defined as the "idea that humans possess an innate tendency to seek connections with nature and other forms of life."[195] The term biophilia was used by psychoanalyst Erich Fromm, where he described biophilia as "the passionate love of life and of all that is alive."[196]

The term "Biophilia hypothesis" has been popularized through Edward Wilson's book *Biophilia*. He describes the term as "the tendency of humans to focus on and to affiliate with nature and other life-forms."[197]

This, perhaps, is a challenge for the modern-day human, as a key for survival for centuries has been to protect oneself against nature and the potential harms of natural scenarios – from weather and the elements to the numerous creatures and organisms that can cause injury.

By creating shelter to remove humans from these harmful natural scenarios, buildings of the past have been more about survival than thriving.

Yet as humans have become more technologically advanced and capable, our architecture has allowed shelter to separate humans from the natural elements. This can be seen in the International Style of architecture, where these buildings are similar in form and function no matter where they are in the world.

Since the early 20th century, the International Style and, in many ways, Modernism and Post-Modernism could provide shelter from any weather conditions. From a hot, dry desert to a cold, snowy climate. Whether it be the rainy tropics or the dry tundra, these buildings provide separation from nature and the natural surroundings and give the required climatized shelter for human survival.

This is also a current day issue in how modern-day architecture, cities, and humanity have developed. The striving for survival in any environmental setting has also removed us from the natural world and segmented us with the illusion that we are no longer connected. To find survival through shelter, humans have created buildings that have given the appearance that we do not need to be concerned about the natural world. In fact, an immense motivation to create modern shelter has been to separate ourselves from the natural world to ensure our survival.

And it is this mentality of overcoming nature that has removed our mindset as being connected to nature. And this is a significant issue in the current world for several reasons.

The first and perhaps most apparent is that we as humans ARE nature. Our bodies are composed of natural elements, from the average 70 percent content of the human body as water to the many natural elements that our bodies use to create our skin, bones, and organs. Elements such as carbon and silica provide the components that we depend upon for life, the same carbon and silica in which much of the natural world is composed of.

While our bodies are literally a part of nature, we also depend on nature's health for life itself. The water we drink, the food we eat, and the environment's quality determine the quality of our health. If we pollute, destroy, or destruct the very nature that supports our lives for survival, then that which we destroy will end up destroying humanity as well.

So What Does This Have to Do With Parametric Design?

You may be wondering what all of this has to do with parametric design. And this is a good question.

If we view parametric design as just a culmination of forms for the purpose of curving shapes, then we are missing the big picture view and the deeper psychology of this topic. This viewpoint is, in my opinion, a short-sided view on parametric and algorithmic design. And what is missing in this short-sided view is the potential for connection to nature, as well as our bodies and our health.

The part that may be missed on this subject is that these curving shapes and designs remind us of our natural origins and our connection to nature. The psychology of being around and living within rectangular shapes and forms as grided streets and developments brings us further away from remembering that we are not only living in nature – we are nature.

By having more curvilinear shapes and parametric forms in our everyday built environments, we are reminded both consciously and subconsciously of our connection to the natural world.

In the mid 20th century, a design style called Googie was common, which is evident in many of the designs of the 1950s in American architecture. While many viewed these curving bubble shapes as a fad, in some ways, it may have prepared us for the current development of parametric architecture. The connections needed today between nature and our technological landscapes have the potential to be bridged using these curving designs. A component missing in the mid 20th century of these Googie designs is a current view of parametric design being researched today. These designs are now seen through the lens of psychology and neuroscience, and not just a fad of curving forms.

As neuroscience shows, these curving shapes and forms can decrease stress and provide less of the fight, flight, and fear modes. This, in turn, allows a less stressful physiological response and a more cognitive capability to recognize and value the natural surroundings that provide us with a healthy life.

When we have these natural forms reminding us of nature's inherent forms, it can also provide a connection to the natural world. And the more that we can feel connected to the natural world and our bodies, the more we can find the importance and empathy for preserving and conserving nature.

The Importance of Curving Designs in the Future

Parametric design may be one of the most important design approaches in the future of architecture for a few reasons.

These curving designs also support several developing fields, such as biomimicry, whose findings show nature's architecture and engineering wisdom. As a result of studying nature's designs and applying this knowledge towards human-created innovations, this can implement wisdom into the future of architecture.

The biomimetic philosophy can be utilized to achieve better design approaches that benefit both the engineering and material life cycle of designs.

As was mentioned in a previous paragraph, I commented that viewing these parametric designs as merely algorithms to create curving designs as an aesthetic is a mistake.

I state this based on the pioneering work that has defined parametric architecture and even organic architecture. I say this because many architects, designers, and engineers who pioneered these developments did so based on emulating nature's curving forms and striving to achieve more optimal engineering solutions.

And this is important because when you view parametric design as a tool created to achieve the applied knowledge of natural forms, you can appreciate the tool as such. Engineers such as Frei Otto created these parametric, curving designs to find optimal engineering forms to decrease material use while increasing the structures' strength. Frei Otto used these curving forms to achieve the goal of spanning large areas without columns, and his tensile-based surfaces and curving shapes accomplished these goals in an optimal format based on mathematical calculations.

Designers such as Buckminster Fuller utilized these curving shapes and design approaches in a similar manner, such as his GeoDesic dome and tensegrity designs. He utilized this wisdom of nature to solve the issue of using fewer materials and optimizing the strength of such designs. The geodesic dome and many of his designs utilize what he called tensegrity, which uses the applied engineering principles and material design to create more with less.

While both Frei Otto and Buckminster Fuller approached the design process differently, they both found that these designs provided a similar aesthetic based on core engineering principles. And these principles are based on a mathematical foundation.

These are some of the same principles that designers such as Santiago Calatrava and Zaha Hadid have found to be optimal in form and function. These principles are based on how nature designs and builds and utilizes the wisdom of these approaches when applied to human-created designs.

These are similar or are the same principles that biomimicry advocates, which is not just to copy nature's curving shapes and forms for purely aesthetic purposes. These shapes result from understanding the core engineering approach of nature's design wisdom. By learning from and implementing this design wisdom, it can yield these forms in an optimal format.

And to view parametric design as just curving forms and shapes for ornamental or purely aesthetic purposes is not entirely correct nor fair. That said, those who are using these calculated designs using random algorithms can be short-sided based on a lack of design principles. Instead of learning from these natural design systems, using curving forms as ornament removes the core wisdom of nature's brilliance. To do so is missing a critical "whole point" of these shapes. And while this can be debated, a more cohesive approach to designing with these shapes and forms should be more deeply understood, if we are to understand these design goals better.

This, of course, is not to criticize designers who are using these new software applications that can create curves as a design aesthetic. Understandably, engineers and designers use algorithms in software, providing random shapes and forms that are curving. However, these random designs may not truly represent the core purpose of such forms instead of utilizing biomimicry and biophilia principles.

And so, what can be defined here is that a cohesive, integrative viewpoint of these different approaches can yield healthier results based on biophilic design. If you are viewing this approach in an integrative format, it can lead to a result as a more cohesive design solution from both an aesthetic and engineering solution.

A good example of viewing these topics in a whole system as a cohesive viewpoint is when the fields of biomimicry and biophilia are combined. Each of these disciplines is studying the benefits of nature yet in different formats and approaches.

And these examples can begin to show connections to health and wellness in terms of parametric architecture and design.

Biomimicry studies the designs, shapes, and functionality of nature. By understanding how nature has solved a particular design issue, humans can then analyze this solution to find the core processes of these designs. This information can then be implemented for a similar design issue that humans are striving to solve. The result is often a solution that can be seen in both function and form, and a design and engineering solution together as a whole.

An example of this is Santiago Calatrava's approach, whose designs are often based on biomorphic shapes. These designs are not necessarily meant to emulate or reconstruct an exact duplicate of shapes found in nature, yet to understand why an organism may be shaped in a certain way and use this knowledge as applied wisdom to solve a design issue.

In Eugene Tsui's book *Evolutionary Architecture*, Dr. Tsui uses anthropomorphic and biomorphic forms in a design process based on the wisdom of nature's designs. By analyzing nature, this knowledge can be applied to utilize fewer materials, yet also provide better structural integrity – for instance, while preparing the structure to handle earthquakes.

Dr. Tsui's house design in San Francisco called "Ojo del Sol" (Eye of the Sun), also known as the "Fish House," according to Tsui is based on the anatomy of a tardigrade.[198] The materials used in making the Ojo del Sol include inexpensive and recycled materials that draw inspiration from the cholla cactus, which is virtually fireproof. Tsui designed the house with the goal of making it the "safest house in the world," intended to survive fires, earthquakes, flooding, and termites.[199]

If you view both of these designer's approaches, you will see that they strive to create beautiful forms with nature's superior engineering. And these designs can provide both a function and form that supports a more advanced approach to architecture.

Combining these design aesthetics with engineering brilliance is also to embrace biomimicry and biophilia in creating architecture that can best support human and biological health for wellness and well being.

Parametric Architecture and Human Wellness

And this brings us to the part of the conversation that involves human health and how these parametric designs also have a great potential for human wellness. Creating curving building shapes can actually provide a more relaxing scenario concerning human physiology.

According to new developments and findings in neuroscience, by reducing sharp, angular forms, the amygdala and brain center, responsible for stress, is less triggered. And when these sections of the brain are less triggered, it supports less stress. This can prevent fear and provide less stress in one's life, either in specific instances or over more extended periods of time.

These curving designs can support better overall health and wellness by decreasing emotional, psychological, and physiological stressors. If specific shapes and forms in a built environment subtly trigger these stress responses, people can become numb to these scenarios by adapting to these reactions or ignoring these sensory responses. The reduction in subtle stress factors over time can prevent prolonged long-term stress.

Many people might not even be aware of these stressors, as, over time, they have consciously ignored these reactions, yet physiologically the stressors are still present.

On the flip side, if there are more curving shapes and forms, it can provide a less stressful experience and offer more support for well being.

These curving designs are not just soothing to the emotions. They have a direct positive impact on the human experience and can support physiological and sensory wellness. And along with providing less toxic building materials and better indoor environmental conditions, these design approaches can offer an improved quality of life.

Chapter: 19   The DNA of Cities & Parametric Architecture

Great Architecture and Curving Spaces

I will also comment that some of the most symbolic Architecture in the world is based on parametric and curving forms.

In the US, there is the oval office of the White House. The highest level of the world's democracy occurs in a room based on a circular or elliptical curving form. For the United Nations, the meetings often gather in a circular or half circle format, and many of the world's most critical discussions are held at a round table.

The circle provides equanimity and balance while providing an equal radian with a core centroid.

Many places of worship in the world are based on circular designs and curving forms, from the arches of churches to the domes of cathedrals and mosques. From the Pantheon in Rome, the Hagia Sophia, and St. Basil's famous onion domes in Moscow to the US Capitol Building, the great stupa at Sanchi in India, and the famous Dome of the Rock on the Temple Mount, all of these great works of architecture are domes and curving forms. Each of these architectural masterpieces embraces life with a view towards that which is beyond comprehension and can lift the spirit.

The Architecture of Life

Another facet of parametric architecture is perhaps less data-driven and more of a silent yet real connection to nature that we as living beings are connected to. From the macro to the micro, nature utilizes particular patterns in the blueprint of life.

In a Scientific American article titled "The Architecture of Life," Dr. Donald Ingber discusses the design of living organisms and how they are constructed in architectural terms.

As architectural structures, he comments that biology can be defined as "a universal set of building rules...to guide the design of organic structures-- from simple carbon compounds to complex cells and tissues".[200] In this writing from 1998, Dr. Ingber talks about the material designs of nature and the architectural designs of all living organisms.

These discussions include the structural integrity of biological forms and highlights the importance of the role of tensegrity in the architecture of organic structures. Tensegrity is a term coined by Buckminster Fuller in the 1960s as a portmanteau of "tensional integrity."[201]

Dr. Ingber's principles of tensegrity show the fundamental blueprint of the skeleton and the mechanics in biochemistry to describe the phenomena observed in molecular biology.

Building upon the concept of tensegrity is the term biotensegrity coined by Dr. Stephen Levin as the application of tensegrity principles to biological structures. It also refers to the "self-assembly of organic structures and the universality of the geodesic form."[202]

As stated previously, according to Schumacher, "parametricism is an autopoiesis, or a self-referential system, in which all the elements are interlinked and an outside influence that changes one alters all the others."[203]

The Common Threads Connecting Biology and the Future of Buildings

This description of parametricism is precisely the same as the architecture of biological life that Dr. Ingber describes as the architecture of cells and tissues.

This nodal interconnectivity is what I defined earlier in the book and provided more in-depth descriptions in chapter 15. This pattern of nodes mirrors the neural networks of neurons, the human brain, anastomosis, and the many living systems and networks of life.

If you look at these design ideas relative to the work of Buckminster Fuller and Frei Otto, you can see a common thread connecting the natural designs of the biological world – as parametric "human-designed" buildings.

Both Otto and Fuller were proponents of tensile structures that created more flowing forms based on this engineering. In the architectural question of form or function, these curving shapes provide an equal response of equanimity balancing design and engineering. As you view their work, you can visually see this thread of commonality.

These designs draw inspiration from the natural world, from the tensile structures of domes to the curving arches and open area spans that their spaces create.

While these designs can show inspiration from nature, their forms have been achieved by reinterpreting this knowledge into their own design language.

And it is this thread of commonality that I believe has an inherent connection to the blueprints of nature and the architecture of human beings.

Resonance and Entrainment

In viewing the designs of structures and architecture that mimic our own human architecture of our biological bodies, it also shows the similarities between the architecture of your cells and that of nature. And perhaps it is this design approach that can inherently connect us or reconnect us to the natural world.

While we don't fully understand how the mechanics of entrainment works, we know that objects often synchronize when placed into the same environment. An article in Science Direct defines *entrainment* as "a process that leads to temporal coordination of two actors' behavior, in particular, synchronization, even in the absence of a direct mechanical coupling."[204]

An example of this is when you put a clock in a room full of clocks, they will eventually synchronize to the same rhythm. "Entrainment is perhaps the most widely studied social motor coordination process. For instance, two people in rocking chairs involuntarily synchronize their rocking frequencies, and audiences in theaters tend to clap in unison."[205 206]

What if entrainment is also impacting humans on an architectural level as well?

For instance, if humans are spending most of the time inside buildings in rectangular, box-like shapes and forms that define most cityscapes, can this attune us to shapes and forms that are less natural? Perhaps these rectangular shapes remove us from our connection to nature?

If most of the natural world is shaped in curving forms, from the flowing designs of streams, rivers, and the shapes of countrysides, to the curving contours of plants and animals, can the built environment's curvilinear forms help to attune us back to nature? Can these curving forms bring us to a more connected future in resonance with the natural world?

Winston Churchill's famous quote, "we shape our buildings; thereafter they shape us," can have an even deeper and profound meaning if indeed it's found that the shapes we reside in can reconnect us to the natural world through entrainment.

Parametric and Curvilinear Architecture and the Future

Drawing on the earlier parametric equations, in 2006, a research paper by Young Hee Geum and Young Ik Kim titled "on the analysis and construction of the butterfly curve using Mathematica" they discussed a very interesting

ParametricPlot[{Sin[t] (E^Cos[t] - 2 Cos[4 t] - Sin[t/12]^5), Cos[t] (E^Cos[t] - 2 Cos[4 t] - Sin[t/12]^5)}, {t, 0, 12 Pi}]

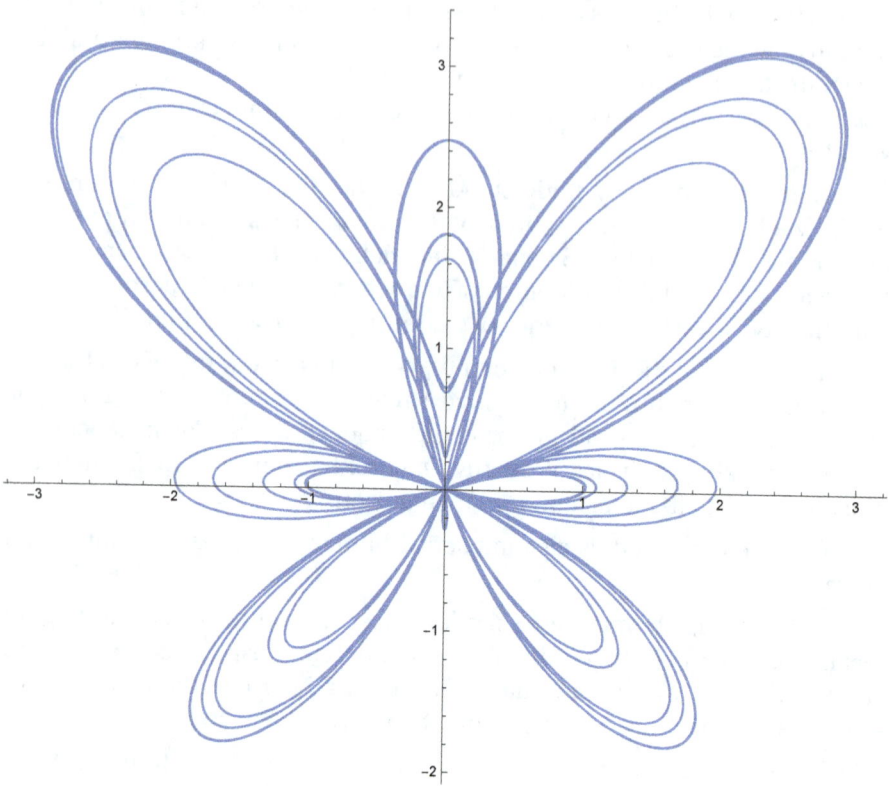

theme. They began with the mathematics of the transcendental plane curve called the "butterfly curve." This parametric equation graphs the shape of a butterfly and is an example of the beauty of mathematics and nature:

In their analysis, when they began to alter the mathematics of the equations, they stated, "these new shapes no longer resemble butterflies. They more closely resemble leafs, flowers or other insects."[207]

Take for example, the adjustment of parameters to the butterfly equation above that was created in Mathematica, you can see the following varying results of this polar equation:

ParametricPlot[{1, Cos[t]} (1 + Sin[t]), {t, 0, 2 \[Pi]}

Chapter: 19 The DNA of Cities & Parametric Architecture

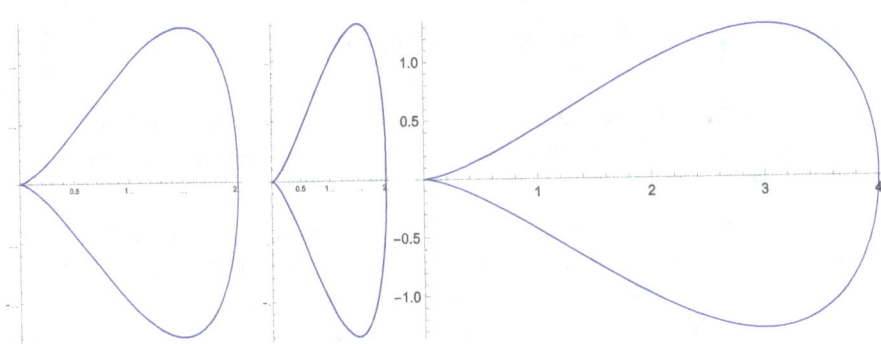

By changing parameters of these equations, the various forms created have similar shapes found in nature. These parametric equations can create simple shapes and forms that can evolve into more complex three-dimentional parametric designs:

For me, this is particularly interesting based on the connection to the forms in nature that these parametric equations create. If new parametric buildings are using similar mathematics to create architecture, perhaps there can be an inherent connection between these parametric designs and nature's architecture. In this manner, is it possible that it can literally reconnect us to nature as a form of biomimicry?

If the blueprints of nature are based on the architecture of math, and parametric equations define how a plant leaf, a flower, or a butterfly wing is architected, the world of human architecture could utilize similar parameters as blueprints. Perhaps this beautiful and efficient architecture can reconnect us to nature and, therefore, back to ourselves and our wholeness or health.

After all, if we are connected to ourselves and our very nature as nature, then perhaps this can help us tune into the processes of building with the earth's systems and have more reverence for our natural environments. This reconnection can provide an easier path to navigate into the future, if humanity is to live in symbiosis with the planet. And this can allow us to live in more harmony with other humans and life forms and be in closer connection with ourselves.

I discuss this topic of symbiosis in the forthcoming book, *Symbiosis Global – Nature is the Most Advanced Technology*, where I outline the integration of technology and ecology.

Essentially, as we advance our research and better understand the inner workings of DNA and the architecture of nature, we become more fluent in the language of life, which is often based on mathematics.

However, to focus on the mathematics, physics, and science of this topic alone is to mistake knowledge for wisdom. To ignore the human spirit and the emotional well being of human existence is, in my opinion, a mistake. The severing of our emotions with a focus on technology and data can leave the nurturing facets of life without empathy and compassion. To do so is to remove a critical facet of the human experience out of life's equation.

By utilizing this knowledge of mathematics and science to focus on human thriving can once again bring us to the topic of health.

And perhaps the process of this reconnection can be seen by revisiting the definition of health:

Health

Old English hælþ "wholeness, a being whole, sound or well," from Proto-Germanic *hailitho, from PIE *kailo- "whole, uninjured, of good omen" (source also of Old English hal "hale, whole;" Old Norse heill "healthy;"[208]

Therefore, the meaning of being un-healthy is based on not being whole or being disconnected and fragmented in some way.

In this manner, part of the process of health and well being is to have this sense of wholeness regained, especially for people in places where life is fragmented. A reconnection back to nature can possibly be provided by this parametric and curving architecture to better support these connections.

While the International Design Style was created at a time when survival was critical and humans were still striving to overcome the potential harmful impacts of the natural world, now that humanity has taken significant strides to achieve a form of survival, the next step would be to strive for thriving. And this includes the return to wholeness and health.

To be clear, this is not to state that all humans on this planet are beyond surviving. It is instead to note that humanity has achieved the potential to accomplish this. It's also a reminder of the importance of human empathy and compassion to recognize that many people are still suffering, and architecture has the capability to provide solutions to the masses — from surviving to thriving.

And using parametric, curvilinear shapes and forms in our everyday architecture and designs in the built environment can help us resonate with nature via entrainment and, in so doing, can reconnect us with our good health for thriving.

These concepts can interconnect subjects such as organic architecture, biomorphic design, biomimicry, biophilia, and many other fields for a fuller human experience. This strives to not only emulate the surroundings in a natural format, yet to understand the design core of its function and form. This can lead to the creation of human-based designs in architecture that both support life and promote health.

Utilizing these more "nature embracing" approaches to design, combined with the knowledge of environmental psychology and evidence-based design, can further enhance the integration process to achieve these wellness goals. Combined with the fields of public health, it can also help reduce pollution and the physical aspects that can cause illness and sickness.

Perhaps much of these concepts are new to the general public. While there are still many unknowns about the outcome and results over time, the process of integrating these multi-faceted topics into a cohesive whole can undoubtedly provide a better connection between humans, the natural world, and the goals of better health.

And this development of healthier built environments can support connections to a life that can be more fully enjoyed.

Parametric Designs to Reduce Stress and Increase Efficient Building Processes

Reflecting on Frei Otto and Buckminster Fuller's designs, these pioneers provided a foundation of building processes focused on reducing materials while benefiting from the methods of nature's wisdom.

Buckminster Fuller spent the second half of his life as Guinea Pig B. He focused all of his efforts on being the guinea pig of innovation to find methods to decrease material use and waste and increase efficiency. His geodesic dome can provide extremely strong structures with limited materials due to tensegrity and curving shapes. His book *Guinea Pig B* defines a human being dedicated to contributing to society's betterment. As he states, "for the first time there exists enough experience-won and experiment verified information current in humanity's spontaneous conceptioning and reasoning for all humanity to carry on in a far more intelligent way than ever before."[209]

These parametric designs can help to reduce the material needs of construction, while providing better engineered structures as one major benefit. This, combined with the decrease in stress levels that curving forms support physiologically, can provide a deeper connection where architecture provides a form of "medicine" to those who live around and within such structures.

These curving shapes and forms can provide less stress and a more relaxed environment on a physiological, emotional, and mental level.

And this should provide a hopefulness of a future that is not easy to find in today's day and age.

These newer designs can bring humanity back to nature while providing a forward momentum utilizing technology for a more positive and healthier future focused on wellness.

And moving forward to this wellness brings us to the next possible step in achieving these goals discussed in the next chapter – *Wellness Centers*...

"Now I see the secret of making the best person; it is to grow with the open air and to eat and sleep with the earth."

– Walt Whitman

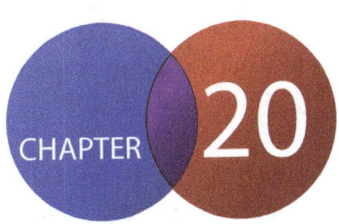

WELLNESS CENTERS

The Future of Health and Wellness in Architecture

There has been a trend, especially in the US, where a main focus is on the aging populations and how younger generations can utilize preventive and integrative medicine for better health and wellness.

This trend includes recognizing better health plans in one's own life, whether it be preventive medicine or preventive care in terms of physical exercise and eating habits.

All of this points in the direction of a lifelong approach to health and wellness, and not just a pill or surgery to fix an ailment. If you follow this trend, it includes exercise, yoga, and other modalities such as meditation and mindfulness practices. It involves better nutrition and supplements, yet perhaps more than anything, it encourages physical, emotional, and psychological care of oneself. It promotes the mantra "know thyself" by taking steps to support your own health and wellbeing.

In addition, there are a growing number of health professionals and coaches supporting whole health and wellness. You can see that the trend points towards a group of professionals and modalities working with your entire being by supporting your process in achieving better health.

What this might look like in the future – in the physical world of architecture – are Wellness Centers. As the hospital is there for fixative measures, the Wellness Center is there as a preventative for long-term health.

What Are Wellness Centers?

While many hospitals are introducing healthier modalities into their process for treatments, including the latest developments of healthy hospital designs, a big factor with hospitals is that many people do not want to go to them. And so there may be a benefit to having these Wellness Centers being in a different location to go to, where one feels more comfortable and empowered, instead of scared to visit a doctor.

In this model, there are places where you go for fixative care in the short term, which is the hospital, and then the places where you regularly go to keep yourself healthy. These are locations where you monitor and evaluate your health while you are healthy and maintain health.

These Wellness Centers can function in many different ways. Yet, perhaps a core functionality with all of these centers is an integrative approach where several health professionals work with you for better health. The Wellness Center supports your whole health, from evaluating and strengthening your physical health to those who can help your emotional and psychological well being.

And because these professionals are all working together, the combination functions synergistically in a comprehensive manner. This includes your exercise evaluations and food providing your best nutrition designed for your body and needs, to the supplements and perhaps prescriptions you need to take, ensuring that it all functions together in unison. Making sure that every modality of care has no contraindications is critical to the future of medicine and health.

These Wellness Centers are places where you can participate in your health, not just in a supplement or a pill. It is your life, and these centers reflect the centrality of this process. It is not about adding some extra component to your life you do on the side or every once in a while. It is a part of your life as a living style. You integrate this into your life as you live from a young age into adulthood and old age. In this manner, you are not just a bystander, and you don't only exercise and eat healthier once during a new year's resolution.

You also have a team of people as professionals supporting your process, physically, mentally, and emotionally. In this process, you can gain the support of a team that also works with each other to ensure that any one modality is not interfering with another. And this can help you throughout your entire life, not just when you get sick or ill.

From "Illness" Support to "Wellness" Support

While hospitals will remain for fixative and emergency care, there will be additional locations, perhaps as centers of towns, villages, and cities, that are there for a lifetime of support, care, and empowerment. These centers provide integrated, multi-disciplinary care and support for the individual to find their formula for wellness and well being. This supports health as a lifelong process and not just something that is considered with the start of each new year or at times of illness. Most important is that it is integrated into one's life and society at large.

Of course, this process also requires the patient to be more involved with their health and not just expect the doctors to "fix" them and know what they need for wholeness. It requires the patient as a citizen to take time to include this process in their lives. It is not some kind of additional, extra component existing outside of their lives when they feel motivated to participate.

It will take some work, yet if this is supported and encouraged from youth to the elderly, perhaps the wellness culture will be more integrated into the towns, villages, and cities where humans live, work, and play. It can become a part of the culture and not some "alternative" lifestyle for the select few.

This also takes an adjusted view on life in general, to invest in health as a part of life. The individual's well-being becomes a greater concern, as the wellness of the individual scales to the wellness of cities and the entire planet.

While many are confused in how the world has become disconnected from sustainable living, and has become less connected to the energy efficiency of green living, it doesn't take long when viewing the big picture to see that most of the planet has become focused on fixative care. Along with the disconnect from health and wellness, it has invested more in solutions of a pill than invested in well being as a part of life.

This, of course, starts as a philosophical view. Yet, if we truly add up the costs of illness, we find that wellness is an inexpensive option and an investment in terms of the population's longevity.

This brings us back to the quote at the start of the chapter:

"Well-being is not just a mere pleasurable sensation. It is a deep sense of serenity and fulfillment." – Matthieu Ricard

This idea of wellness and well being is not just about a pleasurable sensation. It is a physical, mental, and emotional way of living focused on quality of life. It does not promise perfection as an illusion of utopia, yet instead strives for a life worth living in a balanced and deeper sense of serenity.

When the individual can feel more connected to well-being, it may be more probable they will care and have concern for the wellness of others, the planet, and all of its biological inhabitants. This mindfulness and concern are required to utilize the technology of today and tomorrow to ensure that it will be used for the betterment of society and life in general, not a weapon from a lack of inner well being.

It may sound simplistic in its approach, yet if we do not start with this complex picture from both the individual pieces and the collective whole of the puzzle, to think that it will mysteriously and magically fix itself is even more altruistic, utopic, and simplistic.

What Can These Wellness Centers Look Like?

While there are many ways these centers can look and function, a basic premise is that the Wellness Center supports complete wellness, which means that preventive health is a main focus. Wellness is not simply a dataset or measurable process, yet some measurements can help evaluate and guide better health. As such, many forms of illness are not just physical, and can include mental or psychological and emotional illness. If all of these facets of health are not considered, the solutions of wellness and well being can be elusive or impossible to achieve.

Therefore, a basic premise of a Wellness Center is that a person's overall health – physically, mentally, and emotionally – should all be considered for best support. To have all of these professionals in one place may not be a viable solution. Yet, if there is the chance that a center can include all of these professionals in the same location and all working together for a patient's best health, then the potential for synergistic healing can increase.

Chapter: 20   Wellness Centers

How Do We Get There? Reverse Engineering Health and Wellness and Creating Systems to Achieve These Goals

A possible thought or design idea on this concept is the modern-day Mall in the USA. As an example of a transformation of spaces and places, the malls falling apart and are less used could be a perfect fit for a caterpillar to butterfly metamorphosis. While many are shut down and in dormancy at this time across the US, there is potential for these "centers of the past" for material shopping to be transformed into centers of wellness for the communities and cities they exist in. They can emerge from centers of shopping and become centers for well being. Once seen as investments for profit, these locations can be transformed into investment centers for the good health of the people and communities they have served. They can go from service-based places to serving the communities that once utilized them for another benefit.

From Malls to Wellness Centers

A significant benefit of these Malls as Wellness Centers is that they can be transformed from places that are either not used or struggling, to becoming essential centers for many people's quality of life.

Take this idea of Malls converted into Wellness Centers, and think about what could happen. How could these be utilized and designed in a way that could benefit society?

The design itself can be transformed by removing large parking areas and returning these to fields for small farm plots. This would support individuals to be more involved and to have a reason to go to these places for their personal use. The group "Depave," based in the US, has been working to remove parking lot pavements into functional community use.[210]

You can then include places for exercise and keeping fit, both on the inside as gyms and for classes where, for example, yoga can take place while providing exterior environments with walking trails to stay fit. Landscape architecture created to provide beautiful scenery, along with edible plants and small farm plots, can be another reason to wander around to stay active. These outside areas can utilize the design principles of permaculture. And as nature has shown to be helpful for good health, this benefits in a multitude of ways.

In the interior, places can be developed for professionals in different health fields, from the typical doctor as a general practitioner to those such as psychologists supporting emotional and mental health. Then add into the

Architectural Medicine – Building the Bridge to Wellness

BEFORE: THE MALL
AFTER: THE WELLNESS CENTER

WELLNESS CENTERS
FROM MALLS TO WELLNESS CENTERS

FROM DECAYING **MALL**S TO THRIVING **WELL**NESS CENTERS

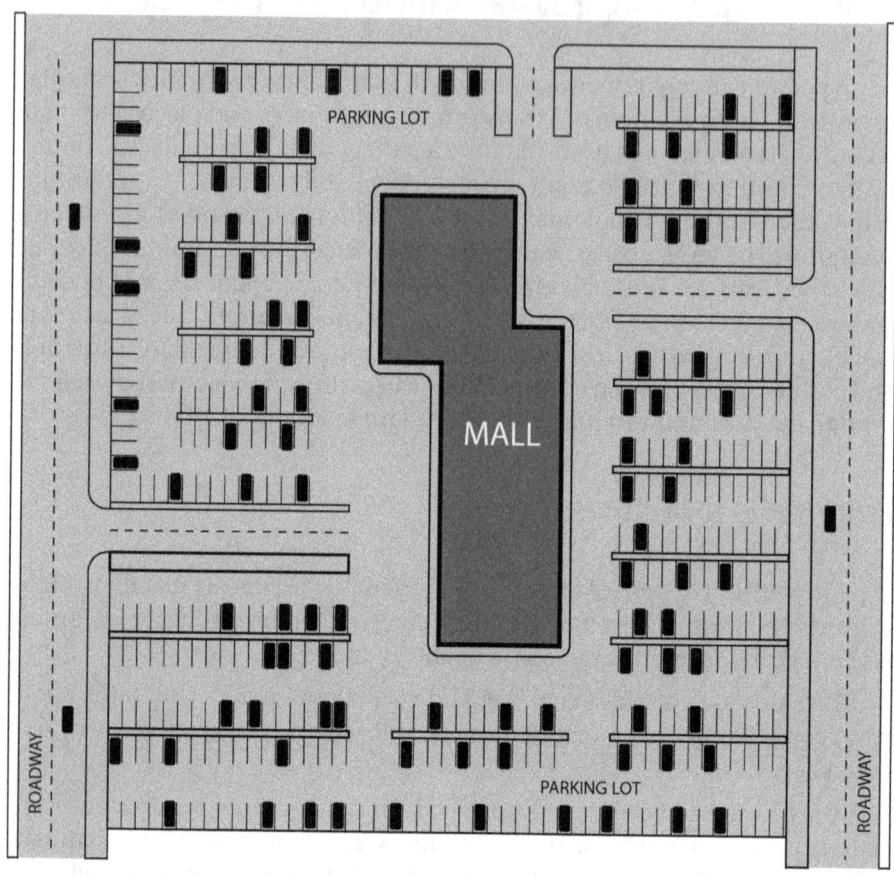

mix restaurants and food stores where healthier cuisine can be accessed and enjoyed. If storefronts were included as places where natural products, such as beneficial medicinal herbs and other healthy foods are provided, then the full circle of support could be offered in one central location.

This blueprint could benefit in a format where restaurants and retail are located on the ground floor, and on the second floor, and higher could exist the business and health professional offices.

A setup of this nature could provide the community with spaces to support places for leisure and enjoyment, while having access to the professional offices on the upper levels.

With gardens replacing the parking lots, those who visit the center can learn about natural medicinals, much like an apothecary of old, yet new once again.

Chapter: 20 — Wellness Centers

BEFORE: THE MALL
AFTER: THE WELLNESS CENTER

WELLNESS CENTERS
FROM MALLS TO WELLNESS CENTERS

FROM DECAYING **MALL**S TO THRIVING **WELL**NESS CENTERS

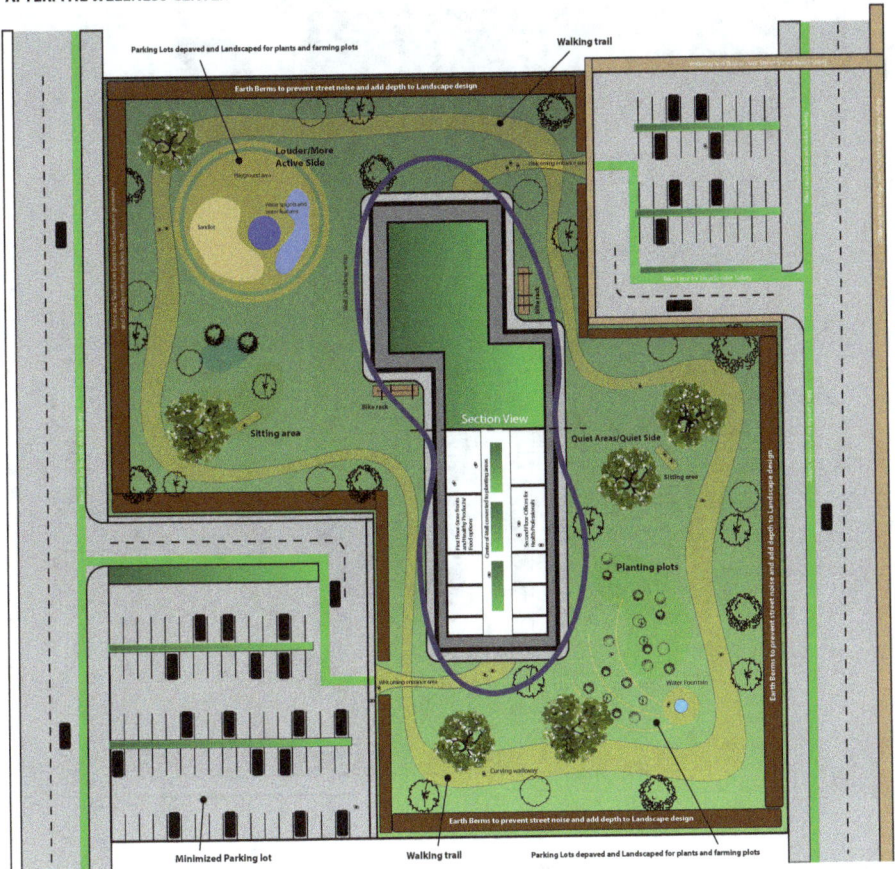

Add the options of acupuncture, massage, and other natural healing and preventive health modalities, and a whole system of services can be provided for wellness.

Perhaps a key ingredient in this approach is to make this form of prescription for health a proper Rx or Recipe for better health, and allow it to be accessible to the entire community. Whereas a hospital is a place to receive immediate emergency treatment, the Wellness Center is a place to provide preventive health into the community life.

These spaces can also include retail businesses for purchasing healthier material goods and provide places to enjoy coffee, tea, or other enjoyable food types. An essential part of this is to have places to spend time in the style of more relaxed cities such as European villages and communities.

It's not striving to replace the European village, yet instead, it's meant to

Architectural Medicine – Building the Bridge to Wellness

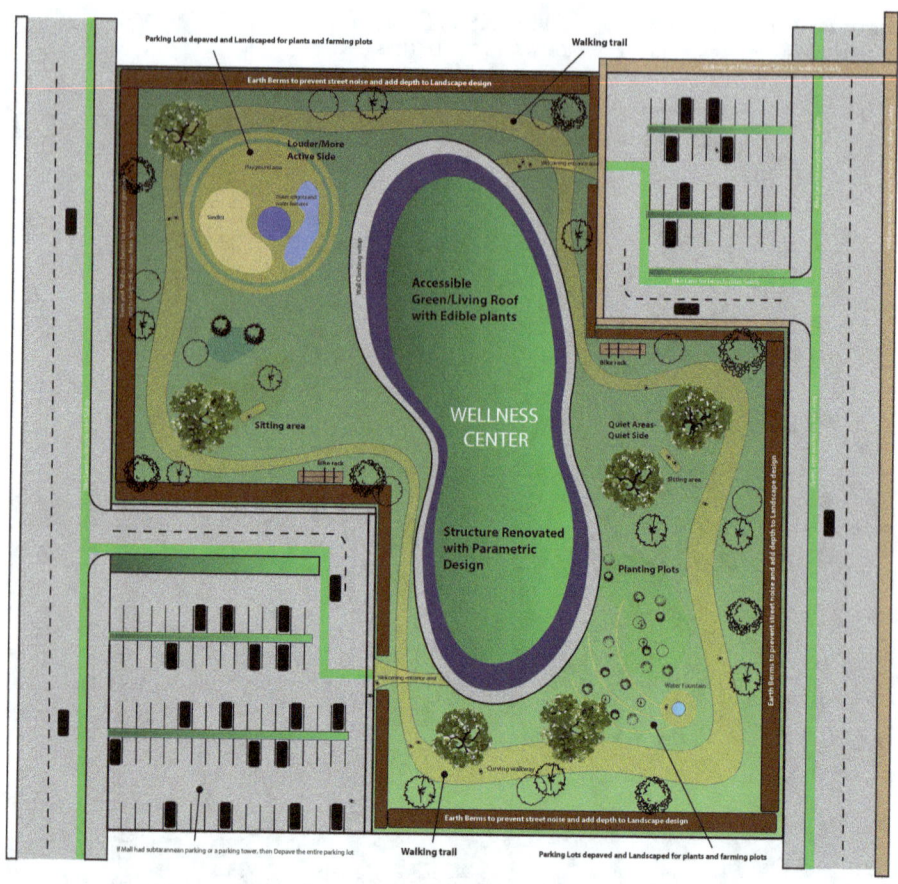

take the benefits of these places and provide new spaces into the fabric of the culture for better health and quality of life. It may utilize the benefits of some of these older towns as models, and includes the best elements while modernizing them. These building ingredients borrow from a global community, from yoga and pilates to Chinese herbs and Mediterranean styles of foods. These can mimic the benefits of worldwide "blue zones" as examples of healthier living.[211]

These are just some examples of converting Malls into Wellness Centers, yet many other variables can transform these spaces into unique locations for each community in the US and worldwide. And even if the rest of the world does not precisely mimic the USA's large Malls, there are still many features that can be applied to places in all areas of the world. Each location can utilize the core blueprint for Wellness Centers, as each site bases the functions on its unique culture, heritage, and people.

Wellness Centers

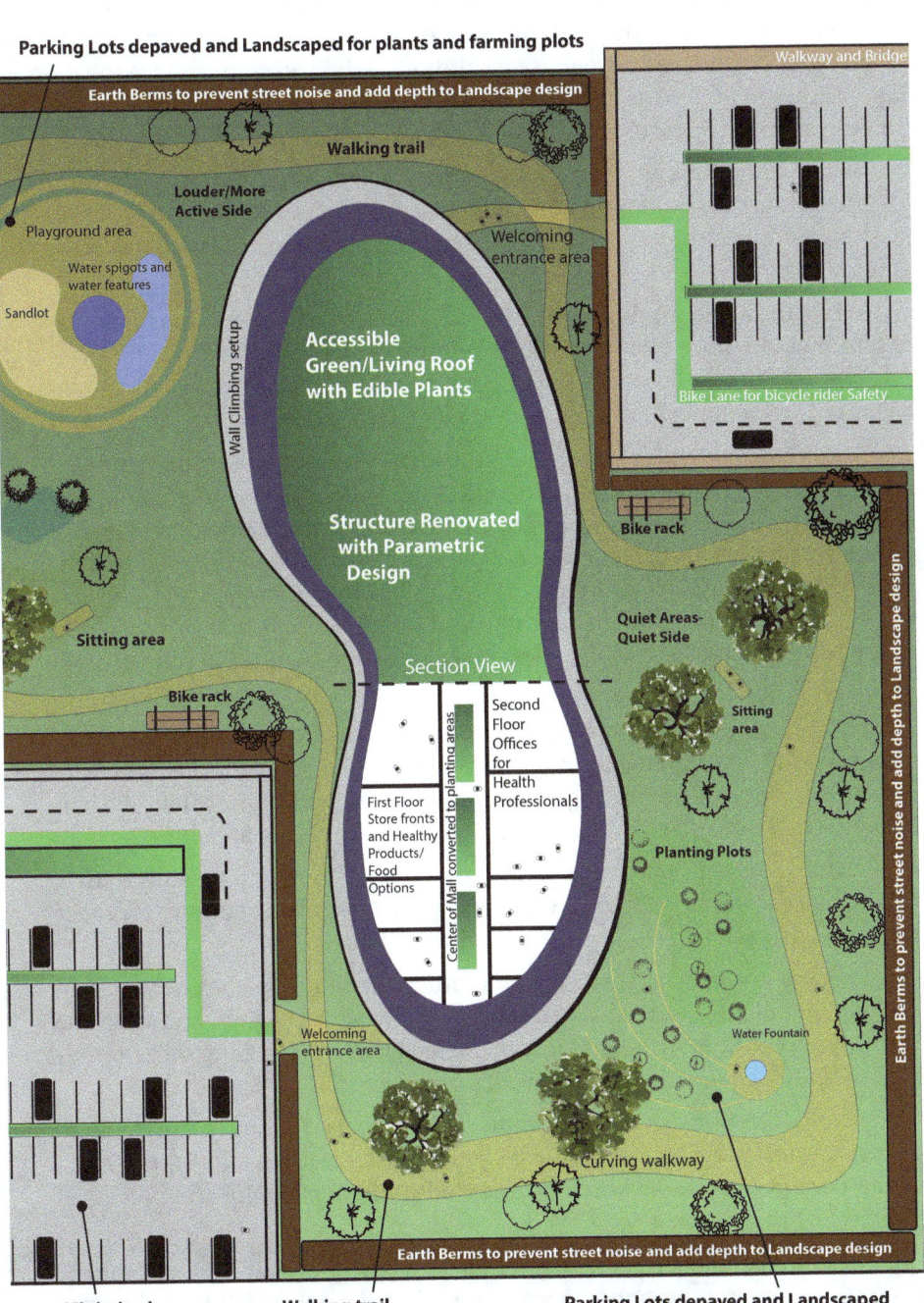

A vital component to the design of these locations, with a multi-disciplinary focus, can include the involvement of many different professions. If you take some time to think about the design requirements, it can include several groups involved for cohesive solutions. It will, of course, have the design process of architects and landscape architects to repurpose the site, and include other professions in the process, such as those in the health fields.

What would happen if you had architects and medical and health professionals working on designs that addressed the needs of these health professionals while also considering the best design strategies for patients as the general public?

While these integrations in the building of hospitals and some health facilities include these two professions working together, what if you took this one step further to include all architecture and built environments be designed in this manner?

Another level to this process is that it can include health practitioners from medical doctors to psychotherapists and others providing healthcare support. So there would be a need to create environments that don't feel like places of the typical medical spaces, yet would have the available functionality and technological requirements available when appropriate. Redesigning medical locations that are less sterile and more comforting can provide a tremendous decrease in stress, especially when the focus of regular visits is based on wellness.

And to include mixed-use spaces for exercise and areas for cuisine, the requirements for both inside spaces and exteriors to enjoy for the public are critical. The use of natural lighting, local plants, and appropriate designs based on local weather must be included to support the local culture.

Yet all of these facets can become a true "center" for society, and as such, can be places people want to go to, as opposed to having no support for these topics of wellness.

Creating spaces that have clean air and are healthier places to be within can also highlight the space as an example of what is possible and what the community can learn through tours of the facilities and teaching the community about health and the various health services.

Having the option of several health professionals working in the same location not only benefits the Wellness Center itself, yet it can allow the sharing of the patient's process where it's accepted professionally for the benefit of patient health.

These locations can also have classes taught on health-related topics. Even topics that can help them create more healing and healthier built environments at their homes and workplaces can be offered.

This is just an example of how a structure that has been a place to go for material goods and commerce in the past or even the current time, can be transformed to support the community. This can be especially important for places where the average population ages are increasing, where elders in the community can achieve and maintain better health.

Three topics that can support the definition of a Wellness Center:

1. The promise of many health professionals working together to support the complete, whole systems health of the patient
2. Utilizing systems approaches to provide the patient and public with processes to support their healing and health over a lifetime of personal development
3. Putting a variety of professionals together for each individual's best health, from physical exercise professionals, psychologists, and health professionals to acupuncture, diet, and yoga practitioners for complete wellness and well being

A recent interview by the publication WIRED posted on youtube highlighted the discussion of the future of Malls and how they are being refurbished. WIRED's Emily Dreyfuss talks with architecture professor Ellen Dunham-Jones about mall culture and the fate of dead malls. She discusses how some are being repurposed, mentioning that some are being used as medical facilities, learning centers, and even places as reconstructed wetlands.[212] If put together into a cohesive whole, this mindset and approach would be a good definition of how these can be transformed into Wellness Centers.

Of course, there are many different paths that these Malls could take, and even the concept of a Wellness Center certainly does not require that it replace a Mall or be rebuilt from a Mall.

It can certainly be a place that is developed in any location or even as a new development.

The key to this is the transformation of public spaces and how the connection can be made as a cohesive whole to provide better health services. This, integrated with opportunities for architecture that supports better health and wellness, is critical, instead of places where health is in decline due to a lack of health support systems.

Wellness Centers can become a center for society as places of self-development, learning about health and preventive health practices, and striving to support communities' health.

These can lead to more integrative developments in local communities to scale up for global wellness.

In taking steps towards global wellness, the next process can consider future developments in terms of architecture in supporting well being. And this is what will be discussed in the next chapter...

"The best way to predict the future is to invent it. "

– Alan Kay

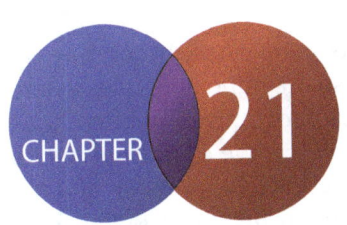

SOME THOUGHTS ON THE FUTURE

Using Technology in Architecture in New and Beneficial Ways

Throughout this book, many of these new approaches embrace more natural solutions, reconnecting humanity back to nature. Whether it be biomimicry or biophilia, there is still the importance of integrating this with the latest technology.

In this process, the focus is more on utilizing technology for better health and wellness, and not depending on technology to achieve and create better health and wellness.

This means that the approach to using technology can be utilized to achieve better health, from creating systems such as the Architectural Medicine Software Solution – ARxMD to emerging technologies such as environmental sensors.

By utilizing personal environmental sensors, and in larger contexts placing sensors in exterior locations in cities, many health-related factors can be analyzed. Personal environmental sensors can range from the Fitbit, and the Apple Watch to devices from the company tzoa. Their initial prototype measured a range of air quality issues such as carbon dioxide and carbon monoxide as a personal sensor device.[213]

When these environmental sensors are installed inside buildings, the quality of the air, temperature, and other metrics can be more readily monitored. Taking this information by itself may not show much benefit, but when this is placed together in big data as bioinformatics, these patterns can lead to exponential insights. This can support the decision-making process or awareness of occurring issues and provide insights and knowledge that can lead to better changes.

These can provide one of the most sophisticated data collections on public health, rivaling the day John Snow utilized data to find solutions to the infamous cholera epidemic.

During the year 2020 of the novel coronavirus, people have become aware of such modern day epidemics. Yet, there are also major health issues where stress has overtaken the leading cause of death. Problems of obesity along with diabetes and ailments such as asthma have become significant health issues on an unprecedented scale. This, combined with depression and the use of opioids, are just a few examples of modern day health problems. They may not all be directly connected with built environments, yet if people are not inspired and feel a sense of fulfillment in their lives, they will seek other sources to fulfill these needs and wants.

It would be unwise to state that the built environment alone can cure these maladies. Yet, it is also foolish to assume that these forms of inspiration and motivation for fulfillment in life are not influenced by places where people live and work. Ignoring the importance of fulfilling goals to work towards, whether personal or societal, is to misunderstand an essential part of human nature.

The Next Steps in Big Data Metrics and Health

The idea of big data evaluated using large anonymous population data may make many people uneasy. The advent of more data collected can conjure "big brother" thinking and can bring people wanting to disconnect from the technological world altogether.

Yet as we've seen the darker side of technology used, we can keep in mind that data being misused and abused are often from those lacking consciousness and mindfulness. However, in terms of the benefits for the masses, there are still many positives.

This doesn't mean there won't be those who want to control and abuse the system, yet we can't really stop the technological developments as this is as human a process as there is. To design, develop, and progress technologically is part of human nature, and as such, we can choose to use this appropriately.

Humans, from the times of using a stick to eat with, or using a rock attached to a stick to use as a hammer, have developed technology. From a fork to computers, the design process is an essential part of human life. We are creatures that mainly utilize ingenuity in providing a better life and living through design.

Whether we use it to build shelters that have morphed into today's architecture or the creativity to develop modern computers, modern medicine, and many other technological developments, they have all been part of human nature to advance.

While many developments in bioinformatics are gathering and analyzing data for primarily personal use, such as the Fitbit or home interior monitors, there is still a lack of truly integrated data collection related to health metrics.

As these environmental sensors become less expensive and easier to connect to one's computing environment, such as the Internet of Things (IOT), there is more possibility of this data gathered and evaluated for human health to benefit humankind.

Companies such as tzoa, Particle, and Purple Air, to name just a few, are at the forefront of devices for personal and large-scale monitoring. By utilizing such devices located around the city, this monitoring of particulates in the air, temperature readings, humidity, carbon monoxide (CO), carbon dioxide (CO_2), and Oxygen levels can bring insights for those in public health in real time.

By monitoring areas at risk for health problems and ensuring good air quality around the city, these pollution metrics can help alert issues when found.

Combining this big city data with personal devices can provide a long term evaluation of personal health. This can offer the individual more tools in their health analysis over time.

This data can then be reviewed with a doctor for yearly analysis, for instance, where the doctor and patient work together in monitoring and maintaining good health.

When this is scaled up to more significant amounts of people and includes personal and city-wide monitoring with geoinformation, the individual and the doctors have a larger scope of data to evaluate. Add epidemiologists for a larger analysis of data, it can provide better evaluations to maintain healthy conditions in both the outside environment in cities and interior built environments.

Artificial Intelligence (AI), Architecture, and Medicine?

Almost everywhere you look these days, there are discussions on how Artificial Intelligence (AI) impacts the world. Can AI impact architecture and medicine as a cohesive whole?

Eric Topol's book *Deep Medicine* discusses the impacts of AI in the field of medicine. He states that AI can reveal patterns in rapid formats, as computers are excellent at evaluating large datasets. Can AI utilize the big data collected in the Architectural Medicine flowchart and data repository collection to help architects and medical professionals have more insights into health related to the built environment?

This would require several groups working together to gather this data, and then work towards developing algorithms to analyze these big datasets for insights. There is certainly the potential for this development to support better health, yet these are more theories than actual current processes. However, there can be quick developments made in this category as more cities utilize sensor devices for "smart cities," and with these datasets from sensors can emerge patterns related to health.

Big Data and SMART Cities for Health

What are "smart" buildings and cities?

As mentioned above, with the advent of more cities utilizing sensor devices to collect temperature, humidity, particulates, chemicals, and data on oxygen, carbon monoxide, carbon dioxide, and many other substances, the collection of pollution metrics can increase over time.

The ability to have this data in real-time can help provide health alerts, such as poor air quality on certain days. This information can be very valuable for older generations, children, and those with sensitive immune systems.

The use of this data in real-time is helpful, yet it can also be beneficial for long-term evaluations. And when these sensors are more common inside buildings, then the potential for both real-time and long-term analysis can be powerful.

These sensors can provide insights into building performance, thereby making them "smarter." The ability to monitor the building's structural integrity and environmental monitoring provides a better understanding of building health. The scaling of these individual building monitors from the inside of buildings to the exteriors of cities, can define the concept of a "smart city."

Smart Homes, Buildings for Health & Personal Environmental Measuring Devices

Over the past ten to fifteen years, the cost of smaller sensors for home use has become a hobby for some and a full-time experience for others. The addition of more personal sensory devices and more common devices to monitor carbon monoxide, radon, and other gases, has become a focus for many interested in their health. Adding these sensors in homes has spurred on the "smart home" movement, whether it be to control lighting with advanced LED lights or sensors to monitor potential issues such as carbon monoxide and radon.

What impact can smart devices and smart homes have on health?

1. Sensors for health, monitoring chemicals, particulates, and gases such as carbon dioxide, carbon monoxide, radon, etc.
2. Data for occupants to utilize for better health, especially during specific time frames such as when people are cooking and sleeping
3. Personal sensors for health and data collection for short and long term monitoring
4. Personal sensors to measure levels of stress to focus on an increase in wellness
5. Public health sensors and data to measure pollution in buildings and cities, showing problem areas in public places (Public Health, Epidemiology, etc.)
6. Big Data, Bioinformatics, Artificial Intelligence (AI), and better metrics over time (Exposome, Social Determinants of Health, etc.)

Smartphones and city-wide environmental measuring devices for big data analysis can also be integrated with population health statistics. Cities, Universities, and other groups can create research stations and sensors in cities to measure environmental conditions. This process can support healthier environments and flag issues when high levels of pollution exists. It can provide information when exposures to chemicals or pollutants are on the rise, providing early warning systems.

These sensors in both exteriors and interiors of the built environment can provide helpful information for the daily life of society, especially as locations are more active where larger groups of people congregate.

The future of bioinformatics and big data can help support healthier built environments by cross-referencing personal data, big city data, and health issues of the individual. This includes topics related to social determinants of health and exposomics.

The Exposome, Exposomics, Biomonitoring, and Big Data

As mentioned in chapters 9 and 17, the term *exposome* has been another topic that has become more common in the discussions of health and environmental exposures.

Why is the topic of exposomics so important?

A primary consideration of this issue is that genetics has been "found to account for only about 10% of diseases, and the remaining causes appear to be from environmental causes." Understanding the 90 percent remainder of diseases, potentially from these environmental causes, is quite a significant reason for critical attention to be focused on this topic.

The promising aspects of personal health relative to the built environment based on behaviors and environment are defined as epigenetic changes affecting the function of your genes. This scientific research, where the long-term impacts of environmental exposures are measured, is defined as the exposome.

As a reminder from chapters 5 and 9, the CDC defines the exposome as "the measure of all the exposures of an individual in a lifetime and how those exposures relate to health."[214] The fact that it strives to map environmental exposure impacts over a lifetime is both interesting and challenging.

Without personal monitoring and a connection to the biomonitoring of built environments and cities, there would be too many gaps of data in providing links to biomarkers and exposures.

These biomarkers and analysis can provide a better understating of the impacts on the genome. The resulting effects that the environment has on the phenotype related to health can provide deeper insights into what Eric Topol defines in his book *Deep Medicine*.[215] The antithesis of this is shallow medicine, where Dr. Topol discusses a lack of depth in analysis with the physician's evaluation process. While *Deep Medicine* focuses on artificial intelligence as helpful data analysis, an essential factor of his writing is stated in his book's subtitle, "how artificial intelligence can make healthcare human again." And this focus on human health is of critical importance, especially as technology advances.

The Architectural Medicine System (AMS), and measuring data as bioinformatics, can provide an exciting potential to help support this exposome and *molecular epidemiology*, which studies the "relationships between occupational exposures and health outcomes."[216]

By utilizing the Architectural Medicine Software Solution – ARxMD for biomonitoring and bioinformatics, these environmental issues, and most notably pollution in built environments, can yield valuable, usable data for better health.

The advent of modern sensor devices becoming more ubiquitous in personal and built environments can provide the potential to utilize all of this data in a helpful format as bioinformatics.

However, as exposomics is the study of the exposome and "relies on the application of internal and external exposure assessment methods," this infers many other fields to include in this analysis. These internal exposures rely on fields of study "such as genomics, metabonomics, lipidomics, transcriptomics and proteomics. Many of the "omics" technologies have the potential to further our understanding of disease causation and progression."[217]

The CDC lists the following as commonalities of these fields:[218]

1. use of biomarkers to determine exposure, effect of exposure, disease progression, and susceptibility factors
2. use of technologies that result in large amounts of data and
3. use of data mining techniques to find statistical associations between exposures, effect of exposures, and other factors such as genetics with disease

A critical factor, and also a challenging issue in describing the exposome, is the "ability to accurately measure exposures and effect of exposures."[219]

An important facet of the Architectural Medicine System (AMS) is collecting this type of data and combining this analysis with health impacts, providing more data for these "omics" fields to research.

This is an example of how the integration between fields can provide deeper insights into health topics. When you view the comments on exposomics, you can see the overlap and similarities of how a Healthy Building Inspector can provide such data by "using direct reading instruments, laboratory-based analysis, and survey instruments."[220] The healthy building inspection utilizes each of these processes when evaluating built environment issues, and can become a strong collaborator in providing these fields with data.

The CDC article on the exposome discusses the importance of "understanding how exposures from our environment, diet, lifestyle, etc. interact with our own unique characteristics such as genetics, physiology, and epigenetics impact our health is how the exposome will be articulated."

When you view epigenetics, the exposome, and the Architectural Medicine System (AMS), you can see the overlap and importance of collecting data for these fields to analyze for better insights into human health in all environments. Without such metrics and data collection, these fields will struggle to find patterns to help iterate building processes for a better future.

IoT – Internet of Things and Advanced CHRs as Comprehensive Health Records

When it comes to thoughts on the future, the key term, in my opinion, is "trajectory" combined with putting the many pieces of a fragmented world together.

Perhaps the most critical part in the future of architectural development is putting these puzzle pieces of buildings, health, and medicine together in integrative formats. Many people are familiar with big data and the increasing amount of devices that each person has in their lives. By putting all of this data together, from smartphones to smart buildings, the result can provide bioinformatics that has never before been possible. This data can answer questions as to how the built environment and newer materials and chemicals impact human health.

Let's also consider the impacts that technology platforms such as Apple's CareKit and ResearchKit, as just two examples of evaluating and processing big data, can have on both personal health and public health. This big data is an example of the concept of weaving together data for a big picture trajectory actualized in a tangible format.

The increase of environmental sensory devices also includes the topic of IoT or the Internet of Things. By utilizing the fabric of cloud services, the world of IoT can provide technological interconnectivity for large-scale data analysis.

And even the increasingly popular Electronic Health Record (EHR) is developing into the CHR as the Comprehensive Health Record. This advancement provides more details or metadata for a more vast scope of measurements. The fact that EHRs have expanded to a more advanced CHR model is an example of how data and metadata are expanding to other facets of the health record. The idea of a more "comprehensive" record, which has evolved from the siloed concept of a simple medical record to other factors in health, is a good example of the trajectory in where the future is headed.

And where is this going? As mentioned above, putting "the puzzle pieces together" may be a path for these developments to have a more synergistic impact on human health informatics.

How will all of these pieces working together make any difference or significant synergistic differences?

Let's use the following graphic, which is theoretical in connectivity, and apply this in real-world formats:

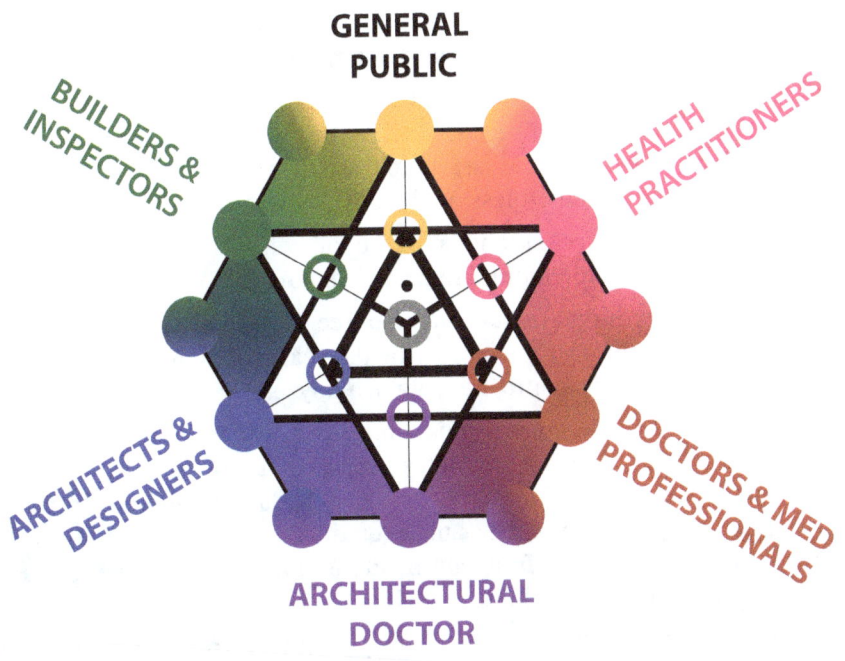

In the diagram above, there are fields listed from the general public, building inspectors and health practitioners to architects, doctors, and builders. It also includes the Architectural Doctor as part of the Architectural Medicine System (AMS).

In chapter 15 on the Architectural Doctor, a flowchart provides details on how the built environment can be included in the evaluation process for the doctor and health professionals.

Throughout the book, several steps can help make these connections in real-world formats using the Architectural Medicine System and ARxMD software.

As shown earlier, including the built environment in the evaluation process provides an opportunity for direct involvement for the medical fields working together with the architecture and building professions.

As can also be seen in this diagram, health researchers and scientists are included, from toxicologists to public health professionals. This is where their involvement directly interfaces with these building and medical professions.

These interconnections include research and evaluation of data to help define health related issues in the built environment. The process of setting standards, protocols, and eventually supporting processes between many moving parts is critical.

These integrations and multi-disciplinary involvements for a more cohesive whole can provide a greater understanding of the built environment's impacts.

These processes can be helpful for the individual as the general public seeking solutions, yet they can also help define new models, standards, and building processes for the professional fields.

A model of this process is shown in the following flowchart, which is the last segment of the Architectural Medicine System (AMS).

The evaluation of data requires a resource of this data to start with. The addition of these building sensors and the data capture of the various types of environmental sensors can provide data to analyze.

As mentioned, these sensors can record a wide range of information such as temperature, humidity, particulates, and a range of gases from carbon monoxide (CO) and carbon dioxide (CO_2) to VOCs and Radon. Areas in cities can also include pollutants such as nitrogen dioxide, methane, and ozone, as a few examples. Other gases from combustible sources and exhaust gases can be valuable to meter and evaluate as well.

This, combined with personal sensors, from smartphones to on-person sensors, can also help in gathering this data. By combining sensor data in

Chapter: 21 — Some Thoughts on the Future

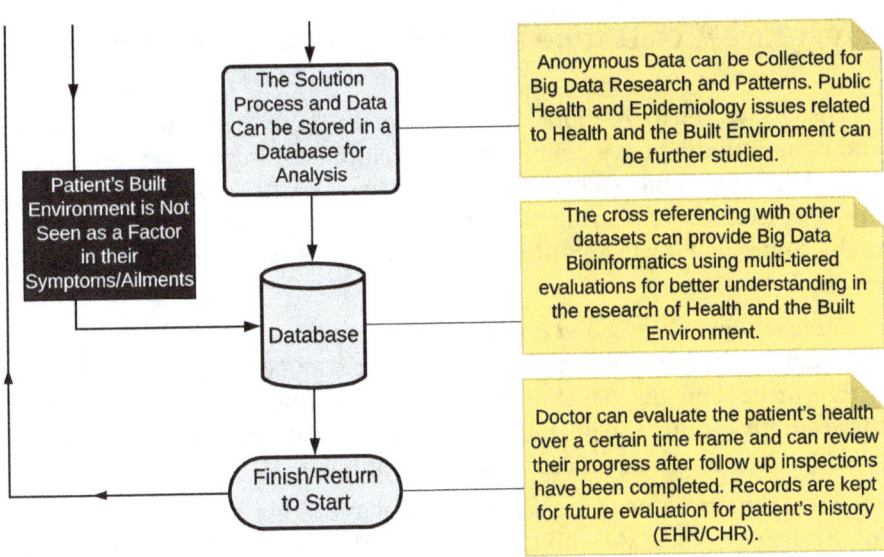

cities using a geographic information system (GIS), this information can be merged with the data of personal sensors.

A geographic information system (GIS) is a "system designed to capture, store, manipulate, analyze, manage, and present spatial or geographic data." Professionals can use the addition of this information layer to see more extensive patterns of health.

As GIS applications are "tools that allow users to create interactive queries, analyze spatial information, edit data in maps, and present the results of all these operations"[221], these processes can all be combined for extensive study.

If you then include epidemiologists, public health professionals, and toxicologists evaluating this information, you now have a large set of data that can be evaluated and analyzed for human health.

An example of utilizing this data are maps on a smartphone. These apps can provide real-time traffic information that can help you navigate when traveling. If you take this real-time data analysis, instead of traffic, you can utilize an app informing you of areas that have health related issues. This can show problems such as high particulate matter or high levels of CO_2 or VOCs. It can guide you to stay away from these areas and be informed when it's ok to be outside in such circumstances.

This data can also be used for the city health professionals to find areas with issues and address them in real time. They can advise the general public and work on resolving these matters.

Integrative Architecture and the Future of Interconnectivity

As I've written in this book, the history of the fields of healthy, sustainable, and green building have been long in development. In the past forty to fifty years, these fields have taken significant steps towards solutions. Sometimes these solutions have been separate from each other, which means that much of the future will involve putting these concepts together to form a cohesive whole.

This whole is based on current and future technological advancements, the latter of which might be premature to write about as an unknown. With all of the current knowns in technological developments and processes, some of these simply require the big picture viewpoint combined with small detailed specifications to provide more complete solutions.

When smart homes can then contribute to a larger dataset and analyzed to include personal data with electronic health records (EHRs), bioinformatics can provide a larger scope of patterns to help better review overall health. These additional facets can be included in Integrative Architecture to ensure whole systems solutions, which I discussed in chapter 10.

These datasets can include on-person metrics, such as temperature, humidity, and other sensory data such as CO_2, CO, VOC levels, and particulates. It can then be coupled with vitals taken from smart devices such as the Apple Watch. Using healthkit and researchkit, the combination can provide a picture of information that has not yet been truly accessible for the professional health fields.

When combining all of this data, there is an enormous amount of information that can be evaluated by public health professions. These bioinformatics and epidemiological studies can help support research to better understand the impacts of the built environment on health, providing insightful patterns in setting better standards.

Of course, when you view this data on health informatics as "before and after" patient health analysis, it can provide valuable metrics to understand health and disease. These insights can be directly applied to preventive health protocols and standards, creating best practices for doctors and architects.

If this data is utilized with advanced sensor devices, it can help evaluate the toxicology of building products and the manufacturing processes, showing impacts on biological and human health. By monitoring these topics, the modern city can help provide deeper insights and flag areas of pollution to support changes and improve conditions. This can be particularly valuable in industrial areas to help provide support for workers and the general public.

All of this data can provide information in electronic health records (EHR) to provide the modern doctor and healthcare provider with better patient insights. This can provide patterns of health with historical datasets from their patient's exposures.

Instead of the doctor evaluating only the patient's current situation, these datasets can help provide the doctor insights into exposures and health impacts over a longer time. This can support a diagnosis based not just on a current evaluation but also on historical information.

These are some potential scenarios as future integrations between the architecture and medical fields. The integration and sharing of this information will be vital for these evaluations to have any meaningful purpose and use. This is a big reason why this integration between architecture and medicine is a driving force in the very name of Architectural Medicine.

Cymatics and Sound Shaping – the Future of Designs

In chapters 12 and 13, emotional and mental wellness topics included the issues of sounds and noises. The quality and types of sounds – from noise to music – can significantly impact human health and well being.

However, what if this was taken a step further by using sound as a design tool?

As many know, sound experiments defined as Chladni plates show a range of shapes and patterns based on frequencies. When a material such as sand is placed on a vibrating plate, different frequencies sent to the plate create specific designs. This can be seen in the following images.

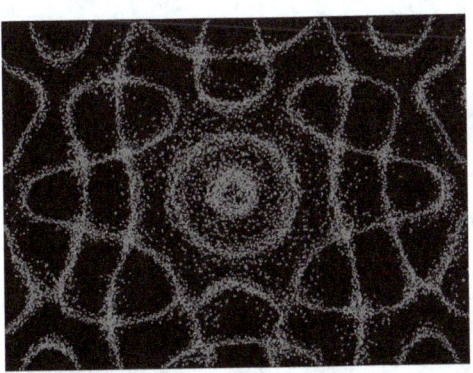
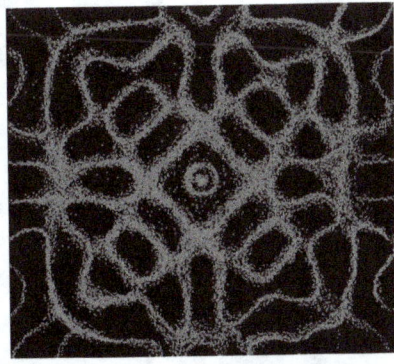

Cymatics is a term coined by Hans Jenny, who wrote about the patterns that these vibrations create based on frequencies in his book *Kymatic*.

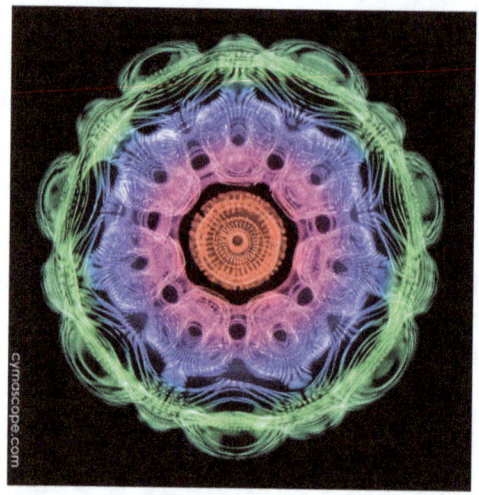

However, most of these experiments are shown in two dimensions on a flat plate. Yet, the world of sound exists in three dimensions, with most sounds looking like a bubble as a sound wave and not a two-dimensional wave. The advanced research of John Stuart Reid, an acoustics engineer who invented the CymaScope, shows the shapes of sound in three dimensions (example on the left) defined as CymaGlyphs. This three-dimensional wave as a bubble could have exciting developments connected to the design world of architecture. If sound waves were tuned to different frequencies creating bubble shapes and forms, could these forms have an impact on human and biological health?

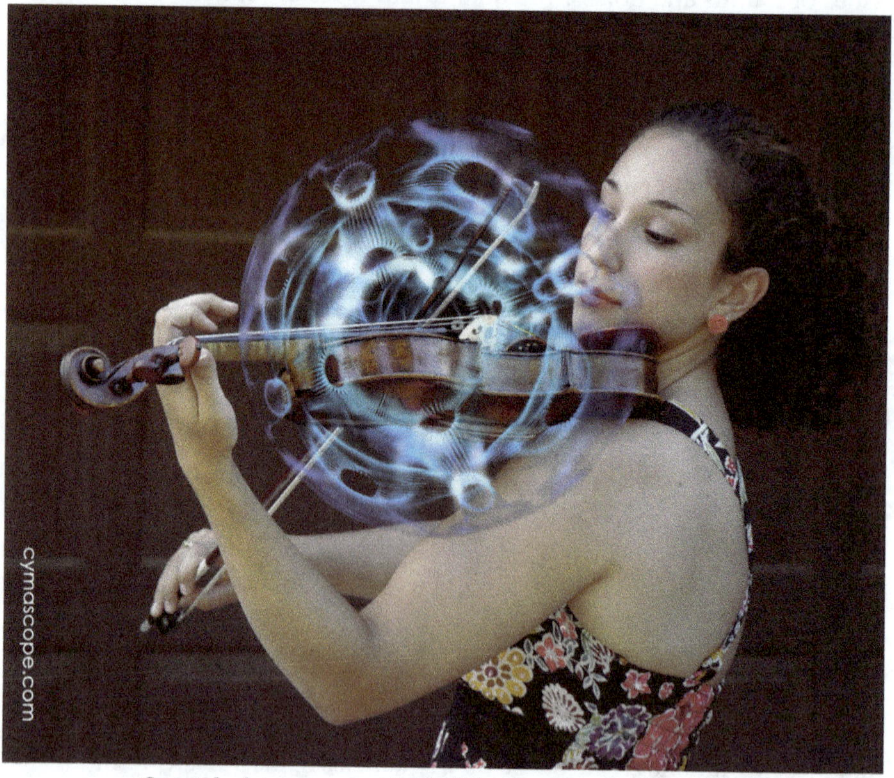

CymaGlyph images provided by John Stuart Reid - Cymascope.com

What if a sound bubble of a particular frequency could be tuned specifically for a form of healing for a specific person. And then, as this shape is created as a building, would the experiences of living within these shapes positively impact human health?

Perhaps it could also be found that certain shapes are not as helpful as others. Could this define places of health for people to spend time within as a healing modality? Perhaps this could be included in the discussions on Wellness Centers from chapter 20.

While it might sound like science fiction, if sound and frequency have such a powerful impact on the world we live in, is it that far-fetched that specific frequencies molded into three-dimensional shapes improve human health?

Of course, only time will tell, yet as we venture into the future, perhaps it's found that certain frequencies designed as physical shapes based on these cymatic, parametric forms can have health benefits.

And perhaps the blueprints of heathier structures can be created utilizing parametric equations tuned to specific frequencies, yielding these shapes as three-dimensional structures.

If we view all of these topics, one common thread between sound and musical shapes is the parametric equations graphed in three dimensions, from the architecture of life as cells, plants, and organisms to these flowing, curving shapes.

These designs can be mathematically created, and in doing so, follow a common blueprint for all life. As more architectural designs implement parametric forms that people will experience, perhaps over time, our human biology will resonate and be more in tune with these forms. Doing so may promote better health and wellness, reconnect us to ourselves and life on this planet, thereby connecting us back to nature.

The benefits of this are many, from a better life experience to connecting to the natural world as biophilia. These connections can provide better personal health and contribute to the conservation and preservation of life on Earth. In so doing, it helps to provide better stewardship of this planet and provides a healthier ecology — benefitting all biological life.

Music and Architecture

There is, in my opinion, an untapped resource of music and the connection to sound in the world of architecture. Music therapy is a subject utilized for many people for healing, and helpful for positive mental and emotional support.

As the topics of the neuroscience of architecture and environmental psychology have begun to develop, there is the physiological component of places that could provide health, healing, and wellness for many people in the future.

This topic is challenging to discuss in objective terms. Yet, perhaps in the future, there will be research to show more congruity in designs that promote health as harmonious built environments.

Music, in terms of harmonies, is created when a composer places different instruments together at the same time with complimentary notes. Architecture, particularly cityscapes, has similarities to these soundscapes by combining many structures in symbolizing the many instruments and sounds of a symphony.

If you've ever heard a symphony out of tune or those playing the wrong notes, what makes them sound bad? How can you tell? Most can tell by the fact that they are expecting notes to fit together, creating harmony. So when there are notes misplayed, these can easily be heard as discordant.

If cityscapes and architecture also have this form of harmonic interconnectivity, can the combination of different forms, shapes, materials, and textures function in a similar fashion? In the future, can architecture be defined in ways that are in harmony with other buildings and also in harmony with the natural surroundings?

As I mentioned in previous chapters, the DNA of the city is defined by the DNA of the single structure. And suppose this single structure is in the form of harmonic balance with the natural surroundings. When scaled up to cities, these cityscapes can also be in tune with the surroundings along with other architectural structures.

And speaking of music composition related to architectural design, another fascinating topic is the connection between musicians, music, and architecture. While I was an architecture student, I learned about an album called "Music for Architectural Students." What surprised me the most about this, at that time, was the album was made by Pink Floyd.

And it was this time in the late 1980s that I first learned the history of Pink Floyd, as the band members met while at architecture school. Roger Waters, Nick Mason, and Richard Wright met at the Royal Polytechnic Institution in London as architecture students. Waters commented about this in a few articles I've read, yet I've always been curious to think what kind of architecture these members would have created.

Of course, they did indeed create architecture – the architecture of music. And the sounds, textures, and emotions of music can be as powerful as beautiful architecture. It moves people in ways that can sometimes be defined as spiritual – being moved in an emotionally powerful way. Perhaps the Pink Floyd album, "The Wall," has another layer of significance with this architectural connection.

When Waters was asked about his architecture school experiences relative to music, he said, "music is only mathematics anyway. It is another way of interpreting maths."[222] To me, this is particularly interesting relative to parametric design and the curving forms of both music and parametric architecture.

Maybe the creative side of architecture, requiring a structural and engineering mindset, is a good overlap for music and musicians. Music, like architecture, requires creativity along with structural integrity for rhythmic and interesting soundscapes. The overlap between music requiring many instruments, each with its layer of sound, can perhaps be mapped in architecture as physical materials create layers as tactile spaces.

Music has space, architecture creates space. And music provides many different moods and emotional responses, while architecture can also offer similar qualities, particularly inspiring forms to uplift society.

David Byrne of the famous group Talking Heads has discussed architecture and sound in many of his interviews. He discusses spaces as integral for certain music, perhaps even influencing music itself, as he noted in his TED talk "How architecture helped music evolve."[223]

The musical artist Björk created an album titled Biophilia, exploring the links between nature, music, and technology.

Of course, Biophilia is a topic we've discussed in this book, defined as a love of nature. With a song titled Crystalline, Björk took inspiration for the song from cities and buildings, stating, "I've sat a lot of my life in buses and taxis from 20 years of touring and somehow all these different types of intersections have gone on file in my brain. Like some have three streets meeting with very tall buildings on all sides while others are complex with like five street meeting but all buildings are low and so on... Seems like each one of them has a different mood, different spatial tension or release. Part of my obsessive nature wants to map out each intersection in the world and match it with a song... To me crystal structures seem to grow in a similar way."[224] Björk included the topic of cymatics in the video for the song Cosmogony, in addition to these connections to architectural spaces.

The long-running radio and online program Hearts of Space (HOS) was developed by a student of architecture, Steven Hill.

My first listening to this ambient or "space music" – as Hill defines it –

many years ago evoked an emotional response that I related to the feelings of spaces and places. Music can often create a visceral experience.

Stephen's bio on the HOS website states, "Hill received a graduate degree in architecture at the University of Pennsylvania in 1969 where he studied and worked with Louis Kahn, Robert Venturi, Romaldo Giurgola, Richard Saul Wurman and other leading architects of the day. Hill's bio ends with the comment, "In retrospect, Hill realizes he never really left architecture. He simply became a sound architect who learned to build his castles on the air."[225]

It seems to me it's not a mistake that this show HOS was developed by an architect. Another long-running radio and internet program with similar ambient sounds and music, is Echoes, hosted by John Diliberto. The show's name was inspired by the song name from Pink Floyd's album Meddle, and fits the ambient, ethereal, and often long playing song lists.

From the members of Pink Floyd and David Byrne to artists such as Björk and the music productions of Stephen Hill and John Diliberto, the fabric of music as an architectural tapestry seems to have a common overlap.

Perhaps this is based on the similar characteristics that sound, as music, and spaces as architecture denote. The frequencies, layers, tones, emotions, and moods of music are akin to the shapes, forms, textures, colors, emotional responses, and moods of architecture.

As music can merge the fabric of many instruments into a cohesive soundscape, the potential for architecture to provide integrative connections between many fields can also provide cohesive and full systems solutions.

3D Printing, Geopolymers, and Mathematical Parametric Design

Another fascinating development occurring in the world of building and architecture is the advent of three-dimensional or 3D printing. With the advancements in Computer-Aided Design and Manufacturing, the possibilities of creating complex mathematical equations as parametric designs, from drawing to construction, are becoming more feasible every year.

What's more, with the ability to utilize different materials in building or printing these designs, the use of more sustainable and green materials is becoming more accessible.

For example, utilizing advancements in geopolymers to replace the enormous energy demands and carbon footprint of manufacturing concrete, can open up possibilities that have not previously existed. The ability to use 3D printing for creating homes and structures can help in housing solutions and provide more ecologically aware developments.

By including in the equation, literally, the use of applications such as Mathematica, formulas can be placed into visual programming language applications such as Grasshopper for Rhino3D or AutoDesk's Revit. These programs can be used to create and update designs using different parameters in real-time.

These three-dimensional forms in the CAD application can be manipulated for different design versions using graphical inputs. As these programs can also provide Computer-Aided Engineering (CAE), the potential for utilizing these equations for both aesthetic purposes and structural assessments can then be actualized in Computer-Aided Manufacturing.

The result can be the manufacturing of these buildings providing more cost-effective housing, while also designing parametric shapes to support healing, health, and well being.

Utilizing these applications, interfaced with 3D printing capabilities and sustainable materials, can provide compelling architecture and building solutions in the 21st century and beyond.

Telemedicine – The Potential to Evaluate Built Environments for Health

As telemedicine advances and becomes more common, there are several benefits that can support patient health in these scenarios. By utilizing advanced hardware that can be sent to the patient for evaluations, there can be additional data captured for analysis.

This hardware can include sensors to monitor building issues, such as indoor air quality monitors. These sensors can be used for both short term and long term monitoring.

The video capabilities can also support the review of the building conditions, from individual rooms to the health care practitioner flagging issues that may be causing problems for the patient.

The patient can be queried as to any smells, such as mold or chemicals. And the visual assessments can also help evaluate interior issues that could provide helpful clues if the building is affecting emotional or psychological conditions.

These telemedicine appointments might be utilized only for preliminary analysis, requiring more involvement and in-person inspections, yet can provide an initial diagnosis for further evaluation.

As telemedicine becomes more advanced, additional services can help the doctor evaluate their patient's health in unique formats that include the built environment for patient analysis.

The initial scope may provide helpful information for the health professionals to request a healthy building inspection or have monitoring devices sent to patients to provide testing and data for review.

Full Systems Solutions – Transcending Knowledge into Wisdom

In chapter 10, I discussed the topic of Integrative Architecture and the synergistic benefits when merging the topics of green, sustainable, and healthy building together.

These topics can form new architectural solutions that can span topics discussed throughout this book, from wellness centers and parametric designs to bioinformatics and big data.

The Architectural Doctor and the Healthy Building Inspector can contribute to missing pieces of the puzzle to bridge these gaps.

And utilizing the Architectural Medicine System (AMS) and the Architectural Medicine Software Solution – ARxMD, a structure can be provided to achieve these goals of wellness in the built environment.

Essentially, many of these topics in the future point to integration between various disconnected fields, along with focusing on whole systems solutions.

And perhaps a key to this better future is the active participation between different professionals that have not previously existed, providing new insights and better design processes with integrated solutions.

This multi-disciplinary approach to viewing issues and finding cohesive solutions provides a more extensive scope of the many pieces. It can provide a vantage point to offer whole-systems solutions.

Instead of facets being resolved that may create new problems, this method can allow for complex challenges to be resolved with more wisdom.

These integrated solutions depend on knowledge and the use of wisdom in navigating these complex processes.

The word origin of wisdom is:

wisdom (n.)

Old English wisdom "knowledge, learning, experience," from wis (see wise (adj.)) + -dom. A common Germanic compound (Old Saxon, Old Frisian wisdom, Old Norse visdomr, Old High German wistuom "wisdom," German Weistum "judicial sentence serving as a precedent").[226]

wise (adj.)

Old English wis "learned, sagacious, cunning; sane; prudent, discreet; experienced; having the power of discerning and judging rightly," from Proto-Germanic *wissaz (source also of Old Saxon, Old Frisian wis, Old Norse viss, Dutch wijs, German weise "wise"), from past-participle adjective *wittos of PIE root *weid- "to see" (hence "to know").[227]

And the definition of wisdom is:

- Ability to discern inner qualities and relationships : INSIGHT
- Good sense : JUDGMENT[228]
- Capacity of judging rightly in matters relating to life and conduct; soundness of judgement in the choice of means and ends[229]

The overall description of wisdom is not just knowledge but "having the power of discerning and judging rightly."

In terms of architecture and medicine, this need to discern and "judge rightly" is critical for a healthier future focused on wellness.

Technological advancements and an increase in knowledge can provide a better ability to navigate in this world. Yet, the wisdom to properly utilize this technology and knowledge is even more essential.

The topics of ethics and balance of power have never been more crucial than this time in recorded history. The decisions that we make as individuals and collectively will impact current and many future generations to come.

The Native American concept of the seventh generation is to consider the impacts that the current generation's actions will have on future generations. Oren Lyons, a Native American Faithkeeper of the Iroquois or Haudenosaunee Confederacy, defines this in the following statement:

"We are looking ahead, as is one of the first mandates given us as chiefs, to make sure and to make every decision that we make relate to the welfare and well-being of the seventh generation to come. ... What about the seventh generation? Where are you taking them? What will they have?"[230]

What decisions will the current architectural creations have on future generations in terms of wellness and well being? And how can the professions of architecture, construction, medicine, and healthcare work together with this goal of better wellness for future generations?

The decisions that humanity chooses in terms of future architectural materials and methods will be critical to help resolve the many topics related to green, sustainable, and healthy building.

I go into more detail on these topics in the forthcoming book *Integrative Architecture* – integrating the processes between green, healthy, and sustainable architecture methodologies for more energy-efficient, ecologically aware, and healthier built environments.

WISDOM Building

If wisdom is to be implemented into future architecture, how can some of these topics be defined? Perhaps using WISDOM as an acronym, the following can be applied with approaches towards architecture and building:

W – Whole/World/Wellness

I – Integration/Inspiring

S – Systems/Solutions

D – Deeper Connections & Meanings

O – Optimum Processes

M – Micro-Macro/Monumental

Whether theoretical concepts or newly developed topics, these ideas can provide several positive benefits to help support healthier built environments into the future.

By analyzing and keeping the focus on the current designs of objects and architecture in the present world, wisdom can be gleaned from what works, what doesn't work, and where there can be modifications to make things better.

If health and wellness is a main focal point of these evaluations, then the result can be a greater understanding of what steps can be taken to arrive at more optimal solutions.

This wisdom can provide new and updated solutions that are iterated over time as a positive spiracycle. And when these are combined, the term "whealth" can define this as an investment in health and wellness.

And the implementation of this wisdom brings us to the subtitle of this book, "Building the Bridge to Wellness."

Perhaps these new integrations and developments can also answer the question "Can Architecture Be Healing?" In my opinion, the answer is yes.

It may take time and require more considerable coordination and cooperation between many fields, professionals, and the general public. Yet, the result can be a win-win for humanity, the planet, and future generations…

"Be the change you wish to see in the world"

– Mahatma Gandhi

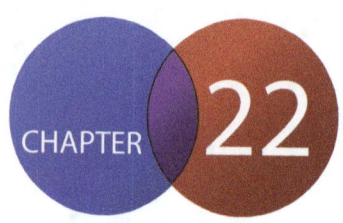

CHAPTER 22

FOLLOW UP AND CONCLUSION

There have been many topics discussed in this book on architecture and medicine, some of which are in process and others that are being independently explored. Some of these are merely ideas, and as such, there cannot be an accurate understanding in forecasting the future.

Yet, forecasting is also an accurate word to use. These puzzle pieces can help inform the future of health in the built environment, just as a weather forecaster uses data and many metrics to understand a trajectory of what might happen in the future.

Another important topic of this book is the many facets of human health, including mental, psychological, and emotional health, which are not typically discussed in the history of architecture.

The modern-day 21st century challenges in human health will have to include these facets of health, as they have increasingly become a topic of concern for the well being of populations.

As mental health and loneliness become more common problems in the world, it will require updated solutions that point towards age-old solutions, dating back to the time of Hippocrates.

Some of these issues can be measured, and others are more challenging to estimate as useful data. Both architecture and medicine have always been considered "fields of science and the arts," and the future will be no different in providing these solutions.

If we are to provide appropriate solutions, many of these topics that are not currently on the radar of these professions will need to be included. The good news is that the involvement of many fields working together is already in progress. And while there are challenges that will be faced and experienced, the participation of so many in this process can produce results that help the individual and scale up to the masses.

This focus on the positive, with an understanding of the challenges involved, can help build a bridge to defining a future with better health and wellness for humanity. The knowledge in which wisdom can be provided, creating solutions for a better world and a better quality of life for humans and biological life on this planet, can offer a hopeful future.

It is this hope with which this book has been written, and with this hope, a better future can be built – both figuratively and literally. This book has been written with this intention, where a blueprint can be created for these solutions for wellness.

In my half-century on this planet, I've noticed a few patterns in how people function or dysfunction on this planet in two major patterns. There are either people in survival mode who are struggling to make ends meet and are therefore less focused on the thriving elements of life or those who have their basic needs met to live a more sophisticated and enjoyable life. In this manner, this can include the ability to have access to professional studies and personal development.

And this can make a big difference in whether one's health is focused on the quality of life and wellness or mere survival. With the increasing number of human populations, humanity will need to decide how we either support human thriving or support systems that do not allow this to easily occur. We've reached a point technologically where we can sustain human survival in terms of shelter, food, and the basic needs for human living. Yet will we as a collective humanity choose to go in this direction of mutual support?

In this manner, these human-created systems, if they are based on human awareness and consciousness of the populations, can provide opportunities for wellness for humanity at large.

After all, if 700 trillion cells in one person's body can all work together in unison as a form of togetherness to support the overall health of the "whole" of the body, then certainly a mere 7 to 8 billion people can work together for the health of humanity.

What Is Old Is New Again

The future of architecture and of human connection to their built environments is not something new. In fact, the history of aboriginal architecture has embraced a mutual interdependence with nature for millennia. All around the world, vernacular architecture has adopted the local materials and factored into their building equation the weather, environment, and site location.

Much of these historic building styles and forms were based on the capabilities of these materials and methods, and since the technological advancements of materials and engineering have provided solutions that can overcome previous limitations, it has also opened up the potential to overrun and overpower the local ecologies.

While previous cultures recognized the value of an integrated, whole systems approach to life and living, this mutual interdependence was part of their way of life. Often it has become the case that Americans and first world countries are typically looking for that "one thing" or a "quick fix" to resolve problems.

The idea that "one pill" can fix everything is the viewpoint of a one-fix solution, where you don't have to change anything else, such as how you eat and exercise to have quality of life. This has come to include the building processes, resulting in the negative impacts of the modern built environment on health.

A good example of this is the history of bau biologie, which began as an investigation to understanding why people were getting sick in post-World War II Europe. Many were trying to figure out why people were getting sick. It took several people's work and investigation process to finally realize that the newer buildings, which were using synthetic materials causing issues from VOCs and other chemical exposures, combined with the newer "tight buildings," were causing illness. As discussed throughout this book, this combination caused a lack of fresh air, and that meant an increase in chemical exposures leading to many health issues. Of course, these newer building processes are beneficial for energy efficiency, but not good for the inhabitants' health.

So this is again is why understanding complete systems is critical, otherwise, the attempt to fix one thing can cause other problems when not adequately evaluated.

Even Feng Shui can provide "common logic" solutions based on science. The very term Feng Shui is literally defined as "Wind Water." Feng is "Wind," and Shui is "Water." The origin of the term developed 5,000 years ago as "Wind Water" focuses on the building's location and ability to site buildings and villages properly. To ensure the elements of nature, both the "wind" and the "water," were properly understood, structures being built could avoid the destructive aspects of nature.

When building, if the location is very windy as when building on top of a hill or mountain, this can cause tremendous challenges for both the structural integrity of the building as well as the general living scenario of these conditions.

And if you build in areas at the bottom of a valley or regions where flooding exists, this would be harsh on the building and the inhabitants. The hurricanes of the southeast US and the below-grade building in New Orleans have shown time and again how detrimental these building choices can become.

These natural elements negatively impact the health of the building, causing distress, sickness, and terrible situations, and possibly death due to the locations of these built environments.

This includes rain and snow and other environmental conditions. So the science part of the approach to building from the beginning of time, was to find places that had a lesser degree of natural environmental impact based on the weather and elements of a region. To reduce exposure to such harsh elements, finding locations and building approaches that could withstand the elements for better shelter was a critical choice.

This points to the vital key to recognizing different needs and different environmental issues in each area in which buildings are constructed. So there is a need to understand the attributes of the location as well as the fundamental building processes.

Without knowledge of both of these facets, there is bound to be issues that are either unplanned or designed incorrectly due to a lack of understanding.

A better shelter meant less stress, and less stress meant better health and wellness and improved quality of life. After all, if your house is being blown away or washed away on a regular basis, it would not lead to a relaxed and enjoyable quality of life.

There are many indigenous aboriginal approaches to building structures around the world, such as Vastu Shastra in India, Geomancy in Europe, and if you look to all of the aboriginal cultures around the world, you will find versions of building for that specific region. These are based on specific weather conditions and utilizing the local materials and methods of the area. While each culture has its customized version of building type and approach, the core of each is based on learning about the patterns of the natural environment and understanding how to build with these natural patterns.

This vernacular architecture can be viewed until around the 20th century worldwide, when the "International Style," as it's called, essentially took over the world of architecture in terms of style and design.

Many designers were happy not to be stuck with the materials and designs of the region and to not be constrained by the natural materials and design process. Instead, they could utilize technological advancements, such as mechanical heating and cooling, that could better control the interior environmental conditioning.

This form of architecture standardized much of the architecture in the 20th century because modern technology and methods allowed the structure to function the same in any climate. And in most conditions, this approach did not have to worry about nature's "wind" and "water" constraints of the past.

Overcoming Nature's Constraints – Navigating the Negatives of Progress

While there are many benefits of not having constraints on where humans can build, there are also issues and concerns with this mindset. The ability to build cities in deserts such as Phoenix and Las Vegas in the US, as two examples, where the natural environment and weather conditions no longer impact the interior conditions of the buildings, can be seen as a victory over nature.

Yet, in this process, there are severe impacts to both the local ecological environments and the many other geo-locations that are negatively impacted. From the borrowing of water, the creation of dams to the extensive infrastructure required for power, waste, and of course, food delivered to these remote areas, each of these poses long-term issues.

Perhaps this has become normal for many, as it's been in process for many decades now, yet if you take the time to analyze the impact this has on the local environments, you may find that there is a long-term impact that will not be experienced for some time.

The Long Now Foundation is an example of a group thinking about these long-term effects, and this includes many generations into the future. And when they state long into the future, they mean 10,000 years. Co-developed by icon and environmental pioneer Stewart Brand, the term was coined by one of the founding board members, Brian Eno. Their mission states the "foundation hopes to provide a counterpoint to today's accelerating culture and help make long-term thinking more common. We hope to foster responsibility in the framework of the next 10,000 years."[231]

The "out of sight, out of mind" process of focusing only on local topics often leads to big picture problems. The Cuyahoga River in Ohio catching on fire in the mid 20th century is a perfect example of just focusing on one facet, while the destructive impacts, on the whole, were ignored. Any time that water spontaneously catches on fire should scare any human into making immediate changes.

This is not to say that humans can not build in more harmony with extreme natural environments, yet it does bring into question the "how" of this process. And this brings up the question of whether or not the time is being taken to analyze and build appropriately for short-and long-term impacts.

This approach to design and building focusing on the impact humans have on the environment, is also interesting to evaluate in terms of stewardship of the earth and its many inhabitants and biological beings.

Humans are not alone here on this planet, and to act as if we can do whatever we want without any recognition of the repercussions is not only unwise, it's dangerous.

There can be an argument, or at least a long philosophical discussion, that this ability to build shelter without being impacted by the natural elements of mother nature was in fact a victory over nature. And, as such, this means that humans are no longer at the mercy of nature's unpredictable ways.

However, while this is neither good nor bad per se, some issues are created when you remove yourself from the natural world as a victory to overcome nature. Especially when you forget that we as humans are not just living in nature – we ARE nature.

So, when we disconnect from the natural world in our built environments, it tells a story that we as humans are also disconnecting from the natural world. And this causes tremendous problems due to a lack of insight, foresight, and a recognition that there is a cause-effect impact on what we do as humans.

So what does all of this have to do with any final conclusions or looking forward to the future?

Much of this leads to questions that are both personal and based on the collective of humanity. When individuals and groups begin to evaluate and analyze both their personal lives and the collective lives of society as a whole, there can be a deeper understanding that can often lead to changes in behaviors and changes in systems.

When more people recognize the importance of being a *global citizen*, then decisions locally become easier to navigate. What's needed are changes in the systems to better support the living standards of the individual, which will ripple out to the collective whole of society. And when these systems are the architecture as buildings and, in particular, the systems of cities, they have huge impacts on large amounts of people. This focus, subsequently, is how we as humans impact a large part of biological life on planet Earth.

This change process requires personal awareness and conscientiousness to want there to be better systems in place for the health of the masses, not just a select few. This awareness is based on consciousness or what's popularly called "mindfulness" in today's time. The Mindfulness movement essentially brings up the topics of how we can all be aware of these issues and how the individual's actions impact the whole of humanity and all other sentient creatures on this planet.

It brings awareness that we have put in place human-developed systems, which impact the life and livelihood of the masses. This is not necessarily a fault of the system but instead is more focused on the fact that life on planet Earth has changed so dramatically in the past one hundred years.

The old systems no longer reflect the current world we live in nor support the masses in a logical and sensible format. And, of course, these developments are also not scalable.

I go into more details on this topic in the forthcoming book *Symbiosis Global: Technology and Ecology Living Together*. Yet the basic premise is that, based on systems processes, the current systems do not support the masses while also respecting the planet.

An important mindset is to view *"Nature as the most advanced technology"* instead of viewing nature as primitive. When viewed in this format, the natural world becomes a place to learn from and conserve for human development. By learning from the natural world's wisdom, we can move forward with human developments for mutual benefit.

I mention the topic of consciousness and mindfulness in this way, and while many may feel that this is inappropriate for a book based on architecture and building as well as medicine, this is also where there is work to be done to make changes in the common mindset.

It's critical to ponder these topics on philosophical levels because architecture and buildings do impact health. Psychological health and mindfulness are very much integral facets of health – if not a critical foundation for good health.

To not talk about the psychological state of humans in terms of health would be akin to not talking about the foundation of a building. You cannot expect to have a successful building without a solid foundation. As such, you cannot ignore or avoid the topic of psychological and mental health if you are discussing wellness, well being, and quality of life.

While there be many disagreements and different viewpoints on how this is defined in some form of standard, to ignore it overall because it has no easy metrics to define is a formula for eventual failure.

And perhaps this lack of attention to these details may help better understand how the current ways of life seem to be falling apart in most parts of the world, especially when these require a scaling up of systems.

Sometimes, a building falls down because it was not built with quality materials and processes. Other times, it falls down because the engineering was not correctly evaluated and performed, resulting in the collapse of the building.

The lack of focus on mindfulness, awareness, and consciousness of these topics does not have to be at the level of a Ph.D., yet to not address them is similar to not having any solid foundation. Not having an engineer properly evaluate and approve of the materials and methods of construction or to not have a doctor assess a condition with basic metrics such as blood tests when appropriate, is an equation set up for failure.

These foundations are both figurative and literal in terms of the medical and health fields, as they are vital for good long-term health.

And now there is a beginning of integration and connectivity between health and the built environment, there must also be awareness and proper follow-through to ensure that this is considered for both current and future solutions in the built environment.

The benefit is that when individual buildings are designed and built with this mindset of mindfulness and consciousness, then the collection of buildings that create a city can then better reflect a mindset of consciousness. This can allow a city that supports a thriving population and supports the health, wellness, and well being of both the individual and the collective society.

The Novel Coronavirus Topic and Responses to Pandemics

In this time of 2020, with the world navigating the novel coronavirus pandemic, there are many topics related to both architecture and medicine that can be analyzed for better responses to pandemics moving forward.

Three main topics can be discussed moving forward.

One is the impact of buildings and how they can be designed to support better health and prevent the spread of such pathogens. The second is the education of the medical professions on how to deal with such built environment facets. And the third is the incredible importance of architecture and medical professionals working together, if and when this occurs again.

In fact, as the world moves forward in this pandemic, it already is requiring professionals to work together to prevent the spread of the virus and provide solutions in the built environment in real-time. To provide solutions for society as preventive measures and allow solutions for the economy and essential working processes to continue, there needs to be collaboration. The Architectural Medicine System (AMS) and the features of the Architectural Medicine Software Solution – ARxMD, can provide processes to achieve such goals. Including the Architectural Doctor and the Healthy Building Inspector in this equation can provide whole systems solutions.

It also requires the general public to re-evaluate life as we know it and recognize that some changes might need to occur in the life of each person. This is also true for creating greener and more sustainable solutions, as the next pandemic that humanity is facing is the crisis of climate change.

The health of many people on the planet is already being impacted negatively. And if we don't make changes to certain ways of life on this planet in the current model, the health of many more on an enormous scale can become catastrophic.

This does not mean that we cannot be positive, but in such optimism, there must be truths to face, and changes to make.

Architectural Medicine is dedicated to doing our part in this process, and I invite you to do your part as well. I encourage collaboration and cooperation on a local scale as well as our role as global citizens.

More information about our involvement and actions can be found on our website:

ArchitecturalMedicine.com

Here's wishing to your good health and wellness...

ABOUT THE AUTHOR

My journey into this field of Architectural Medicine began many decades ago, and while at the time I may not have recognized that "this" is what I was working towards, the process has been a trajectory that, when looking backward, is both logical and sensible in many ways.

I began my professional life as an Architectural Engineering student in the late 1980s, where my questions about the core components of how I viewed architecture first met the reality of the building mindset at that time. For me, architecture included the designing and building of spaces and places focused on energy efficiency, environmental awareness, and places to support health as nurturing spaces where people would want to spend time.

At the time, these topics were not a main focus during my studies in the field of architecture, so I went out into the big world seeking to find these answers. Along the way, I did find some of these answers, along with the people who developed these great solutions. I have had the great honor to learn from them and work with many of them.

My meeting and working with many pioneers in these fields allowed me to keep asking questions. Eventually, I asked the questions enough times, and with enough professionals, I realized that some of the answers did not exist.

And based on this, I decided a few decades ago to work towards defining these ideas in a way that seemed common sense to me, yet was and is currently not very common in the building world. Although I am happy to see this is changing in the world of architecture every year.

Because these concepts are complex, it has taken me many years to work towards a core understanding of these ideas to manifest. Today, I define them as necessary "systems" required for proper development moving forward.

As many people know, when you are dealing with systems, there are many different moving parts and processes that need to work together. This is akin to an analog clock with gears that need to fit into the correct places and timing for the entire system to work for the end goal. If they don't all fit or work together, you end up with grinding gears to bring the process to a halt.

This has been true for me in my process, as the original idea of these basic systems occurred in the late 1990s. It's been 20 plus years of work toward these goals, and this book is the result of the blood, sweat, and tears to achieve what I initially sought out to achieve – solutions for creating healthier, greener, and more sustainable architecture.

About the Author

One of the first green, eco-building events I attended was in 1993 at the Eco-Design, Environmental Building event in New York City with William McDonough, James Wines, Paul Bierman-Little, Mary Cordaro, and Katherine Metz. All of these pioneers in various fields of the healthy, green, and sustainable building movement. This is where I first met healthy building consultant Mary Cordaro, with whom I spent many years discussing and working to create solutions to these issues in the built environment.

My early involvement also included attending the Professional Design/Build course and the inaugural Sustainable Building course in 1995 at the Yestermorrow Design/Build School. It was a great honor and experience where John Connell, Bill Maclay, Bill Bialosky, Dave Sellers, Sylvia Smith, and many other leading architects and designers taught topics on sustainable building. This course was a milestone on my path. It was the first time I was around other architecture students and sustainable building advocates with similar interests and concerns for the state of architecture and the future of construction.

And to make that summer as complete as could be in this milestone learning, it was also where I first met James Hubble, where he was teaching his Soil and Soul course at Yestermorrow. I was so impressed by his lectures and overall approach to building that I attended a month-long event later that summer. This event in southern California and Mexico was a fantastic experience as Mr. Hubble taught Organic Architecture and Permaculture with other great architects and instructors, including Kyle Bergman and permaculture pioneers Penny Livingston and Bill Roley. This small group of architecture students gathered to help build a school in Tijuana, Mexico, based on these principles.

The ability to attend several Eco-Expos from the early 1990s onward also helped me to learn about the topics of sustainability and life cycle assessment.

In 1996 I began my studies with Helmut Ziehe at the International Institute of Building Biology and Ecology, a course he translated from the original German-based Bau Biologie program. Several years later, I then had the great fortune to study and work with Bosco Büeler, an important pioneer in the international field of healthy, green, and sustainable building. It was also where I met Christi Graham, an amazing person who created the West Coast Green conferences that have led to many beneficial green developments.

Through the years, I have been involved with ecological and sustainable building, as well as green and healthy building. In 1999 I co-formed the company Integrated Environmental Solutions and then H3Environmental with other professionals and pioneers in the healthy, environmental building fields.

Architectural Medicine – Building the Bridge to Wellness

During this time of the late 90s and early 2000s, I worked with noted Environmental Inspector Richard Scarborough and learned building science concepts from Joe Lstiburek's in-person courses.

My integration of building and health was also highly influenced by my time working at a health center in New York called Body, Mind, and Soul in the early 1990s. This was a first of its kind integrated health center where a healthy food cafe was combined with a book store focused on healthy living topics. The center also included a natural supplements section, offering many natural healing modalities that have become more commonplace today.

This center included lectures and classes on many health topics and offered meditation, yoga, tai chi, chi gong, and other natural living classes. There were services provided, such as acupuncture, that have become part of the integrative medicine process that people are familiar with today. Yet back then, in the early 90s in suburban New York, these were primarily foreign to both the general public and the medical and health professions.

My time spent at this center provided a wide-ranging group of topics in which to learn. From the far east to the far west, this knowledge planted seeds for a future of contemplation that gave me insights into health and wellness.

This experience led to many questions and insights into the "medicine" facet of Architectural Medicine. And it also allowed me to ponder the topics of health and medicine in ways that were very uncommon at that time, providing a foundation for my exploration of these topics related to the built environment.

My Path and Journey to Architectural Medicine

Reflecting on the Stanford commencement speech by Steve Jobs who said, "you can't connect the dots looking forward, you can only connect the dots looking back," I have taken time to review my life path and found it to ebb and flow to where I am today – and that quote reflects this well.

In truth, while my path began as a child when I look back at my influences growing up, it was my work in construction and as a student of architecture in the late 1980s when it all started to come together. When I attended the Eco-Design event in NYC with William McDonough and James Wines in 1993, it confirmed for me that I was on the right path.

My learning path often happened in small portions, yet as I've weaved each thread together, it has created a synergistic fabric.

In 1996, I began working with a natural, eco-building group focused on healthy building led by Cedar Rose Guelberth in Colorado. My introduction to health in building studies began with this group and the inaugural Building for Health conference with Paula Baker-LaPorte (at that time just Paula Baker), Carol Venolia, Cedar Rose Guelberth, and others in the early fall of 1996.

This was another big event in my life's journey. Before this, in the summer of 1996, I had attended several hands-on courses focused on ecological, sustainable, and natural building. These natural building events took place in Colorado and Washington state with eco-building pioneers such as Linda Smiley, Ianto Evans, Sun Ray Kelly, and Robert LaPorte, which led to my working for Cedar Rose.

This occurred right after my time working for Paolo Soleri at Cosanti, where I was inspired by his parametric, curving architecture and sculptures. Mr. Soleri's writings were inspirational, especially his book *Arcology: The City in the Image of Man*.[232]

All of these experiences led me to attend the 1998 Environ Design conference in California, and a unique, extended continuing education course at the Metropolitan Institute of Interior Design on topics related to Sacred Architecture during 1998.

I continued my studies attending a Bau Biologie event in Europe in the summer of 1998, learning about the various facets of natural and healthy building in Europe. And this is where I met the Swiss architect and mentor, Bosco Büeler.

In a moment of serendipity, it was also the trip that reunited me with Mary Cordaro, whom I had met in 1993 as she taught a segment at the Eco-Design Event in NYC.

This led to my collaboration as co-founder of Integrated Environmental Solutions and the eventual co-creation of H3 Environmental. This was a company focused on supporting the training and education for healthy, green, and sustainable building for professionals.

In those times, I developed the systems architecture to provide systems that most of us involved in the environmental or healthy inspection and consulting field were struggling with. These struggles included a lack of integration between the many professionals to provide greener, healthier building solutions.

In late 1999 into the early 2000s, I began to put my many years involved in technology and computer work into professional practice. I was responsible for the systems architecture, company systems setup, and operations, as many of these solutions required technological systems for integrated solutions. My work included infrastructure setup, technical systems development, database development, video production, web development, and the many Information Technology (IT) needs of a business.

Back in the early 2000s, the technology was more basic and was beginning to become more accessible. Back then, outside of large companies, smaller businesses had fewer options to provide more robust solutions.

It was also where I began to put the many courses of study into practice that I had been working towards in the decade of the 1990s. In retrospect, this multi-disciplinary span of classes and subjects was a self-designed program of study crafted from my curiosity and desire to learn more about these various subjects.

Since that time of the late 90s, I've spent the past 20 plus years involved with IT, technology, and systems architecture. This experience has provided a greater understanding of systems and digital developments.

I continue to learn more on this wide-range of topics, including advancements in systems architecture and digital systems integrations. I have also stayed involved in these green, eco, healthy building developments, keeping my skills and abilities agile and relevant.

All of these steps have led to the development of Architectural Medicine, which was created in 2011. And since that time, I've worked to develop the Architectural Medicine System (AMS) and the Architectural Medicine Software Solution – ARxMD. This also includes the development of the Architectural Doctor and the concept of the Healthy Building Inspector. In my opinion, all are vital to these ideas in providing whole systems integrations.

All of this has led me to the development of Architectural Medicine, including this book.

My hope is that this book can offer insights into these topics, provide clarity on the importance of multi-disciplinary systems, and contribute to integrative solutions moving forward.

It has been a long journey, yet in many ways, it is also just the beginning...

Timothy D. Rossi

About the Author

NOTES - BIBLIOGRAPHY

1. "The Project Gutenberg EBook of Ten Books on Architecture, by Vitruvius.," https://www.gutenberg.org/files/20239/20239-h/20239-h.htm.
2. "Healing | Origin and Meaning of Healing by Online Etymology Dictionary," https://www.etymonline.com/word/healing.
3. "Heal | Origin and Meaning of Heal by Online Etymology Dictionary," https://www.etymonline.com/word/heal.
4. Lacey Robinson and Rachel Miller, "The Impact of Bisphenol A and Phthalates on Allergy, Asthma, and Immune Function: A Review of Latest Findings," Current Environmental Health Reports 2, no. 4 (December 2015): 379–87, https://doi.org/10.1007/s40572-015-0066-8.
5. "Architecture, n.," in OED Online (Oxford University Press), https://www.oed.com/view/Entry/10408.
6. "Edifice, n.," in OED Online (Oxford University Press), https://www.oed.com/view/Entry/59535.
7. "Architecture | Origin and Meaning of Architecture by Online Etymology Dictionary," https://www.etymonline.com/word/architecture.
8. "Architect | Origin and Meaning of Architect by Online Etymology Dictionary," https://www.etymonline.com/word/architect.
9. "Medicine, n.1," in OED Online (Oxford University Press), https://www.oed.com/view/Entry/115715.
10. "Medicine, n.1."
11. "Medicine | Origin and Meaning of Medicine by Online Etymology Dictionary," https://www.etymonline.com/word/medicine.
12. "Healing | Origin and Meaning of Healing by Online Etymology Dictionary."
13. "Heal | Origin and Meaning of Heal by Online Etymology Dictionary."
14. "Health | Origin and Meaning of Health by Online Etymology Dictionary," https://www.etymonline.com/word/health.
15. "Medicine | Origin and Meaning of Medicine by Online Etymology Dictionary."
16. "Healing | Origin and Meaning of Healing by Online Etymology Dictionary."
17. "Integration | Origin and Meaning of Integration by Online Etymology Dictionary," https://www.etymonline.com/word/integration.

18. "Optimum Health - Dr. Andrew Weil," DrWeil.Com (blog), September 8, 2006, https://www.drweil.com/diet-nutrition/nutrition/optimum-health/.

19. Max Roser, Hannah Ritchie, and Esteban Ortiz-Ospina, "World Population Growth," Our World in Data, May 9, 2013, https://ourworldindata.org/world-population-growth.

20. CDC, "What Is Epigenetics? | CDC," Centers for Disease Control and Prevention, August 3, 2020, https://www.cdc.gov/genomics/disease/epigenetics.htm.

21. CDC.

22. "CDC - Exposome and Exposomics - NIOSH Workplace Safety and Health Topic," November 9, 2018, https://www.cdc.gov/niosh/topics/exposome/default.html.

23. "CDC - Exposome and Exposomics - NIOSH Workplace Safety and Health Topic."

24. "Deoxyribonucleic Acid (DNA) Fact Sheet," Genome.gov, https://www.genome.gov/about-genomics/fact-sheets/Deoxyribonucleic-Acid-Fact-Sheet.

25. "Buildings," Alliance to Save Energy, July 22, 2013, https://www.ase.org/initiatives/buildings.

26. "Circular Economy Schools Of Thought," https://www.ellenmacarthurfoundation.org/circular-economy/concept/schools-of-thought.

27. Michael Braungart and William McDonough, Cradle to Cradle: Remaking the Way We Make Things, 2019.

28. William E. Rees, "Ecological Footprints and Appropriated Carrying Capacity: What Urban Economics Leaves Out," Environment and Urbanization 4, no. 2 (October 1, 1992): 121–30, https://doi.org/10.1177/095624789200400212.

29. "Glaze, v.1," in OED Online (Oxford University Press), https://www.oed.com/view/Entry/78821.

30. "Sick Building Syndrome and the Problem of Uncertainty : Environmental Politics, Technoscience, and Women Workers (Book, 2006) [WorldCat.Org]," https://www.worldcat.org/title/sick-building-syndrome-and-the-problem-of-uncertainty-environmental-politics-technoscience-and-women-workers/oclc/1064988081&referer=brief_results.

31. "About Legionnaires Disease and Pontiac Fever | Legionella | CDC," October 31, 2019, https://www.cdc.gov/legionella/about/index.html.

32. "Legionnaire Disease | Britannica," https://www.britannica.com/science/Legionnaire-disease.

33. Lorraine Boissoneault, "The Cuyahoga River Caught Fire at Least a Dozen Times, but No One Cared Until 1969," Smithsonian Magazine, https://www.smithsonianmag.com/history/cuyahoga-river-caught-fire-least-dozen-times-no-one-cared-until-1969-180972444/.
34. OA US EPA, "The Origins of EPA," Collections and Lists, US EPA, January 29, 2013, https://www.epa.gov/history/origins-epa.
35. National Geographic Society (U.S.), Energy: Facing up to the Problem, Getting down to Solutions : A Special Report in the Public Interest. (Washington, D.C.: National Geographic Society, 1981).
36. "Amory Lovins," Rocky Mountain Institute, https://rmi.org/people/amory-lovins/.
37. Braungart and McDonough, Cradle to Cradle.
38. ORD US EPA, "Indoor Air Quality," Reports and Assessments, US EPA, November 2, 2017, https://www.epa.gov/report-environment/indoor-air-quality.
39. "Resource Efficiency," in Wikipedia, https://en.wikipedia.org/w/index.php?title=Resource_efficiency&oldid=997288927.
40. "Green, Adj. and n.1," in OED Online (Oxford University Press), https://www.oed.com/view/Entry/81167#eid2426583.
41. "What Is Green Building?," World Green Building Council, https://www.worldgbc.org/what-green-building.
42. "International Energy Outlook 2016," 2016, 290.
43. "Chapter 5: Increasing Efficiency of Building Systems and Technologies," n.d., 39.
44. "International Energy Outlook 2016."
45. Whole Earth Catalog. (San Rafael, CA: Point Foundation, 1998).
46. "Basic Information | Green Building |US EPA," https://archive.epa.gov/greenbuilding/web/html/about.html.
47. Sim Van der Ryn and Stuart Cowan, Ecological Design (Washington, D.C.: Island Press, 2007).
48. "The Burning River That Sparked a Revolution," Time, https://time.com/3921976/cuyahoga-fire/.
49. US EPA, "The Origins of EPA."
50. Robert Deitch, Hemp: American History Revisited: The Plant with a Divided History (New York: Algora Pub., 2003).
51. "Sustainable, Adj.," in OED Online (Oxford University Press), https://www.oed.com/view/Entry/195210.
52. "Sustainability, n.," in OED Online (Oxford University Press), https://www.oed.com/view/Entry/299890#eid225085209.

53. "John T. Lyle," in Wikipedia, September 23, 2019, https://en.wikipedia.org/w/index.php?title=John_T._Lyle&oldid=917458325.
54. "Regenerative Design," in Wikipedia, https://en.wikipedia.org/w/index.php?title=Regenerative_design&oldid=992860942.
55. B. C Mollison, Reny Mia Slay, and Andrew Jeeves, Introduction to Permaculture (Tyalgum, Australia: Tagari Publications, 1991).
56. Ryn and Cowan, Ecological Design.
57. "Definition of VERNACULAR," https://www.merriam-webster.com/dictionary/vernacular.
58. Roger W Caves, Encyclopedia of the City, 2013.
59. V. Kanellou, "Ancient Greek Medicine as the Foundation of Contemporary Medicine," Techniques in Coloproctology 8 Suppl 1 (November 2004): s3-4, https://doi.org/10.1007/s10151-004-0095-z.
60. Geraldine Perriam, "Sacred Spaces, Healing Places: Therapeutic Landscapes of Spiritual Significance," The Journal of Medical Humanities 36, no. 1 (2015): 19–33, https://doi.org/10.1007/s10912-014-9318-0.
61. Guenter B Risse, Mending Bodies, Saving Souls: A History of Hospitals (New York: Oxford University Press, 2011).
62. Hubert Palm, Das gesunde Haus (Konstanz: Ordo-Verl., 1979).
63. Perri Klass and M.D, "How to Minimize Exposures to Hormone Disrupters," The New York Times, April 1, 2019, sec. Well, https://www.nytimes.com/2019/04/01/well/family/how-to-minimize-exposures-to-hormone-disrupters.html.
64. Bao-Liang Sun et al., "Lymphatic Drainage System of the Brain: A Novel Target for Intervention of Neurological Diseases," Progress in Neurobiology, Neurobiology of Stroke: advances, challenges, and future directions, 163–164 (April 1, 2018): 118–43, https://doi.org/10.1016/j.pneurobio.2017.08.007.
65. "About AIHA," AIHA, https://www.aiha.org/about-aiha.
66. "Industrial Hygiene: Keeping Workers Healthy and Safe | Executive and Continuing Professional Education | Harvard T.H. Chan School of Public Health," https://www.hsph.harvard.edu/ecpe/industrial-hygiene-keeping-workers-healthy-and-safe/.
67. "About AIHA."
68. "About AIHA."
69. "CDC - Exposome and Exposomics - NIOSH Workplace Safety and Health Topic."
70. "CDC - Exposome and Exposomics - NIOSH Workplace Safety and Health Topic."
71. "Optimum Health - Dr. Andrew Weil."

72. "Welcome | Yestermorrow Design/Build School," https://yestermorrow.org/about/welcome.
73. "What Is Integrative Medicine?," The Andrew Weil Center for Integrative Medicine, https://integrativemedicine.arizona.edu/about/definition.html.
74. "What Is Integrative Medicine? - Andrew Weil, M.D.," http://www.drweil.com/drw/u/ART02054/Andrew-Weil-Integrative-Medicine.html.
75. "What Is Integrative Medicine?"
76. Andrew Weil, M.D., What Is Integrative Medicine? | Andrew Weil, M.D., 2010, https://www.youtube.com/watch?v=4pXsm3qaFIk&feature=youtu.be.
77. Andrew Weil, M.D.
78. Andrew Weil, M.D.
79. "Environmental Health: An Integrative Approach - Andrew Weil Center for Integrative Medicine," The Andrew Weil Center for Integrative Medicine, https://integrativemedicine.arizona.edu/education/online_courses/enviro-med.html.
80. Andrew Weil et al., 8 weeks to optimum health: spontaneous healing, 2004.
81. "Integrate | Origin and Meaning of Integrate by Online Etymology Dictionary," https://www.etymonline.com/word/integrate.
82. "Health, n.," in OED Online (Oxford University Press), https://www.oed.com/view/Entry/85020.
83. "Wellness, n.," in OED Online (Oxford University Press), https://www.oed.com/view/Entry/227459.
84. "Six Dimensions of Wellness | National Wellness Institute," https://nationalwellness.org/resources/six-dimensions-of-wellness/.
85. R. S. Ulrich, "View through a Window May Influence Recovery from Surgery," Science (New York, N.Y.) 224, no. 4647 (April 27, 1984): 420–21, https://doi.org/10.1126/science.6143402.
86. Moshe Bar and Maital Neta, "Visual Elements of Subjective Preference Modulate Amygdala Activation," Neuropsychologia 45, no. 10 (2007): 2191–2200, https://doi.org/10.1016/j.neuropsychologia.2007.03.008.
87. "Lead Poisoning and Health," https://www.who.int/news-room/fact-sheets/detail/lead-poisoning-and-health.
88. Center for Food Safety and Applied Nutrition, "Lead in Food, Foodwares, and Dietary Supplements," FDA, June 19, 2020, https://www.fda.gov/food/metals-and-your-food/lead-food-foodwares-and-dietary-supplements.

89. A. Trevor Hodge, Roman Aqueducts & Water Supply (London: Bristol Classical Press, 2012).
90. "What Is Integrative Medicine?"
91. "The American Academy of Environmental Medicine (AAEM)," American Academy of Environmental Medicine, https://www.aaemonline.org/.
92. "Environmental Health," https://www.who.int/westernpacific/health-topics/environmental-health.
93. "Environmental Health."
94. "Challenges," The Andrew Weil Center for Integrative Medicine, https://integrativemedicine.arizona.edu/enviro2016/challenges.html.
95. "Environmental Health Course Overview," The Andrew Weil Center for Integrative Medicine, https://integrativemedicine.arizona.edu/enviro2016/overview.html.
96. Joshua Cubista, "The Practice of Biophilia," Biophilia Foundation (blog), February 20, 2018, https://www.biophiliafoundation.org/practice-biophilia/.
97. "Biophilia Hypothesis | Description, Nature, & Human Behavior," Encyclopedia Britannica, https://www.britannica.com/science/biophilia-hypothesis.
98. Edward Osborne Wilson, Biophilia (Cambridge, Mass.: Harvard University Press, 1996).
99. Wilson.
100. Aaron Antonovsky, Health, Stress and Coping (San Francisco: Jossey-Bass, 1991).
101. Antonovsky.
102. Bar and Neta, "Visual Elements of Subjective Preference Modulate Amygdala Activation."
103. Antonovsky, Health, Stress and Coping.
104. "Healing | Origin and Meaning of Healing by Online Etymology Dictionary."
105. "Phenomenology (Architecture)," in Wikipedia, October 4, 2020, https://en.wikipedia.org/w/index.php?title=Phenomenology_(architecture)&oldid=981799344.
106. "The Eyes of the Skin: Architecture and the Senses, 3rd Edition | Wiley," Wiley.com, https://www.wiley.com/en-us/The+Eyes+of+the+Skin%3A+Architecture+and+the+Senses%2C+3rd+Edition-p-9781119941286.

107. "Environmental Psychology," in Wikipedia, https://en.wikipedia.org/w/index.php?title=Environmental_psychology&oldid=998456175.
108. "Environmental Psychology."
109. "Environmental Psychology - PPD151 / PSYBEH171S / PUBHLTH151 on Apple Podcasts," Apple Podcasts, https://podcasts.apple.com/us/podcast/environmental-psychology-ppd151-psybeh171s-pubhlth151/id516983549.
110. Minding Design (Symposium) et al., Mind in Architecture: Neuroscience, Embodiment, and the Future of Design, 2017, https://library.dctabudhabi.ae/sirsi/detail/1246037.
111. Minding Design (Symposium) et al.
112. Minding Design (Symposium) et al.
113. Bar and Neta, "Visual Elements of Subjective Preference Modulate Amygdala Activation."
114. Bar and Neta.
115. Sarah Williams Goldhagen, Welcome to Your World: How the Built Environment Shapes Our Lives, 2019.
116. Goldhagen.
117. "WHO | Social Determinants of Health," WHO (World Health Organization), https://www.who.int/gender-equity-rights/understanding/sdh-definition/en/.
118. "Social Determinants of Health | NCHHSTP | CDC," https://www.cdc.gov/nchhstp/socialdeterminants/index.html.
119. "Social Determinants of Health - Healthy People 2030 | Health.Gov," https://health.gov/healthypeople/objectives-and-data/social-determinants-health.
120. "A Brief Guide to Genomics," Genome.gov, https://www.genome.gov/about-genomics/fact-sheets/A-Brief-Guide-to-Genomics.
121. Jeremy M. Berg, John L. Tymoczko, and Lubert Stryer, "A Pair of Nucleic Acid Chains with Complementary Sequences Can Form a Double-Helical Structure," Biochemistry. 5th Edition, 2002, https://www.ncbi.nlm.nih.gov/books/NBK22386/.
122. Shelley L. Berger et al., "An Operational Definition of Epigenetics," Genes & Development 23, no. 7 (April 1, 2009): 781–83, https://doi.org/10.1101/gad.1787609.
123. CDC, "What Is Epigenetics?"
124. "The Skill of Happiness - Matthieu Ricard," https://www.matthieuricard.org/en/books/the-skill-of-happiness.
125. Mohd. Razali Salleh, "Life Event, Stress and Illness," The Malaysian Journal of Medical Sciences : MJMS 15, no. 4 (October 2008): 9–18.

126. Antonovsky, Health, Stress and Coping.
127. "Definition of SALUTOGENESIS," https://www.merriam-webster.com/dictionary/salutogenesis.
128. Jan A. Golembiewski, "Salutogenic Architecture in Healthcare Settings," in The Handbook of Salutogenesis, ed. Maurice B. Mittelmark et al. (Cham (CH): Springer, 2017), http://www.ncbi.nlm.nih.gov/books/NBK435851/.
129. Golembiewski.
130. Ulrich, "View through a Window May Influence Recovery from Surgery."
131. Randel L. Swanson, "Biotensegrity: A Unifying Theory of Biological Architecture With Applications to Osteopathic Practice, Education, and Research—A Review and Analysis," The Journal of the American Osteopathic Association 113, no. 1 (January 1, 2013): 34–52, https://doi.org/10.7556/jaoa.2013.113.1.34.
132. "Optimum Health - Dr. Andrew Weil."
133. "Medicine | Origin and Meaning of Medicine by Online Etymology Dictionary."
134. "Healing | Origin and Meaning of Healing by Online Etymology Dictionary."
135. "Heal | Origin and Meaning of Heal by Online Etymology Dictionary."
136. "Health | Origin and Meaning of Health by Online Etymology Dictionary."
137. "Medicine, n.1."
138. "Rx | Search Online Etymology Dictionary," https://www.etymonline.com/search?q=Rx.
139. "Definition of ANASTOMOSIS," https://www.merriam-webster.com/dictionary/anastomosis.
140. "Anastomosis | Origin and Meaning of Anastomosis by Online Etymology Dictionary," https://www.etymonline.com/word/anastomosis.
141. "Anastomosis, n.," in OED Online (Oxford University Press), https://www.oed.com/view/Entry/7139.
142. "WHO | Social Determinants of Health."
143. "Social Determinants of Health," in Wikipedia, https://en.wikipedia.org/w/index.php?title=Social_determinants_of_health&oldid=992923740.
144. Goinvo/HealthDeterminants, HTML (2016; repr., GoInvo, 2020), https://github.com/goinvo/HealthDeterminants.

145. "System | Origin and Meaning of System by Online Etymology Dictionary," https://www.etymonline.com/word/system.
146. "System, n.," in OED Online (Oxford University Press), https://www.oed.com/view/Entry/196665.
147. "Eco- | Origin and Meaning of Prefix Eco- by Online Etymology Dictionary," https://www.etymonline.com/word/eco-.
148. "Ecology | Origin and Meaning of Ecology by Online Etymology Dictionary," https://www.etymonline.com/word/ecology.
149. "Ecology | Origin and Meaning of Ecology by Online Etymology Dictionary."
150. "Phenomenology (Architecture)."
151. Bar and Neta, "Visual Elements of Subjective Preference Modulate Amygdala Activation."
152. Bar and Neta.
153. Bar and Neta.
154. "About OSHA | Occupational Safety and Health Administration," https://www.osha.gov/aboutosha.
155. "Discover IH," AIHA, https://www.aiha.org/ih-careers/discover-industrial-hygiene.
156. ioha-admin, "Our Vision & Mission," IOHA (blog), https://www.ioha.net/about/vision-mission/.
157. "CDC - Exposome and Exposomics - NIOSH Workplace Safety and Health Topic."
158. "CDC - Exposome and Exposomics - NIOSH Workplace Safety and Health Topic."
159. Nadine Steckling et al., "Biomarkers of Exposure in Environment-Wide Association Studies – Opportunities to Decode the Exposome Using Human Biomonitoring Data," Environmental Research 164 (July 1, 2018): 597–624, https://doi.org/10.1016/j.envres.2018.02.041.
160. Steckling et al.
161. "Evidence-Based Design Accreditation and Certification (EDAC) | The Center for Health Design," https://www.healthdesign.org/certification-outreach/edac.
162. "Rx | Search Online Etymology Dictionary."
163. "Introduction | Meaningful Use | CDC," https://www.cdc.gov/ehrmeaningfuluse/introduction.html.
164. "Introduction | Meaningful Use | CDC."
165. "Industry Foundation Classes (IFC)," buildingSMART International, https://www.buildingsmart.org/standards/bsi-standards/indus-

try-foundation-classes/.
166. 14:00-17:00, "ISO 16739-1:2018," ISO, https://www.iso.org/cms/render/live/en/sites/isoorg/contents/data/standard/07/03/70303.html.
167. "Industry Foundation Classes (IFC)."
168. "Overview-Dev - FHIR v4.0.1," https://www.hl7.org/fhir/overview-dev.html.
169. "Health Information Privacy," Text, HHS.gov, August 26, 2015, https://www.hhs.gov/hipaa/index.html.
170. "Classification of Diseases (ICD)," 11, https://www.who.int/standards/classifications/classification-of-diseases.
171. admin, "Mission," Academy of Neuroscience for Architecture (blog), https://www.anfarch.org/about/mission/.
172. "The Internet Classics Archive | Of the Epidemics by Hippocrates," http://classics.mit.edu/Hippocrates/epidemics.1.i.html.
173. "The Internet Classics Archive | Of the Epidemics by Hippocrates."
174. Stanford, Steve Jobs' 2005 Stanford Commencement Address, 2008, https://www.youtube.com/watch?v=UF8uR6Z6KLc&feature=youtu.be.
175. "Definition of TACK," https://www.merriam-webster.com/dictionary/tack.
176. Ulrich, "View through a Window May Influence Recovery from Surgery."
177. Salleh, "Life Event, Stress and Illness."
178. "Stress Effects on the Body," https://www.apa.org, https://www.apa.org/helpcenter/stress.
179. "The Project Gutenberg EBook of Ten Books on Architecture, by Vitruvius."
180. "The Project Gutenberg EBook of Ten Books on Architecture, by Vitruvius."
181. "The Project Gutenberg EBook of Ten Books on Architecture, by Vitruvius."
182. "Eero Saarinen," in Wikipedia, https://en.wikipedia.org/w/index.php?title=Eero_Saarinen&oldid=996519128.
183. "Parameter | Mathematics and Statistics | Britannica," https://www.britannica.com/topic/parameter.
184. "Parameter, n.," in OED Online (Oxford University Press), https://www.oed.com/view/Entry/137519.
185. "Definition of ALGORITHM," https://www.merriam-webster.com/dictionary/algorithm.

186. "Parameter," in Wikipedia, https://en.wikipedia.org/w/index.php?title=Parameter&oldid=998744646.
187. "Parameter."
188. "Parameter."
189. Eric W. Weisstein, "Parameter," Text (Wolfram Research, Inc.), https://mathworld.wolfram.com/Parameter.html.
190. "Parametricism," in Wikipedia, https://en.wikipedia.org/w/index.php?title=Parametricism&oldid=999669568.
191. Patrik Schumacher, Parametricism. (John Wiley & Sons, 2016).
192. "Parametricism."
193. Eric W. Weisstein, "Parametric Equations," Text (Wolfram Research, Inc.), https://mathworld.wolfram.com/ParametricEquations.html.
194. "Parametricism."
195. "Biophilia Hypothesis | Description, Nature, & Human Behavior."
196. "Biophilia Hypothesis | Description, Nature, & Human Behavior."
197. "Biophilia Hypothesis | Description, Nature, & Human Behavior."
198. Eugene Tsui, Evolutionary Architecture: Nature as a Basis for Design (New York [etc.]: J. Wiley & Sons, 1999).
199. Tsui.
200. D. E. Ingber, "The Architecture of Life," Scientific American 278, no. 1 (January 1998): 48–57, https://doi.org/10.1038/scientificamerican0198-48.
201. "Tensegrity, n.," in OED Online (Oxford University Press), https://www.oed.com/view/Entry/199174.
202. Ingber, "The Architecture of Life."
203. Schumacher, Parametricism.
204. "Entrainment - an Overview | ScienceDirect Topics," https://www.sciencedirect.com/topics/psychology/entrainment.
205. "Entrainment - an Overview | ScienceDirect Topics."
206. Günther Knoblich, Stephen Butterfill, and Natalie Sebanz, "Chapter Three - Psychological Research on Joint Action: Theory and Data," in Psychology of Learning and Motivation, ed. Brian H. Ross, vol. 54, Advances in Research and Theory (Academic Press, 2011), 59–101, https://doi.org/10.1016/B978-0-12-385527-5.00003-6.
207. Young Hee Geum and Young Kim, "On the Analysis and Construction of the Butterfly Curve Using Mathematica®," International Journal of Mathematical Education in Science and Technology 39 (July 1, 2008): 670–78, https://doi.org/10.1080/00207390801923240.
208. "Health | Origin and Meaning of Health by Online Etymology Dictionary."

209. R. Buckminster Fuller, Guinea Pig B: The 56 Year Experiment (Summertown, Tenn.: Book Publishing, 2004).
210. "Depave | From Parking Lots to Paradise," https://depave.org/.
211. "1. Blue Zones Life: Why, What, Where, Who, How?," Blue Zones (blog), https://www.bluezones.com/1-blue-zones-life-why-what-where-who-how/.
212. WIRED, Architecture Professor Explains Why Malls Are Dying | WIRED, 2019, https://www.youtube.com/watch?v=sBEajQWy-LU.
213. "Our Story » TZOA," TZOA, https://tzoa.com/our-story/.
214. "CDC - Exposome and Exposomics - NIOSH Workplace Safety and Health Topic."
215. Eric J Topol and Abraham Verghese, Deep Medicine: How Artificial Intelligence Can Make Healthcare Human Again (New York: Basic Books, 2019).
216. "CDC - Exposome and Exposomics - NIOSH Workplace Safety and Health Topic."
217. "CDC - Exposome and Exposomics - NIOSH Workplace Safety and Health Topic."
218. "CDC - Exposome and Exposomics - NIOSH Workplace Safety and Health Topic."
219. "CDC - Exposome and Exposomics - NIOSH Workplace Safety and Health Topic."
220. "CDC - Exposome and Exposomics - NIOSH Workplace Safety and Health Topic."
221. Vida Maliene et al., "Geographic Information System: Old Principles with New Capabilities," URBAN DESIGN International 16, no. 1 (January 1, 2011): 1–6, https://doi.org/10.1057/udi.2010.25.
222. "Roger Waters Interview w/Chris Salewicz, June 1987," http://www.pink-floyd.org/artint/wat1987.htm.
223. David Byrne, "Transcript of 'How Architecture Helped Music Evolve,'" https://www.ted.com/talks/david_byrne_how_architecture_helped_music_evolve/transcript.
224. "Crystalline (Song)," in Wikipedia, https://en.wikipedia.org/w/index.php?title=Crystalline_(song)&oldid=1005256742.
225. "The Hearts of Space - Stephen Hill," https://www.hos.com/shbio.html.
226. "Wisdom | Origin and Meaning of Wisdom by Online Etymology Dictionary," https://www.etymonline.com/word/wisdom.
227. "Wise | Origin and Meaning of Wise by Online Etymology Dictionary," https://www.etymonline.com/word/wise.

228. "Definition of WISDOM," https://www.merriam-webster.com/dictionary/wisdom.
229. "Wisdom, n.," in OED Online (Oxford University Press), https://www.oed.com/view/Entry/229491.
230. Christopher T Vecsey and Robert W Venables, American Indian Environments: Ecological Issues in Native American History (Syracuse, N.Y.: Syracuse University, 1994).
231. "About - The Long Now," https://longnow.org/about/.
232. Paulo Soleri, Arcology: The City in the Image of Man (Cambridge: MIT Press, 1969).

Notes – Bibliography

ARCHITECTURAL MEDICINE℠

BUILDING THE BRIDGE TO WELLNESS

CAN ARCHITECTURE BE HEALING?

TIMOTHY D. ROSSI

OTHER BOOKS BY THE AUTHOR

THE ARCHITECTURAL DOCTOR℠

Creating integrated solutions and systems for the fields of Architecture and Medicine to create healthy and healing places to live, work, and play. The Architectural Doctor – the liaison between Architecture and Medicine.

(Forthcoming)

INTEGRATIVE ARCHITECTURE

Integrating the processes between green, healthy, and sustainable Architecture methodologies for energy efficient, ecologically aware, and healthier built environments.

(Forthcoming)

SYMBIOSIS GLOBAL
NATURE IS THE MOST ADVANCED TECHNOLOGY
TECHNOLOGY & ECOLOGY : LIVING TOGETHER

How can we navigate the challenges of humanity while also striving for progress in the world of Technology? How can we create a future more aligned to the planet's Ecological systems?

Symbiosis Global outlines these topics with a focus on the premise "Nature is the Most Advanced Technology."

(Forthcoming)

www.ingramcontent.com/pod-product-compliance
Lightning Source LLC
Chambersburg PA
CBHW050258010526
44107CB00055B/2085